P9-ECZ-572

Human Services
in
Contemporary
America

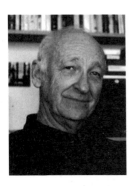

Paul Schmolling, Jr., is a clinical psychologist trained at the NYU Graduate School of Arts and Science. His clinical experience includes 10 years as a psychologist at a child guidance center, and he has also worked as a ward psychologist at New York City's Bellevue Hospital. Currently he teaches at Kingsborough Community College of the City University of New York, where he is associated with the Mental Health and Human Services Program. Paul is an active researcher and has published a number of articles on cognitive processes in schizophrenia. He has a special interest in stress and is studying the long-range psychological impact of confinement to Nazi concentration camps. He is also interested in the effects of family destabilization on the mental and physical health of college students.

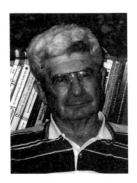

Merrill Youkeles is a certified social worker who received his MSW degree from the University of Pennsylvania. He received his doctoral degree in studies on aging at Columbia University with the aid of a grant from the Administration on Aging. Merrill has more than 30 years of experience as a practitioner, consultant, and educator. His work in agencies, clinics, hospitals, and community organizations has given him a broad and realistic view of the human services field. He is presently on the faculty of the Mental Health and Human Services Program at Kingsborough Community College of the City University of New York. Merrill is a staunch advocate of prevention in the human services field and of human services training programs.

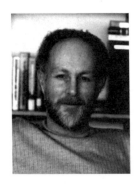

William R. Burger received his doctorate in social psychology, but his academic background also encompasses the fields of educational psychology and philosophy of education. While attending graduate school at Harvard University, he was awarded a research assistantship for his work in the area of community decision making. Bill is presently director of the Mental Health and Human Services Program and chairperson of the Department of Behavioral Sciences and Human Services at Kingsborough Community College of the City University of New York. He has served as a consultant to a variety of human services programs in New York and Massachusetts, has lectured at various colleges and universities, and has written a number of guest editorial articles for various newspapers.

Human Services in Contemporary America

Paul Schmolling, Jr.
Merrill Youkeles
William R. Burger

*Kingsborough Community College
of the City University of New York*

Brooks/Cole Publishing Company

I(T)P® An International Thomson Publishing Company

*Pacific Grove • Albany • Belmont • Bonn • Boston • Cincinnati • Detroit
Johannesburg • London • Madrid • Melbourne • Mexico City • New York • Paris • Singapore
Tokyo • Toronto • Washington*

Sponsoring Editor: *Lisa Gebo*
Marketing Team: *Jean Thompson, Deborah Petit*
Editorial Assistant: *Lisa Blanton*
Production Editor: *Keith Faivre*
Manuscript Editor: *Frank Hubert*
Permissions Editor: *May Clark*
Interior Design: *E. Kelly Shoemaker*
Cover Design: *Laurie Albrecht*

Cover Art: *Laura Militzer Bryant*
Art Editor: *Lisa Torri*
Photo Editor: *Bob Western*
Typesetting: *Shepard Poorman Communications, Inc.*
Cover Printing: *Phoenix Color Corporation, Inc.*
Printing and Binding: *Quebecor Printing–Fairfield*

COPYRIGHT © 1997 by Brooks/Cole Publishing Company
A Division of International Thomson Publishing Inc.
I(T)P The ITP logo is a registered trademark under license.

For more information, contact:

BROOKS/COLE PUBLISHING COMPANY
511 Forest Lodge Road
Pacific Grove, CA 93950
USA

International Thomson Editores
Seneca 53
Col. Polanco
México, D. F., México
C. P. 11560

International Thomson Publishing Europe
Berkshire House 168-173
High Holborn
London WC1V 7AA
England

International Thomson Publishing GmbH
Königswinterer Strasse 418
53227 Bonn
Germany

International Thomson Publishing Asia
221 Henderson Road
#05-10 Henderson Building
Singapore 0315

Thomas Nelson Australia
102 Dodds Street
South Melbourne, 3205
Victoria, Australia

Nelson Canada
1120 Birchmount Road
Scarborough, Ontario
Canada M1K 5G4

International Thomson Publishing Japan
Hirakawacho Kyowa Building, 3F
2-2-1 Hirakawacho
Chiyoda-ku, Tokyo 102
Japan

All rights reserved. No part of this work may be reproduced, stored in a retrieval system, or transcribed, in any form or by any means—electronic, mechanical, photocopying, recording, or otherwise—without the prior written permission of the publisher, Brooks/Cole Publishing Company, Pacific Grove, California 93950.

Printed in the United States of America

10   9   8   7   6   5   4   3

Library of Congress Cataloging-in-Publication Data

Schmolling, Paul.
    Human services in contemporary America / Paul Schmolling, Jr.,
Merrill Youkeles, William R. Burger. — 4th ed.
        p.   cm.
    Includes bibliographical references and index.
    ISBN 0-534-34571-9 (alk. paper)
    1. Human services—United States. 2. Human services—Vocational
guidance—United States. 3. United States—Social
policy—1980–1993.   I. Youkeles, Merrill.   II. Burger, William.
III. Title.
HV91.S294 1997
361.973—dc20   96-25502
                                                  CIP

To Patricia, and to Paul and Rosemary,
who recently presented us with Justin, a new addition to the family.
P.S.

To the memory of my wife, Marcia,
who is with me always.
M.Y.

To my wife, Mary, and my daughter, Kim,
who help me maintain a balanced perspective
and keep my priorities in order.
W. R. B.

FOREWORD

In the best of all possible worlds, good intentions would invariably compel their desired positive results. But the reality of contemporary American society produces a road to social improvement fraught with detours, hazards, and delays that good intentions alone cannot successfully overcome. Since human services are formulated, devised, and implemented within a social milieu in which human needs are but one of many policy considerations, the value of *Human Services in Contemporary America* lies in the realism it fosters in its readers. As a sociologist, I welcome the authors' approach because it departs from the often simplistic cause-and-effect characterizations and "how to help" syndrome of many standard introductory human services texts. Optimism and idealism are not enough. They are, at best, necessary but insufficient prerequisites to progress. That recognition, coupled with the careful explanation of its implications, is perhaps the greatest strength of the book you are about to read.

Social scientists are sometimes criticized (and often rightfully so) by human services professionals for the distance they seek to maintain from the issues they research. It is as if the dispassionate, objective nature of the research process demanded an aloof neutrality of spirit on the part of the researcher. Similarly, human services professionals are sometimes criticized (and, again, often rightfully so) by social scientists for plunging headfirst into action programs without benefit of careful, reasoned analysis. This tension between researcher and activist, between analysis and action, can engender an unproductive stalemate in which the real losers are those among us who are genuinely in need of assistance. Perhaps the best way to avoid such an impasse is to promote meaningful dialogue instead of indulge the tendency of each group to bemoan among themselves the misguided efforts of "those other folks," whether "those other folks" are academics with their heads in the clouds or human services workers with their hearts in their hands. But how do we bridge this gap I've noted and transcend the limitations of too narrow academic training? How do we go beyond a trained incapacity to respect the validity of another's point of view?

Although I am not so naively optimistic to believe that there is a single, easy solution to this dilemma, I do see reasons for at least a cautious optimism. *Human Services in Contemporary America* is a rare text in that it genuinely seeks to cross traditional disciplinary boundaries. The interrelatedness of personal troubles and public issues and the interplay of analysis and action are prominent themes of the book. Such themes do, in my view, encourage that meaningful dialogue across disciplinary lines that I mentioned earlier. An exemplary introductory-level text in any field provides more than a cursory survey of accumulated knowledge in a subject matter. It is an invitation to adopt a new perspective, to enhance your vision in that you might see in a new light things you merely looked at before but didn't truly see.

As do most good books, *Human Services in Contemporary America* raises far more questions than it answers. But having read it, you will likely ask more perceptive questions, be less satisfied with simplistic, pat answers, and be ready to tackle new intellectual challenges, armed not simply with more information but with a broader, more critical perspective on the real issues before us. For both students and teachers, this might well be more than they've bargained for. Certainly, it is more than we've come to expect in an introductory text. But perhaps we should learn to accept nothing less. For, if beginning students in human services fields continue to find in their texts a "cookbook" approach detailing simple solutions to complex social problems, they will be impotent to effect change in a political world they scarcely comprehend. And, similarly, if beginning students in the social sciences continue to find in their texts theories and abstractions divorced from a consideration of their practical application, they too will be unable to play an active role in the improvement of our society. *Human Services in Contemporary America,* in striking a balance between realism and idealism, pessimism and optimism, theory and application, and analysis and action, sheds welcome light on some of our most pressing social issues.

In the years that have passed since this foreword was originally written for the first edition of *Human Services in Contemporary America,* so many dramatic cultural, political, and economic changes have reshaped the contours of our social landscape. As a consequence, the context in which human services are provided has similarly reconfigured the task of helping people. Concepts and trends such as downsizing, privatization, and managed care (just to name a few), which just a few short years ago held little or no meaning as arcane theoretical constructs, now are inexorable forces with profound impact on our careers and lives. For those of us who, in our own chosen way, accept the challenge of trying to create a more humane future, that calling has become more bewildering than ever. But if we throw up our hands in confused desperation, then we are defeated before we have even begun. *Human Services in Contemporary America* offers to its readers an intellectual road map to the knowledge and understandings that must be the bedrock of any social improvement efforts with a realistic chance of success.

My choice of the "road map" metaphor to characterize this book's pedagogical stance does, I believe, capture the authors' intentions. Furthermore, it demonstrates their awareness of and sensitivity to the latest research in the field of education on the learning process. One of the potential benefits of the increased emphasis on outcome assessment in educational programs is a heightened concern with what, how, and how much students actually learn in their classes. This renewed concern is substantially altering the criteria by which instructors choose their textbooks. "Informational" type texts with their barrage of tables, charts, graphs, and findings often overload students with a wealth of disconnected social facts. Cast adrift in a sea of minutiae, students do not often truly learn. What they need to truly experience the excitement of real learning is just the sort of intellectual road map that *Human Services in Contemporary America* provides.

An exemplary "interpretive" text does not allow the motivated student to remain in the role of passive recipient of information. Rather, it fosters active learning by introducing ideas as tools for further exploration. Readers of this book are invited to utilize intellectual tools for acquiring, evaluating, and integrating information. The skillful application of these tools will enable students to differentiate between the trivial and the significant, to evaluate opposing viewpoints, and to construct empirically based arguments and interpretations. They will, in essence, have begun to build the intellectual foundation upon which meaningful efforts to maximize the human serviceability of this society must rest.

Stephen L. Markson
University of Hartford

CONTENTS

Human Services in the United States Today   1

Groups in Need   65

Human Services in Historical Perspective   137

Theoretical Perspectives   163

The Human Services Worker   211

Careers in Human Services   247

Social Policy   275

Prevention in Human Services   305

Current Controversies and Issues   327

PREFACE

In future societies, the most valuable people might be, not those with the greatest ability to produce material goods, but rather those who have the gift to spread good will and happiness through empathy and understanding. Such a gift may be innate in part but could certainly be enhanced by experience and education. (René Dubos, *Celebrations of Life.* New York: McGraw-Hill, 1981, p. 229)

We wrote this text in the hope of enhancing the student's capacity to facilitate the lives of others. We believe, along with Dubos, that this capacity can, to a large extent, be taught and learned. The ability to help others in a professional context requires a base of knowledge along with a range of helping skills. We intend this text to help the beginning student take the first steps toward acquiring the needed knowledge and skills.

This book provides a general introduction to the field of human services and is designed for introductory college courses in human services, mental-health technology, social work, community mental health, and other human services programs. We expect that most students who read this text are headed toward careers that involve direct contact with people. However, the book would also be useful to those considering administrative work in the human services.

Students in the human services typically begin their training with hopes of helping other people lead more fulfilling lives. Unfortunately, these hopes are sometimes dampened by the realities of the outside world. The humanistic society of the future described by Dubos is not yet here. Although humanistic values do play an important role in present-day America, they must compete with other motives such as profit, power, and self-aggrandizement. In order to be effective, the human services worker must be able to face the harsh realities of our complex, imperfect society. Of course, the worker can keep the ideal society in mind and work toward it in a realistic way.

In the pages that follow, we have sought a balance between idealism and realism. We certainly do not intend to dampen the idealistic feelings of students. However, our collective experience as teachers has shown us that the students who become discouraged are often those who expect too much of clients, helping agencies, and themselves. This disillusionment can be avoided if the student develops a realistic idea of what to expect.

Aside from these aims, we offer a great deal of valuable information about human services, a field whose scope and complexity have greatly increased in recent decades. The material is presented in a provocative manner, raising issues not usually addressed in introductory texts. The impact of political, economic, and social pressures on human services is explored.

The text begins with an account of the goals, functions, and organization of human services seen in the context of contemporary social problems, followed by a description of the groups of people who receive help from human services. A historical survey of human services provides a background against which current efforts can be viewed. There is also coverage of the major theories that govern helping efforts, as well as a review of the techniques and methods of helping. The student is also provided with practical information about career options in the human services field.

The final chapters are certainly unusual in an introductory text. We feel it is important for students to know something about how social policies are developed and about how human services workers might influence policies. These policies, which determine who receives what kind of help, have a great impact on worker and client alike. It is undeniable that today's student is the policymaker of tomorrow.

In the chapter on prevention, we demonstrate a strong bias in favor of programs aimed at preventing problems and dysfunctions from developing in the first place. Frankly, we try to persuade students, instructors, and human services agencies that prevention programs should play a major role in the future of human services.

The text concludes with a sampling of current controversies affecting human services. We offer this selection with the intent of fostering a realistic understanding of conflicts and issues that confront human services workers. In addition, we also discuss the issues of the various titles by which human services workers are identified.

The introductory course in human services is perhaps the most important a student will take. It is here that the student's attitudes and philosophy are developed. We believe that a humanistic perspective, combined with a realistic awareness of societal problems, provides the best foundation for creative and effecting helping.

New to the Fourth Edition

In our preface to the third edition, we noted that many human service agencies are struggling to meet increasing needs with limited resources and predicted a challenging time ahead for workers in the field. Certainly, this prophecy has come true. However, we did not anticipate the dramatic changes in the political atmosphere that have taken place in the last few years. Social programs have become the focus of intense political controversy. Once viewed as attempts to solve problems, some programs, especially welfare, are being condemned as the cause of problems. Charles Murray,* a well-known conservative spokesman, argued that federal welfare policy has been a disaster and is indirectly responsible for the large number of fatherless families found in the inner cities; he added that children of immature, irresponsible parents are stunted in ways that no

*Murray, C. (1995, November 14). Welfare hysteria. *The New York Times*, p. 21.

amount of money for schools or services can remedy. Economist John Kenneth Galbraith,** however, pointed out that liberal social policies did not come out of the blue but were designed to ameliorate great social upheavals. According to Galbraith, the poor were mostly hidden away in rural communities, unseen and unheard, until the mid-1960s. Only when they came to the cities in large numbers did welfare and related services become essential. We might add that these rural workers who came to the cities in search of jobs were soon caught in another development: the decline of American industry and consequent loss of factory jobs. It seems to us that simply cutting welfare benefits will not solve the underlying problem. The need for decent paying jobs will still be there.

The trend to hold the line on government expenditures that we pointed out in the previous edition is, if anything, even more pronounced than before. Plans are underway to balance the federal budget by the year 2002. We don't know if this objective will be achieved, but it seems certain that serious efforts to contain federal spending will be made. It is also certain that the states of the union will be given more responsibility for managing welfare and other programs. We recognize the need to reduce the huge federal deficit, but we are concerned that human services will be curtailed at a time of increasing need. Recent data on crime, drug abuse, homelessness, and other social ills, presented in this edition, reinforce our conviction that more persons than ever are in need of help from human services.

We feel it is important that workers understand the new social and political landscape in which human services will operate. Accordingly, we have added material on the Clinton administration and have described the nation's swing toward conservatism as shown by the so-called Republican Revolution of 1994. In addition, we have described important economic and technological changes that affect human services, including the erosion of our industrial base and the emergence of information technology. Also highlighted in this edition are the data showing a disturbing trend in income distribution in this country; the rich are getting richer and more numerous while the incomes of middle- and working-class persons are stagnating. At the same time, recent political and geographic changes may result in reduced attention to the needs of poor persons in the inner cities. We also document the increasingly hostile attitudes toward illegal immigrants that are currently quite obvious. As before, we have updated the current status of various groups in need of help, including the homeless, persons with mental retardation, juvenile offenders, and others.

Also new to this edition is an examination of the law as it relates to human services. In particular, we emphasize issues around human rights and patient rights. As society becomes increasingly complex, a basic knowledge of the legal issues confronting human services becomes more essential. We have also added a section on the media and how they affect social

**Galbraith, J. K. (1995, September 19). Blame history, not the liberals. *The New York Times*, p. 21.

policies and human services. Some new teaching aids also appear in this edition, including material designed to sharpen the students' capacity to think critically about social and political issues.

Most existing texts in human services now seem dated and obsolete. There have been so many dramatic changes during the last few years that human services are operating in a new climate. We have attempted to provide a realistic picture of this new situation. We repeat what we said in our first preface: In order to be effective, the human service worker must be able to face the harsh realities of our complex, imperfect society.

In closing, we would like to thank the instructors and students who have helped this text achieve its present state of eminence in the field. We believe that this is the best short introduction to human services that is currently available. It is gratifying to know that so many of you agree with our immodest assessment.

Acknowledgments

We wish to express our gratitude to the many individuals who provided input, advice, and support during the preparation of this text. In particular, we appreciate the contributions of Dr. Sam Goldstein, former Dean of the Wurzweiler School of Social Work, Dr. Arthur Schwartz, former Director of Consultation of Education of the Sound View Throggs Neck Community Mental Health Center, and Ellen Gorman, former President of New York City Coalition for Prevention in Mental Health.

In preparation of our fourth edition, we must single out Barbara Manzo for our special thanks. She not only typed numerous rewrites for us, but kept us going with her delightful sense of humor and unconditional support. We also wish to thank Dean Fred Malamet for his editorial contributions to the fourth edition. We also wish to acknowledge Janice Strizever for her expert help in preparing the final manuscript of this edition. In addition, we want to thank Ellen Singer for her efforts on our behalf.

To Claire Verduin, who launched previous editions of this text, goes our appreciation for her support and encouragement, along with our best wishes on her retirement. We also deeply appreciate the efforts of our new sponsoring editor, Lisa Gebo, who handled the fourth edition with style and grace.

Finally, we give thanks to the reviewers of the manuscript for their helpful comments and suggestions: James F. Carroll, Tacoma Community College; Catherine Collins, SUNY—Empire State College; Susan A. Farrell, Kingsborough Community College; Charles O. Jaap, Pasco-Hernando Community College; Kathleen Perkins, Louisiana State University; David Siddle, Assumption College; Douglas A. Whyte, Community College of Philadelphia; Dick Wilson, Saddleback College.

Paul Schmolling, Jr.
Merrill Youkeles
William R. Burger

Human Services
in the United States Today

INTRODUCTION

Over the years, human services in the United States have evolved into a network of programs and agencies that provide an array of services to millions of Americans. The one feature shared by all of these services is that they are designed to meet human needs. Since services are invariably linked to needs, it is important to understand the full range of human needs. Thus, this chapter begins with a consideration of human needs and the kinds of services that seek to meet them. Some service agencies are devoted mainly to helping people meet basic survival needs such as food and shelter, whereas some are concerned with helping clients achieve more satisfying relationships or attain other kinds of personal fulfillment. Primary social supports, such as family and friends, also play a role in meeting human needs, and we examine that role in this first chapter.

There is controversy about just what needs should be met by agencies supported by public funds. There is, in fact, a great deal of controversy about questions involving the scope and quality of human services. In this chapter, we provide an overview of the human services that raises some of these questions. Critics argue that human services are wasteful and inefficient, whereas supporters are convinced that more should be done to meet people's needs. Some social planners want to cut funds for services, but others demand increased funding. Because these conflicts are fought out primarily in the political arena, it is vital to grasp the liberal and conservative positions that underlie the countless debates about specific programs. We outline these positions in this chapter.

This chapter also includes a survey of some contemporary problems that may affect the ability of Americans to meet their own needs. For example, a person involved in a natural disaster such as a hurricane or earthquake is very likely to need help from human services on an emergency basis. Social problems such as discrimination, poverty, and unemployment may also reduce a person's ability to be self-supporting. Some victims of these problems need help only temporarily, but others receive help for an extended period.

So this chapter introduces some of the topics basic to a study of contemporary human services. At first glance, they may appear to be simple topics, but closer examination shows them to be very complex—so much so that the brief preliminary information given in this introductory chapter is elaborated throughout the book.

HUMAN NEEDS: FOCUS OF HUMAN SERVICES

A number of schemes have been proposed for conceptualizing human needs. The one suggested by Maslow (1968) is useful for present purposes. He conceived of needs as existing in a kind of pyramid or hierarchy, as shown in Figure 1–1.

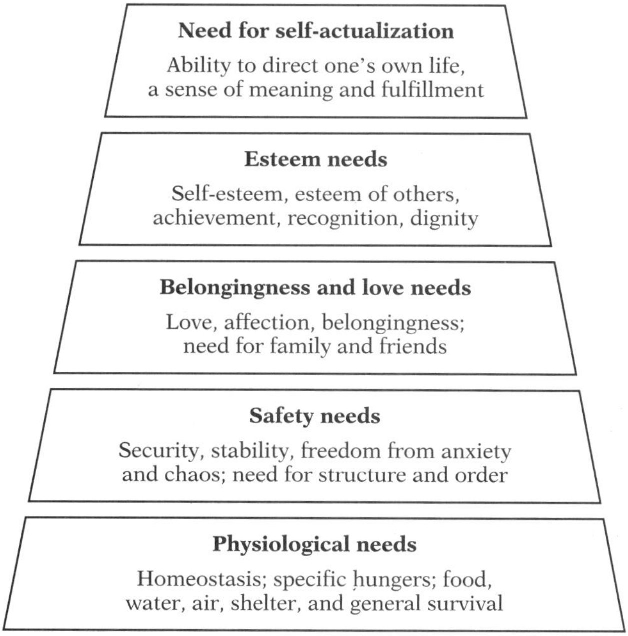

Need for self-actualization

Ability to direct one's own life,
a sense of meaning and fulfillment

Esteem needs

Self-esteem, esteem of others,
achievement, recognition, dignity

Belongingness and love needs

Love, affection, belongingness;
need for family and friends

Safety needs

Security, stability, freedom from anxiety
and chaos; need for structure and order

Physiological needs

Homeostasis; specific hungers; food,
water, air, shelter, and general survival

FIGURE 1–1   Maslow's hierarchy of needs

At the base of the pyramid are the basic **physiological needs** such as hunger, thirst, and the need for oxygen. These are matters of life and death. It is only when survival needs are satisfied that the individual focuses on **safety needs,** which involve the need for a stable, predictable, and secure environment. Clearly, this includes decent housing in a safe neighborhood.

Once partial satisfaction of safety needs has been attained, the need for **belongingness and love** begins to emerge, expressed by a desire for affectionate relations with others. This includes acceptance by one's family, lover, or some larger group. Once the three lower needs have been partly satisfied, **esteem needs** come to the fore, such as the need to be respected as a competent or even a superior person. Most of us desire the recognition and appreciation of others.

The highest need, that for **self-actualization,** has to do with fulfilling one's innate tendencies and potentials. This need involves expressing one's inner nature and talents. For one person, the path to self-actualization might be artistic creativity; for another, it might be studying Eastern religions. This highest level of motivation generally becomes prominent in later life. Young adults are generally preoccupied with making a living and winning the love and approval of others. Maslow (1970) estimated that the average American adult has satisfied about 85% of physiological needs and that the percentage of needs satisfied declines at each step up the hierarchy. At the top step, only 10% have attained satisfaction of self-actualization needs.

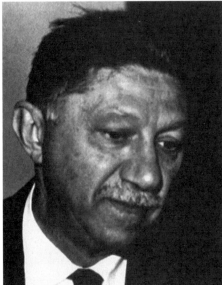

Archives of the History of American Psychology

Abraham Maslow

Maslow (1987) believed that needs arrange themselves in a hierarchy in terms of potency—that is, physiological needs are stronger than safety needs, which in turn are stronger than love needs, and so on. The higher the need, the less imperative its fulfillment is for sheer survival and the longer gratification can be postponed. Deprivation of higher needs does not produce the kind of desperate emergency reaction triggered by deprivation of lower needs. For example, needs for belongingness are a luxury when food or safety is denied.

Maslow (1987) also pointed out that for higher needs to be satisfied, environmental conditions must be favorable. By this he meant that a person must have a supportive family, a decent income, opportunities for a good education, and so on. People without these kinds of advantages face an uphill struggle to attain the higher levels of need satisfaction. In general, Maslow stated, counseling and psychotherapy are more appropriate and effective in helping people achieve higher needs than lower needs. At the lowest need levels, psychotherapy is not much use at all. People who are struggling for basic survival are too worried and preoccupied to give much thought to higher needs. Social planners agree that society must offer tangible kinds of help like food and shelter and medical care to the truly disadvantaged.

Some human services devote themselves to safety needs. The criminal justice system, which includes law enforcement and corrections, is designed to meet safety needs. Citizens want to live in secure communities and go about their daily activities without fear of being threatened, robbed, or assaulted. To this end, the public spends millions for police, courts, and corrections. In Chapter 2, we discuss some reasons for the partial failure of the criminal justice system to create a safe environment.

One of the most consistent findings of social research is that the risk of physical or mental illness is greatest when the individual cannot find a place in the social order. Persons who have been deprived of meaningful social contact for any of a number of reasons are at relatively greater risk of developing tuberculosis, alcoholism, accident proneness, severe mental illness, and suicidal tendencies (Cassel, 1990). Some human services help people to feel that they belong and are valued members of a group. It is expected that such membership may help keep a person out of an institution and, therefore, serve an important preventive purpose. For example, some agencies set up senior clubs for elderly people who would otherwise be living a lonely, isolated life. Another example is the establishment of psychiatric residences for former mental patients who have no family.

Some human services agencies are primarily concerned with meeting the higher needs for esteem and self-actualization. Others help indirectly by meeting basic needs, thus allowing the individual to pursue higher needs on his or her own initiative. Education, particularly at the higher levels, is attuned to helping students attain fulfillment and satisfaction through pursuit of a career. In general, human services workers encourage people to function at their highest possible level. More tangible kinds of help are provided in the form of scholarships and grants offered by a number of governmental and private agencies.

Criticisms of Maslow's Theory. Although Maslow is revered as one of the founders of humanistic psychology, we should not overlook the criticisms that have been leveled against his theory of motivation. At first glance, the theory seems reasonable and fits some observations of everyday life. For example, it seems obvious that people who are starving must first satisfy the need for food before they pursue higher goals. But, on closer examination, we find that Maslow's theory is beset by problems.

The idea that our lower needs must be satisfied before we move to the next higher ones is contradicted by several kinds of evidence. In some societies, for example, people periodically go hungry but, at the same time, exhibit strong social ties and a strong sense of self. In fact, a certain degree of hardship in meeting basic needs can bring people together and give them a sense of purpose in working together to overcome adversity (Neher, 1991). Similarly, many couples in our own society report that a strong bond was formed during a period of early struggles that was weakened by later affluence. Contrary to Maslow's theory, these examples suggest that deprivation of basic physiological needs may sometimes facilitate satisfaction of higher needs, such as the need for intimacy. Aside from anecdotal evidence, there are a number of research studies that have attempted to test Maslow's concepts. The results, according to Neher's (1991) review, have been mixed: Some support and others refute various hypotheses.

In general, the research conducted in work settings has not supported Maslow's theory. For example, Wahba and Bridwell (1976) asked workers to list their needs in order of importance and found that the rankings did not fit Maslow's hierarchy. Other investigators suggested that more than one need may be operating at a time (Geen, Beatty, & Arkin, 1984). In other words, a person may be striving to fulfill simultaneously both basic and growth needs. Still other studies have suggested that moderate levels of deprivation stimulate creative potential, ward off boredom, and enhance a sense of competence (Neher, 1991). This idea runs counter to Maslow's notion that higher needs emerge only after complete satisfaction of lower needs. It may be that some need deprivation is experienced as a challenge and, ultimately, is growth enhancing.

THE ROLE OF PRIMARY SOCIAL SUPPORTS IN MEETING NEEDS

Most people seek gratification of needs through a network of social relationships. For example, needs for nurturance and intimacy can be met by family, friends, and peer groups. Religious and social groups help meet needs for belongingness, esteem, and spiritual enrichment. A job satisfies crucial economic needs and also provides a setting for social interaction with co-workers. Additional support may also come from informal social contacts. For example, bartenders and hairdressers are well known for listening sympathetically to the problems of their customers. This network of relationships, which makes up the primary social support system, is the traditional source of need satisfaction in our culture. One important feature of this support system is that there is usually some sense of mutual obligation underlying the transactions. In other words, a person is expected to give something, to meet certain needs of others, in exchange for what is received. Sometimes, it is enough to simply let others know that one is ready to help if the need arises.

The importance of this primary network to a person's well-being can hardly be overestimated. A study of the Chinese-American community in Washington, DC, showed that psychiatric symptoms were more commonly reported among unmarried people, those with low-paying jobs, and those with weak social supports (Lin, Simeone, Ensel, & Kuo, 1979). Another study showed that social supports can help people to counteract the effects of a difficult or challenging situation (Sarason, 1980). Lack of a support system can also increase the chances of serious illness, including coronary artery disease (Lynch, 1977). These are just a few of the many studies that have shown that the availability of a social support system can help a person to maintain good health in both emotional and physical areas.

Many people in this country are sadly lacking in primary social supports. They may have no friends, no family, no job, and therefore, no way to meet important needs. In some cases, a person may have family and friends who would be willing to help but who lack the means to do so. As detailed in Chapter 3, certain human services came into being to meet the needs of people who have nowhere to turn for help. Over the years, human services have expanded greatly and now go far beyond helping the poor, sick, and disabled. Gradually, they have taken over some of the functions of primary social supports. For example, the task of caring for poor elderly persons, once assumed by the family, is increasingly being accepted by governmental human services agencies.

Self Help Groups

These are basically mutual-help groups made up of people who have similar problems. They occupy a position somewhere between traditional social supports and formal agencies that provide services. The increasing popularity of these groups may be due partly to the decline of the extended family and other traditional sources of support in our society (Bloch, Croch, & Reibstein, 1982). Whatever the cause, these groups have grown from 300 in 1963 to 500,000 in 1992 with 15 million current members. What distinguishes these groups from formal service organizations is that they operate without professional leadership. Many professional therapists view self-help groups as useful adjuncts to treatment and urge clients to participate in them (Comer, 1996).

A wide variety of problems or disorders may be the focus of a self-help group. Alcoholism, drug abuse, compulsive gambling, bereavement, overeating, phobias, rape victimization, unemployment and physical illnesses (e.g., heart disease, diabetes, and cancer) are some examples of issues that may be addressed in support groups. Some advantages of self-help groups are that they are less expensive and less threatening than a professionally led group. Of course, they are designed to offer the support that comes from people who share a problem. A number of self-help groups are mentioned or described in various sections of this book.

The Effects of Social Programs on Primary Supports

During the 1960s, there was a vigorous expansion of social programs designed to eliminate poverty, remove slums, and improve the health and education of poor people. By the end of the decade, some social planners had come to realize that (a) the programs were not always having the desired effect and (b) new problems were being created. Nathan Glazer (1988), employed as an urban sociologist by the Kennedy administration, described his growing disillusionment with the government's reform efforts. For example, it appeared that welfare programs were having the unintended effect of breaking up families and sometimes leading to family nonformation. The programs were administered in such a way that a mother with limited income received not only cash but also a package of other benefits including medical insurance, food stamps, and rent subsidies. If there were a father present, he was usually a low-paid worker at risk of being laid off. He could jeopardize the entire benefits package if he attempted to support the family alone. If he left, little effort was made by the welfare program to require him to support the family in any way. In fact, the family was more economically secure without him. Clearly, the system provided little incentive for the family unit to stay together.

Although we cannot go into great detail about the possible impact of government programs on other primary supports, we can note the evidence, reviewed by Butler and Kondratas (1987, p. 105), that well-intentioned government efforts had the effect of weakening neighborhood associations: "there can be little doubt that the erosion of America's poor communities stems in large part from the explicit attempt of . . . reformers to fold them into the larger 'national' community." There was a tendency, the authors assert, on the part of federal planners to view poor communities as pockets of pathology and to see nothing of value in them. Too often, they failed to recognize and support church, civic, and neighborhood groups that were supportive to the community.

The lesson to be drawn from this part of our national experience is that programs designed to help, however well intended, may have perverse or unexpected consequences. When these programs weaken the family and the neighborhood, there is good reason to be concerned. The strength of such primary supports is essential if individuals are to cope with a complex society. They are the basic linkage of one person to another. We agree with Butler and Kondratas (1987), who argued that America has a strong public interest in government programs that strengthen families; when the family is fragmented, what often follows is poor education, poor skills, and poor performance. This in turn causes the perpetuation of poverty, and the vicious cycle continues.

AN OVERVIEW OF HUMAN SERVICES

"What are human services, anyway?" is one of the questions most frequently asked by students. We would like to provide an "official" or generally accepted definition, but there is no such thing. Actually, ideas about human services have changed over the course of time. As discussed in Chapter 3, early approaches to human services were centered around the hazards of illness, disability, and economic dependence. Programs were designed to help people who were unable to take care of their own needs. It was recognized that people with little or no income in increasingly complex industrial societies were at risk of starvation or serious distress. This view, which equates human services with providing services to the economically dependent, now seems rather narrow.

Another approach is to define human services in terms of the activities of modern society that enhance the well-being of its citizens. Hasenfeld (1983), for example, suggested that human services are designed to "protect or enhance the personal well-being of individuals" (p. 1). This is a broad definition that might include a wide spectrum of services, ranging from job creation to maintaining a clean, safe, and pleasant environment for efforts to help people achieve the highest possible level of self-sufficiency.

Experts do not agree on the range or type of helping activities that should be included in human services. We prefer a definition that falls between the very narrow and the very broad ones just discussed. Human services are organized activities that help people in the areas of health care; mental health, including care for persons with retardation; disability and physical handicap; social welfare; child care; criminal justice; housing; recreation; and education. Another type of service that might be included is income maintenance, a term that refers to programs, like unemployment insurance and social security, that provide income to people who are unemployed or retired (Schmolling, 1995).

It should be noted that human services do not include the help given by family, friends, or other primary supports. The help is provided by some type of formal organization, be it a clinic, hospital, nursing home, agency, bureau, or other service institution.

Obviously, human services cover a lot of ground. During recent decades, human services have increased greatly in size and scope in the United States. This increase is reflected by the fact that the total cost of social welfare went up from $23.5 billion in 1950 to over $1162.2 billion in 1991. This means that social welfare expenses, which were 8.8% of the gross national product in 1950, now consume 20.5% of the value of all goods and services produced in the country (Social Security Administration, 1994). Included in social welfare are expenses for social security, welfare, veteran's programs, education, housing, and other public programs. The federal government is the major provider of social welfare benefits. In fact, most of the huge federal budget goes for social programs of one kind or another. About 12% of all employed people in this country work in human services, either providing direct services or administering them (Hasenfeld, 1983). By any standard, human services is one of the largest industries in the United States.

Human Services Workers

The personnel at human services agencies can be divided into four general categories: (a) those who provide help to recipients, (b) supervisory personnel, (c) administrators who determine the policies of the agency, and (d) support personnel who do clerical, maintenance, and security work. In addition, some settings, such as hospitals and nursing homes, require kitchen, housekeeping, and other support workers. In smaller agencies, workers sometimes have to do work in several of these categories.

A great many job titles, positions, and professions are included under the general heading of human services worker. These range from positions that require relatively little formal training, such as mental hospital aide and teacher assistant, to those that require extensive formal training and education. Clinical and counseling psychologists, psychiatrists, social workers, and nurses are included in the latter category. Chapter 6 goes into detail about a wide range of career options in the field.

There is considerable variation in the extent to which different professionals identify themselves as human services workers. Social workers, for example, have generally been more accepting of the term than have psychologists or psychiatrists. The term *human services worker* is more than a way of identifying workers in a particular field; it carries with it a certain attitude or philosophy about the field. The underlying idea is that the separate disciplines should emphasize what they have in common—serving people's needs—rather than emphasize their differences.

Some activists would like to phase out specialty training in favor of generalist training in human services. However, there is considerable resistance to this idea from professionals who wish to preserve separate identities as psychologists, social workers, psychiatrists, and so on. We apologize if all this sounds confusing; it *is* confusing because the field of human services is undergoing rapid change. It is not possible to know for certain how human services workers of the future will be trained or what their job titles will be.

Kinds of Help Provided

Human services provide many kinds of aid and services. Perhaps the most basic kind of direct aid consists of *tangible items* such as food, clothing, shelter, tools, and other useful articles. Victims of natural disasters and homeless poor persons may be in dire need of this kind of help. The Salvation Army and the Red Cross are well known for providing hot meals and shelter to homeless people.

In most situations, *cash transfers* can readily be exchanged for needed goods and services. Social security, welfare, and unemployment insurance are among the most important benefits of this kind because millions depend on them for economic survival. These cash benefits can be used in any way the recipient sees fit. This freedom worries some politicians who fear that the money will be used for nonessential or even destructive items. This explains why some benefits are offered with strings attached—in other words, the benefits can be used only for some specified purpose. Food stamps, for example, are given to eligible poor persons but can be used only to buy food. Another example is a housing subsidy paid directly to the landlord for a welfare recipient's rent.

In addition to these forms of aid, there are services designed to increase clients' capacities to gain satisfaction of needs by their own efforts. The next few paragraphs give brief preliminary definitions of some of the major kinds of services offered by human service workers.

Primary prevention refers to services designed to prevent people from developing an illness or psychological problem. These services are usually offered to healthy or relatively well-functioning individuals and often have an educational or informative component. A school program designed to inform teenagers of the hazards of alcohol abuse is an example of primary prevention.

Counseling helps people to consider their choices and options in life. Counseling may focus on career choice, budgeting, legal matters, or marital problems. Career counseling, for example, may help a client to select a suitable occupation, whereas marital counseling may focus on a decision about continuing a marriage. Some forms of counseling become involved in helping a client deal with personal problems and, therefore, overlap with psychotherapy.

Psychotherapy has the general goal of changing a client's behavior or emotional responses to improve psychological well-being. Typical goals of therapy are to reduce anxiety, to improve social relationships, and to control undesirable behavior patterns. There is an implication that the client suffers from some degree of psychological impairment.

Crisis intervention is a special form of help designed to meet the needs of a person faced with an unusually difficult life situation. The word *crisis* implies that the person's usual coping mechanisms may not be enough to handle the situation. There is a risk of severe emotional upset or even disorganization. Situations that might trigger a crisis include loss of a loved one or being the victim of rape, assault, serious accident, or large-scale disaster. The helper provides support and suggests effective ways of coping with the crisis. The goal is not to change the person's personality but to restore the client to the precrisis level of functioning. Crisis intervention may be done in the context of face-to-face meetings or by means of a hotline. The latter is a telephone service that allows the caller to get in touch with a counselor at any time of the night or day. The most familiar hotlines are designed to help suicidal individuals. Hotline services are also available to battered women, to rape victims, and to people actively struggling with alcoholism or other chemical dependence.

Rehabilitation is designed to help people with disabilities achieve the highest possible level of productive functioning. Some experts make a distinction between habilitative and rehabilitative programs: The former aim to help those who have never been productive, whereas the latter focus on restoring skills to those who were once capable. In either case, the emphasis tends to be on practical skills such as those involved in self-care and earning a living. The type of disability may be physical, emotional, or developmental.

Social support may be offered in various forms to those who can benefit from a strengthening of social ties. An example is a club for senior citizens that enables them to get together with peers once or twice a week.

Other familiar examples are the athletic and social programs for teens provided by many Ys and community centers. In addition, many self-help programs such as Alcoholics Anonymous emphasize social support in their therapeutic approach.

Community organizing represents another indirect form of support for those in need. The general idea is that the human services worker works with community leaders to provide some program needed by an unserved population in the community. For example, the worker may help the community set up a training school for persons with delayed intellectual development.

Many human services agencies provide a mix of aid and services to clients. Both mental hospitals and prisons, for example, provide aid in the form of food and shelter and may also provide counseling, therapy, or rehabilitation. The employment services of some states link direct cash benefits to job and career counseling. At the other end of the scale are smaller programs that offer only one or a limited range of services to clients.

Sponsors of Human Services

Human services organizations may be sponsored—that is, organized and funded—by private citizens, by religious and other groups, and by government.

Private agencies may be operated on either a profit-making or nonprofit basis. Nursing homes, rehabilitation hospitals, and agencies providing home nursing care are often private profit-making corporations that are run in basically the same way as other businesses. This means that management is under pressure by owners to keep costs down and to show a profit at the end of the year.

Many other private agencies are organized on a not-for-profit basis. Youth employment and child care agencies are sometimes nonprofit. The Red cross and the March of Dimes are examples of large nationwide private human services agencies operated on a nonprofit basis. Typically, such agencies are controlled by a board of directors that lays down general policies and selects the administrative officers who are responsible for the day-to-day operation of the agency. These agencies raise money by appealing to the general public for donations. An important advantage of nonprofit status is that it exempts the agency from certain taxes, which, in effect, allows more of the income to be used for helping consumers of the service.

Religious and other groups also sponsor nonprofit helping agencies. The Federation of Jewish Philanthropies, Catholic Charities, and the Lutheran Brotherhood are supported by major organized religions. In addition, unions, fraternal organizations, and ethnic groups sponsor countless helping agencies all across the country. The necessary funds are raised by appealing to parishioners and members for donations. Increasingly, both private and religious agencies are making use of professional fund-raisers who are paid on the basis of a percentage of the income they raise.

There have been steady increases in voluntary giving during recent years (AAFRC, 1990). In 1988, Americans broke the $100 billion mark in donations to charitable causes and followed that up by a 10% increase the next year. For every $5 we spent on food, we gave more than 80 cents to a worthy cause. For every $2 we spent on shoes and clothing, we gave $1 to philanthropy. Individuals provided about 84% of the total funds, with foundations and corporations far behind.

Who receives this money? Religion gets the largest share, with the remaining funds divided by education, health, human services, the arts, and other causes. Not all of this private giving goes to help poor people. Much of the money goes to groups active in environmental issues, civil liberties, women's rights, pro- and antiabortion issues, museums, and symphony orchestras.

Without minimizing the importance of private and religious human services agencies, it is certain that governments (local, state, and federal) have become the major providers of direct and indirect aid to those in need. The scope and purpose of huge federal programs like social security will be discussed in the next chapter. State governments play a major role in education, administer employment insurance, and manage most of the nation's mental hospitals. Local governments are responsible for actual administration of welfare programs, and they also provide many other kinds of help such as programs for seniors and teens.

Studying Human Services Firsthand

One of the best ways to learn about human services is to identify and study the different agencies and facilities within your geographical area. This kind of study readily lends itself to a team approach because students can divide the work and share information with one another. The information can come from many sources, including literature available at agencies, onsite visits, and meetings with staff members.

Your class might list all of the human services agencies, programs, and facilities in your area and provide answers to the following questions:

- What are the *stated* goals of the agency?
- What needs does the agency attempt to meet?
- What population is served? Roughly how many people does the organization serve? Hundreds? Thousands?
- What does the service cost the consumers? What are the eligibility criteria?
- Where does the money come from? If several sources are involved, list them in order of contribution.
- How many and what kinds of human services workers are employed by the human services agency?

Students can also share their subjective impressions of the agencies they visited. Did they feel welcome? Did the service seem to be well organized? How were clients treated by staff?

Human Service Workers and Bureaucracy

Students beginning their training in human services rarely express the ambition to become bureaucrats. Nevertheless, the great majority of them will eventually find themselves working in the type of organization called a bureau or a bureaucracy. The fact is that welfare agencies, hospitals, employment services, nursing homes, and psychiatric clinics are all examples of this kind of organization. Bureaucracies, which may be small or large, public or private, are defined by certain formal arrangements including some form of central control and a clear division of labor among administrators, supervisors, workers, and clerical staff. The employees are usually arranged in a hierarchy from higher to lower, and exchanges between the lower and upper levels without "going through channels" are often discouraged (Macht & Ashford, 1990, p. 227). One of the frustrating features of the large bureaucracy is the difficulty a worker may experience in feeling that he or she makes a difference. Each person may feel like a small cog in a big machine. Despite the shortcomings of these kind of organizations, they have adapted and survived. No one has developed a more efficient means of providing services on a large scale.

We agree with Macht and Ashford (1990) that educators often fail to prepare students to become effective bureaucrats. When bureaucracy is discussed in class, it is often in terms of the potential conflict between agency goals on the one hand and between client or worker goals on the other. Or the discussion may focus on the organization as a cause of low morale among workers. It is all too easy to lose sight of the fact that specialization of workers, clear lines of command, and other features of the bureaucracy enable it to deliver services on a large scale and in an efficient manner. Rather than focus on the negative aspects, it is more productive to help students develop the knowledge and skills to work effectively within the bureaucracy. To this end, the student should be acquainted with the patterns of organization in human services organizations. We think so highly of this idea that we initiated a course in human services organizations taught at the undergraduate college level (rather than at the graduate level). Some of the topics explored are the use of power, funding sources, specialization, and delivery of services. Also discussed is the important topic of how to bring about constructive changes in the organization.

It has been suggested that use of systems theory may be useful when working with bureaucracies that have become rigid and unresponsive to client needs. The input of new energy, knowledge, skills, technology, and personnel into the system can only be facilitated by workers who fully understand how the agency is organized (Brill, 1990, p. 114). Here is a list of characteristics of human services organizations, some of which were suggested by Caplow (1976) in his book *How to Run Any Organization*.

- ◆ Every organization has an identity of its own, with its own territory, program, rules and procedures, history, and vocabulary.
- ◆ Every organization has its own supporters and antagonists in the community and in other agencies.

- Every organization was established to achieve definite purposes and goals in providing human services.
- Most organizations have subsystems whose interests are not always compatible with the larger system. The subsystem may, for example, be a unit that is not in fact serving any useful purpose but whose members are determined to preserve their jobs.
- At a given point in time, an organization will be growing, stable, or declining, and this tendency will affect all parts of the organization.
- Organizations may develop crises, based on conflicts around policy, that have the potential either to destroy the agency or to bring about its reorganization in positive ways.

The Trend Toward Privatization

The process of arranging for private companies to do certain jobs formerly done by government is called privatizing or privatization. Recent decades have seen an increase in the trend to privatize government services along with an increasing role for profit-making companies. David Linowes (1995, p. 86), who served as chairman of President Reagan's Commission on Privatization, supported this trend: The push to privatize, he argued, is a reaction against "the fact that much of government has become entangled in its own power, stifling creativity and productivity. Government agencies responsible for serving the people have become muscle bound, almost to the point of paralysis when it comes to considering more effective performance." He added that government agencies are trying to solve social problems with outmoded designs and solutions. Clearly, Linowes is giving voice to the dislike of government bureaucracies shared by many conservatives.

Opposition to the trend to privatize has come from government employees, including many human service workers. Perhaps the best organized resistance has come from the nation's unions of public employees. Although industrial unions have declined in influence since the end of World War II, unions of government employees have increased in size and power. By the end of 1992, and for the first time in American history, more people were employed by governments than in manufacturing (Peterson, 1994, p. 190). Many government workers are organized into civil service employee unions. Like other special interest groups, these unions lobby state and local legislators, contribute to campaign funds, and may deliver a sizable block of votes in elections. The purpose of this lobbying is, of course, to secure the kinds of benefits unions have always sought for their members: decent pay, job security, and fringe benefits such as pensions and medical insurance. During recent years, an increasing number of taxpayers began to resent the favorable contracts won by these unions. As we show in a later section, the wages of most nongovernment workers stagnated during recent decades, and employers became more reluctant to give fringe benefits. At the same time, there were pressures to cut the costs of government. By contracting with private companies to do certain jobs, it was possible to cut costs while weakening the power of the unions. How are private companies able to achieve significant savings? They hire nonunion workers at salaries lower than those of union workers, and they typically provide limited (or no) fringe benefits.

The Westchester Experience.   The county executive of Westchester, a suburban community in New York, was quoted by Wilson (1995, p. 1A) as saying: "Our [county] workers have priced themselves out of existence. The government has a right to save money. Taxpayers are important people, and if there is a better way to do things, we should do it." In previous years, this same county executive had accepted the endorsement of the county worker's union and had agreed to generous contractual benefits for the members. Now, there was concern that hospital laundry and housekeeping workers were earning $12–15 an hour when the going rate in nonunionized facilities was closer to $5 an hour. Union officials complained angrily that the move to privatize was intended to "bust" the union. Union workers were very much afraid of losing their jobs and predicted that privatization would result in a decline in the quality of the services provided. They wondered how workers could live and support a family on $5 an hour.

This drama is being enacted in many other communities across the nation. It is of great importance to the reader for the obvious reason that government provides most human services. Here is a list of some of the services that have been privatized in some communities:

Housekeeping, laundry, and food services for hospitals and prisons.
Transportation services to and from schools and other facilities.
Shelters and housing for the homeless.
Computer services for various human service agencies.
Jails for illegal immigrants.
Halfway houses and day hospitals for persons with mental illness.
Halfway houses for released prisoners.
Recovery homes for alcoholics and drug addicts.
Fire protection.

These examples show that parts of larger operations may be privatized by government. More ambitious efforts to privatize may involve entire programs and facilities. For example, Brown County, Wisconsin, has turned over its welfare program to an outside private organization, and Corrections Corporation of America has more than $100 million in contracts for prisons and detention centers in nine states (Linowes, 1995).

There are potential dangers involved in either government-run or privatized services. Programs run by government are at risk of becoming job programs for union employees and political appointees. The needs of the workers may take precedence over the needs of recipients. The danger of privatization, on the other hand, is that the profit motive may come to dominate all other considerations. For example, one firm providing halfway houses for prisoners was charged with hiring low-paid, untrained employees and with allowing living conditions in the facility to deteriorate markedly. Fire hazards such as exposed electrical wires went unrepaired, and vermin were permitted free run of the place (Sullivan & Purdy, 1995).

Suggestion for a class report or term paper:

Examine the effects of a specific program or service that has been privatized in your county or state. What was the effect on the government workers who previously provided the service? Describe the new workers in terms of salary and qualifications. Was there any change in the quality of the services provided? Interview some people who were directly affected by the change and report their reactions.

Education for Human Service Careers

During the 1960s, the federal government greatly increased its support for human services. The rapid expansion of mental health and other facilities translated into a demand for additional trained workers. To meet the need, the National Institute for Mental Health provided funds to various professional groups such as the Southern Regional Education Board (SREB) to develop human service training programs. These training programs, most of which were offered by community colleges, continued to grow during subsequent decades. A 1993 survey of 2-year human services programs revealed some important trends in program growth, student composition, and career paths (Schindler & Brawley, 1993). Here are some results of the survey:

◆ Of the 837 colleges that responded to an initial inquiry, 532 (64%) reported that they had a human service education program with human services defined as social services, mental health, child care, youth work, corrections, counseling, and similar descriptions.

◆ After a period of stabilization in the number of programs through the mid-1980s, a period of increased growth during the 1988–1991 period was reported.

◆ Twenty-three different titles of programs were reported, with human services and early childhood being the most common. Criminal justice, substance abuse, mental health, social services, gerontology, family services, and interpreter training for the hearing impaired were also reported.

◆ There was a significant increase during recent years in the number of people seeking higher education after graduation as opposed to seeking employment at the 2-year level.

◆ The findings suggested that the total enrollment nationwide in such programs was in the 65,000–75,000 range. Most colleges reported that enrollments had increased or remained the same for the past 5 years.

◆ The great majority of programs provided fieldwork or practicum training for students. This means the student comes into contact with clients in a community setting.

◆ Social work was the most popular choice of transfer students, followed very closely by psychology. Next in popularity were careers in child development and education, followed by criminal justice, sociology, human services, counseling, and others.

◆ About 44% of the programs reported that 75–100% of their graduates found appropriate jobs in human services, and 20% reported that 50–75% found suitable jobs. The remaining programs found that fewer than 25% found suitable jobs. It was not known if the wide variation in placement success was due to the vagaries of the job market in a given area or to other factors.

◆ A great many job titles were cited by graduates who did obtain work in human services. These included social worker, social work technician, caseworker, case manager, human services worker, and various kinds of aides. Specialized designations such as gerontology worker, substance abuse counselor, and corrections worker were also mentioned.

◆ About half of all programs in the survey reported they offered in-service and continuing education for employed workers. Obviously, many programs were sensitive to the need for skills renewal, updating knowledge, and lifelong learning.

◆ Looking ahead, faculty members see a need for an increased number of workers with specialized knowledge and skills to work with new client populations such as those with HIV infection, the homeless, and youngsters at risk of teenage pregnancy.

◆ Some programs are modifying curricula in the direction of greater specialization. This shift away from the generalist approach is sometimes driven by the availability of grant money given to help specific population groups such as abused women or drug addicts.

It appears obvious that the notion of training a generalist human service worker has not made much headway in recent years. This kind of worker draws from all the major mental-health fields and uses ideas from psychology, social work, counseling, and related areas. Consequently, he or she is well equipped to work side by side with a wide variety of mental-health workers (Neukrug, 1994). As we have seen, however, the current trend is toward greater specialization in human service training.

SOURCES OF NEED SATISFACTION

Figure 1–2 is a flowchart that illustrates the relationship between needs, primary sources of help, and human services. A person in need often seeks help from primary sources such as family and friends before going to a human services agency. For example, a person with financial difficulties may seek help from the family before applying for welfare. Similarly, a person with emotional problems may seek advice from a priest, minister, or rabbi before going to a psychiatric clinic. It is often more comfortable to

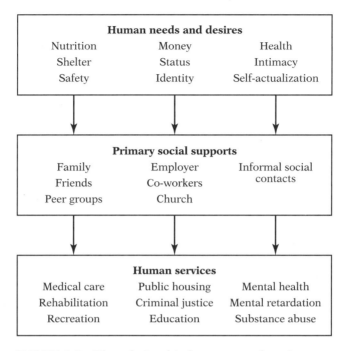

FIGURE 1–2   The relationship between needs, primary social supports, and human services

appeal to familiar persons than to an impersonal agency for help. The bureaucratic procedures of some agencies make people hesitate to go to them: Some agencies make clients wait for hours, require that complicated forms be filled out, and process the claims in a cold, perfunctory manner.

In some circumstances, however, a person may prefer to go to a human services agency rather than to primary sources. For example, an individual may want to conceal an unwanted pregnancy from family and friends. Others may feel too embarrassed about certain behaviors to even discuss them with friends or family. Child abusers, gamblers, and drug addicts may well fall into this category. In these cases, the human services agency offers the opportunity to deal with the problem in a confidential manner. And to those lacking in primary social supports, the human services often represent the last defense against personal disaster.

FALLING THROUGH THE SAFETY NET

An unknown number of people need help from human services but don't get it. These are the people who fall through the safety net provided by basic services. Some needy people are not eligible for help based on the criteria of the agency in question. For example, a worker may not be eligible for unemployment benefits if he or she did not work for a specified number of months during the previous year. Other needy people may simply be unaware of existing programs. For example, some illegal immigrants do not know about programs designed to help them. Still other needy people may be fully aware of programs but are too proud to accept the help available.

What happens to these people who are not helped by either primary social supports or by human services? Many thousands of them end up in the streets. The story of America's homeless is told in detail in Chapter 2. Runaway children, long-term alcoholics, and former mental hospital inmates may be included in the ranks of "street people." During severe weather, some of them try to secure admission to jails or mental hospitals. Some depend on handouts from passersby, and many take meals provided by soup kitchens or shelters. There is continuing debate about what to do with these people, usually with one agency or level of government trying to shift the responsibility elsewhere.

Up to this point, we have emphasized the role of human services in attempting to meet needs. However, human needs are only one consideration in the design and delivery of services. Let's examine some other potent factors that influence human services in the United States.

POLITICAL CONTROVERSY AND HUMAN SERVICES

The magnitude, scope, and purpose of human services are shaped only in part by the needs of people. Other considerations are the resources available for helping and the attitudes of various groups toward human services. Unfortunately, there is no consensus of opinion about the issue of who should receive what kind of help. The ultraconservative view is that government support for human services should be cut to the barest minimum. Liberals see the need for increases in all human services. In our society, there is constant conflict between those who would cut and those who would increase expenditures for human services. This has resulted in an ebb and flow of governmental support for human services. One unfortunate consequence is that human services have not been allowed to develop in an orderly, rational manner. Services are initiated under one administration only to be limited or eliminated by the next administration. The political forces underlying these conflicts are generally labeled *liberal* and *conservative*. Of course, people are not consistent within these frameworks. A particular individual may take a liberal position about one kind of service but a conservative position on another. Let's look more closely at these positions.

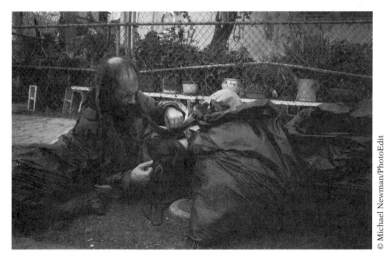

One of thousands of homeless people living in the streets of our cities

A Conservative Point of View

Conservatives wish to preserve traditional American values, including a strict adherence to the Constitution and respect for the rights and property of others. They profess a deep respect for the values of the American pioneer with a strong emphasis on hard work, perseverance, and self-reliance. Jealous of their personal liberty, conservatives tend to distrust big government and wish to limit its role to the barest essentials. This resentment against interference extends into the economic sphere. Generally, conservatives favor a free market and maintain that free enterprise and the pursuit of private profit have made the United States the richest nation on earth.

Conservatives perceive liberals as sentimentalists who spend billions of dollars of taxpayers' money on ill-devised and ineffective social programs. For example, Barry Goldwater (1978), a leading conservative spokesman, attacked the liberal political movements for offering federal financing as the answer for every problem that had ever confronted the American people. Federal spending for housing, health, education, civil rights, equal employment opportunities, urban renewal, and revamping farms had totaled billions of dollars in recent decades. Yet, Goldwater argued, all this government expenditure had solved no domestic problems and in some cases had made things worse. Goldwater expressed the conviction that the individual is often ignored in all of this liberal organizational activity. Conservatives place great value on the concept of Americans as rugged individualists who believe in pulling themselves up by their bootstraps.

Conservatives no longer oppose social programs in an automatic, reflexive fashion. They recognize that there are some circumstances when people, through no fault of their own, require help from government. Few, if any, conservatives now favor elimination of the social security program, although some would favor a reorganization along the lines of a voluntary insurance program. Conservatives also accept the need for some form of welfare benefits for those who are unable to meet immediate needs. However, they would like to see built into the system incentives that would induce individuals to become self-supporting. They are horrified by the specter of long-term welfare dependence extending from one generation to the next. Conservatives also generally favor unemployment insurance, partly in recognition of the fact that workers are often caught up in economic problems far beyond their individual control. It must also be recognized that all of these programs are beneficial to the economy because they help individuals maintain purchasing power.

Conservatives are likely to oppose programs that go beyond meeting basic survival needs. They express concern that help from the government tends to weaken the initiative of the recipient, creating an attitude of passive dependence. They also believe that the federal government has assumed excessive control over our lives through its massive programs and that power and control should be returned to the individual states.

A Liberal Perspective

Liberals see themselves as champions of the disadvantaged. They are convinced that conservative rhetoric about liberty and self-reliance doesn't mean very much to a person who is hungry, broke, and unemployed. Arthur Schlesinger (1962), the noted historian and liberal spokesman, suggested that American conservatism began on a lofty idealistic plane but degenerated into a concern about immediate class interest—that is, it became increasingly concerned with the profits of the business community. The control of government by big business, Schlesinger continued, drove the country to the brink of revolution. In fact, the Great Depression of the 1930s followed about 50 years during which business interests were predominant in American political life (Ebenstein, Pritchett, Turner, & Mann, 1970). The Depression was an economic disaster during which nearly one out of every three workers was unemployed; there was no money to borrow and no real opportunity to begin any kind of new enterprise. The frontier with its opportunities had vanished. Millions were helpless victims of a complex industrial society beyond their control or comprehension.

The New Deal of the Franklin Delano Roosevelt administration initiated a period of liberal dominance of our country's political life. The basic premise of the New Deal was that government must help people do what they cannot do by their own individual efforts. The principles of FDR and the New Deal were soon translated into ambitious governmental programs. Slum clearance and public health programs were put into effect along with insurance programs for the aged, disabled, and unemployed. Assistance programs for families with dependent children and for blind people were

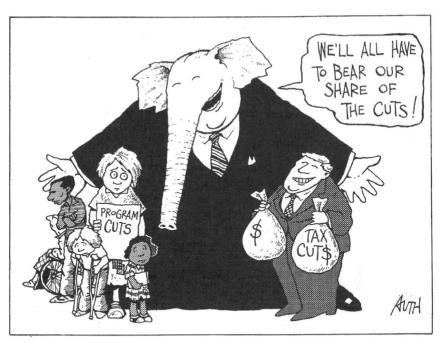

AUTH © The Philadelphia Inquirer. Reprinted with permission of UNIVERSAL PRESS SYNDICATE. All rights reserved.

created in the mid-1930s, along with an array of other kinds of help for those in need. There was a basic shift of political power from big business to big government. The liberal tradition was carried on by the administrations of Harry Truman, John F. Kennedy, and Lyndon Johnson. All perceived that government must take a leading and responsible role in working for the health, safety, and welfare of the people.

During periods of liberal ascendancy, conservatives have been alarmed by the vast increase in the size of government, by the increased taxation needed to support wide-ranging social programs, and by the tendency of liberals to spend more money than they raise. The financial near collapse of New York City during the late 1970s was seen by conservatives as the inevitable result of liberal mismanagement. Political momentum began to swing in a conservative direction.

Mario Cuomo (1994) contrasted the liberal and conservative positions in the following way: Liberals accept the idea of collective responsibility, a sense of we are all in this together, whereas conservatives are more reluctant to get involved in sharing benefits or burdens. Cuomo argued that people don't have to love their needy neighbors, but they should at least consider their own self-interest. "If we bring children into this world and let them go hungry and uneducated, if we are indifferent to the drugs and squalor that surround them . . . , then all of us will share the outcome," wrote Cuomo (1994, p. 9), adding that we will all be obliged to spend more on jails and police while we live in fear.

Conservatism Under Ronald Reagan

Ronald Reagan was carried into office by the nation's swing toward conservatism. Once in office, he put into effect a conservative economic program that eventually achieved considerable success in lowering the rate of inflation. Also enacted were tax cuts designed to increase the purchasing power of consumers, thereby stimulating the economy. The tax cuts were also designed to put more money into the hands of wealthy individuals and corporations. Conservative economic theory held that this excess capital would be invested and create a climate of vigorous business activity. The poor and working class would eventually benefit because new jobs would be made available. Some liberal critics denigrated this theory as a "trickle down" approach to helping the poor. Nevertheless, the administration's economic policies did result in a significant reduction in unemployment. Although many benefited from the active economy of the mid-1980s, the fact remains that millions of people were still poor and/or unemployed as the Reagan administration came to a close. One difficulty was that many of the newly created jobs were low paying dead-end positions in service industries such as fast-food operations.

During the 1980 elections, Reagan criticized the previous administration for lagging behind Russia and the communist bloc nations in overall military strength. Once in office, President Reagan acted promptly to increase spending for national defense. To the dismay of some conservatives, the Reagan administration began spending more money than it received, eventually creating the largest budget deficit in U. S. history. Conservative notions of fiscal responsibility, which stress a balanced budget, were ignored. The spending for weapons systems and the growing deficit intensified pressure to cut spending for social programs. There were reductions in school lunch programs, more stringent criteria for aid to disabled persons, cuts in medical insurance benefits, and so on.

In line with conservative policies, the Reagan administration increased the freedom of each state to deal with social programs in its own way. This was done by giving federal money to the states in the form of block grants that allowed each state considerable leeway in deciding how to spend the money (Bloom, 1984). The states were provided with block grants for health services, including specific funds for mental health and for alcohol and drug abuse programs. However, these grants were accompanied by an overall reduction in spending for social programs. It was expected that state and local governments would take up the slack. There *was* growth in spending by local governments during the Reagan years, but most of the increase was used to satisfy an outcry from middle-class people for better schools and police protection. Many of the federal programs for the poor were not picked up by the states and localities (Uchitelle, 1987). It appeared that the needs of those with the greatest political influence were given top priority.

Liberalism in Decline

During the 1980s, conservative ideas became widely accepted among policy-makers at the federal level. They viewed the war on poverty as a giant failure and suspected that the social-welfare policies of previous decades had increased crime, illegitimate births, drug use, teenage pregnancies, family breakup, and other social ills. Charles Murray (1984, p. 45), an influential policy analyst, was applauded for his view that the expanded social-welfare measures of the '60s created poverty by undermining the "fragile assumption . . . that adults are responsible for the state in which they find themselves." He suggested doing away with the entire federal welfare and income-support structure. In this climate, according to liberal spokeswoman Barbara Ehrenreich (1989, p. 191), the "liberal response to . . . Reagan's domestic policies was, for the most part, a shameful silence." There was no serious rebuttal to conservative ideas, and liberals seemed to distance themselves from the concerns that had defined liberalism since the days of the New Deal. Humorist Russell Baker, himself a liberal, declared the breed near extinction: "The last official count . . . showed 20 female liberals and 17 males"—some of whom he identified as "white-wine and brie" liberals. There was a feeling that many liberals were doing well in the 1980s and had lost some of their zeal for helping the disadvantaged. It came as no great surprise when George Bush, the Republican nominee, easily defeated Michael Dukakis, the Democratic nominee, in the presidential election of 1988.

The Bush Administration: A Kinder, Gentler America?

Although President Bush generally adhered to the conservative principles of his predecessor, he was often viewed as a more practical and less doctrinaire leader than was President Reagan. Bush's speeches suggested that he wanted to be seen as a man who was deeply concerned about the needs of the nation's downtrodden. The "points of light" campaign was central to the domestic policy of the Bush administration. The phrase entered political consciousness when George Bush accepted the nomination of his party at the 1988 Republican convention. He spoke of "a brilliant diversity spread like the stars, like a thousand points of light in a broad and peaceful sky." Each point of light was a volunteer group or individual who provided service to someone in need. This approach is very much in line with the conservative idea that, whenever possible, private efforts are to be preferred over the expansion of government programs. According to a White House aide, such volunteers bring something that the sick and needy value: a purity of motivation that government workers lack (DeParle, 1991). Social healing is turned into a daily part of life. A privately managed Points of Light Foundation, near the White House, presented commercials on radio and television. A point of light coordinator in the White House designated a daily "point of light" for providing outstanding volunteer service.

Sweden: A Study in Contrast

◆ Sweden's approach to human services provides a sharp contrast to that of the United States. It may be viewed as the ultimate welfare state. Sweden puts about 30% of its entire national wealth into human services, compared to 14% for the United States. That money is used to provide paternal leave from work; day care for children between ages 2 and 7; free education, including university and continuing education; large-scale public housing; health care; and worker benefits including job placement, training, and sheltered employment for the disabled (Barkan, 1991). Furthermore, the Swedes deliberately act to equalize the distribution of income between workers in different industries. They also use taxes to further equalize income between individuals. The proportion of families living in poverty is about 5% compared to a much higher rate for the United States. The great disparity in health between children of different social classes found in the United States does not exist in Sweden. The rate of violent crime is much lower than in most other industrialized nations. Although other factors may be involved, it seems fair to say that social services contribute to the high level of personal security that Swedes enjoy.

Of course, there is a downside to all of this government nurturing. Swedes pay much higher rates of taxation than do U. S. citizens. It seems doubtful that Americans would sit still for a 50% rate of income tax. They would prefer fewer government services and more money in their pockets. The Swedes themselves are having second thoughts about the costs of their welfare state. Recent political developments in that country suggest that some reduction in benefits is now favored by a majority of citizens.   ◆

This Bush initiative was subjected to scathing criticism by the political opposition. Some commentators charged that the "points of light" campaign was designed to cover up the callous indifference of the administration to glaring social problems: It was a public relations effort that allowed the government to shirk its responsibility (DeParle, 1991). Cartoons of devastated communities were identified as "a thousand points of blight." By placing the burden on the private nonprofit section, the critics said, the administration avoided the task of raising revenue to finance the large-scale government efforts that alone can solve our problems.

The Clinton Administration

In 1991, George Bush appeared certain to be reelected. He had led a brilliantly successful war against the unpopular Saddam Hussein, crushing the Iraqi army in a matter of weeks. Running against Bush was likened by the popular press to a suicide mission. However, Bush was hurt by a downturn in the economy in the months before the election and by the entry of billionaire industrialist Ross Perot into the race as a third party candidate. Perot, who amazingly was to win 19% of the vote, focused on reforming a corrupt political system that was a captive of lobbyists and special interest groups. He urged voters to take back control of their government and also highlighted the huge federal deficit which was to unfairly impose a great burden on future generations.

When Bill Clinton announced his candidacy for president of the United States, he presented himself as a champion of the middle class, stressing the values of work, family, self-responsibility, and community. He promised to fight for the "forgotten" middle class: "Middle class people are spending more hours on the job, spending less time with their children, bringing home a smaller paycheck to pay more for health care and housing and education." He would not stand by "and let our children become part of the first generation to do worse than their parents" (quoted in Greenberg, 1995, pp. 182–183).

During the campaign, Clinton ran as a "new" Democrat, carefully distancing himself from the liberal policies of the failed Dukakis campaign during which Republicans had portrayed Democrats as weak on defense, soft on criminals, catering to minorities, and incapable of balancing a budget. Clinton moved close to the political center as he battled his two opponents. He won the election of 1992 but with only 43% of the vote. He was a minority president without a strong mandate for his policies.

The Clinton administration quickly became embroiled in controversies. Administration support for gays in the military, the strong leadership role assumed by First Lady Hillary Rodham Clinton, and the preference shown to women and minorities in appointments to high positions not only generated criticism by conservatives but suggested a commitment to an agenda that had been concealed from the voters. Scandals and vacillating foreign policies created further difficulties for the administration. Successes were passage through Congress of a gun control bill, an anticrime bill that would put more police officers on the street, and a family leave bill. The major initiative was reform of the nation's health care system. The failure of this attempt, to be described in a subsequent section, was a serious blow to the Clinton presidency.

The Election of 1994—A Political Revolution?

The election of 1994 signaled a shift in public opinion toward conservative policies. What was surprising was the decisive nature of the victory for conservative forces represented by the Republican party. For the first time in 40 years, Republicans won control of both the House and Senate. The new congressional majority leaders were Representative Newt Gingrich of the House and Senator Bob Dole of the Senate. The strength of the victory was shown by the fact that no sitting Republican governor, senator, or representative was defeated. Republicans spoke of a political revolution and of a strong mandate to balance the federal budget. The voters seemed to be calling for smaller government, lower taxes, and more individual freedom and personal responsibility instead of more government power (Clymer, 1994).

The Contract with America.   This is the name of a document that was signed in September 1994 by the members of the Republican party in the House of Representatives. Here are some of its provisions:

Pass a constitutional amendment requiring a balanced budget.

Give the president a line-item veto, meaning the power to eliminate expenditures for dubious projects that are embedded within larger bills.

Require convicted offenders to pay full restitution to victims.

Relax rules of evidence at trials so that the guilty will not get off on minor technicalities.

Limit death penalty appeals.

Streamline deportation of criminal aliens.

Increase penalties for child pornography.

Provide tax relief to families with children.

Give tax breaks for adoption and elder care.

Restrict unfunded mandates (i.e., requirements by the federal government that the states provide certain services that are not accompanied by federal funding).

Reduce federal regulations and accompanying paperwork.

Limit punitive damages awarded in lawsuits.

Impose term limits in the form of a constitutional amendment to limit the number of terms someone can serve in Congress.

Provide for a sweeping revision of welfare programs including aid to families with dependent children, child nutrition, food stamps, and supplemental security income (Toner, 1995).

Leading Democrats conceded that the Republicans at least knew what they wanted to do. As Senator Moynihan, Democrat of New York, said, the Republicans did not find themselves in the majority asking, "What now?" Senator Moynihan was also quoted as saying that the contract with America represented "the harshest, most regressive legislation in our history" (Toner, 1995, p. 18). Mario Cuomo (1994) also expressed concern that Americans were heading back to an earlier historical period when exploitation of the poor was the rule. In his view, we must not let the safety net woven by the New Deal and the Great Society become unraveled.

The Ebb and Flow of Support for Human Services

One factor that determines the degree of public support for human services is the state of the economy. In good times, tax revenues increase and more money is made available for human services. During economic downturns, funding for services is likely to be reduced.

Changes in the public's attitude toward government also affect funding for services. In recent years, the public's confidence in government seems to have reached a low point. Some people feel that the less money we send to government, the less it will have to waste. Taxpayers periodically rebel against the relentless pressure for increased tax revenues. A case in point was the victory in 1978 of California's Proposition 13, a referendum that restricted the taxing of property.

Supporters of human services argue that it is futile to attempt to save money by cutting funds for human services programs. For example, if we pay less for child care services now, we will have to spend more later for supporting people in mental hospitals and correctional facilities. If we cut back on funds for probation, we reduce our chances of rehabilitating offenders. Overcrowding in our prisons coupled with a lack of therapeutic programs is responsible for the high rate of recidivism. Is there really any long-run saving to be derived from "dumping" former mental patients into communities that are unable or unwilling to provide supportive services for them? By shortchanging human services agencies, we prevent them from reducing the number of dependent and dysfunctional people.

Human services programs need sufficient funding and an orderly, predictable flow of funds from one year to the next to fulfill their missions. In fact, government seems to provide for human services on a hand-to-mouth basis with the threat or actuality of significant cutbacks always possible. These variations in funding are usually related to political and economic factors that have little to do with the needs of the agency or its clients. It is difficult to do an effective job, maintain employee morale, and keep the confidence of the clients under such unstable conditions. This is why human services workers are increasingly seeing the need to organize effective lobbying groups. They recognize that well-organized groups such as the gun lobby, the tobacco lobby, and other special interest groups are often successful in securing favorable legislation. On a practical level, the political system works through the application of this kind of direct pressure. Unrepresented groups, no matter how worthy their cause, are likely to be overlooked.

THE IMPACT OF
CONTEMPORARY PROBLEMS ON NEEDS

Human services do not operate in a vacuum; they are shaped by social, environmental, political, and economic conditions that prevail in a given time and place. The purpose of this section is to pinpoint some contemporary problems that affect the ability of Americans to meet their own needs.

In recent years, there have been decreases in population in both farming areas and in the centers of our large cities. Many people have left the northern, industrial states for the Sun Belt—that is, the tier of southern states ranging from California to Florida. This is also a time of rapid social and technological change. Whereas all of these changes may bring opportunities for some, they create problems for others. To be fully effective, human services need to be based on an up-to-date grasp of the obstacles confronting people. Services need to be constantly modified to keep pace with changing needs.

Natural Disasters

Although natural disasters have occurred since antiquity, this topic is included in a discussion of contemporary problems because the rate of casualties from natural disasters is increasing sharply and will continue to go up in the foreseeable future. A disaster is a phenomenon that can have devastating social consequences when the awesome forces of nature come into contact with people. On a worldwide basis, nearly a quarter of a million people die in natural disasters each year (Frazier, 1979). Earthquakes, floods, hurricanes, tornadoes, and volcanic eruptions are among the natural hazards with the greatest potential for destruction.

In the United States, several trends are acting to increase disaster tolls. One is the vulnerability brought about by increasing dependence on interlinked computer systems and surface electrical power lines. The New York City power blackout of 1977 was triggered by a lightning strike on electronic switching equipment. Another trend that increases the potential for disaster in this country is the shift in population. More and more people are moving into floodplains, seismic risk zones, and coastal areas exposed to hurricane winds, storms, and erosion. There is also an increased risk due to the spread of population to California where landslides and earthquakes are serious hazards. More than half the population now live in places highly susceptible to natural disasters (Frazier, 1979).

In the event of a disaster, people usually first seek help from family, friends, and neighbors. However, if the disaster is severe, local service agencies are called upon to help the sick and homeless. The police, fire department, church organizations, social welfare groups, and medical services may all play important roles, depending on the nature of the disaster. Restoring communication, effecting evacuations, rescuing survivors, and providing temporary shelter and emergency first aid are just some of the important jobs that may need to be done. It is obvious that well-trained, well-organized service workers function more effectively than untrained ones. People tend to turn to large disaster relief organizations such as the Red Cross or Civil Defense only as a last resort (Quarantelli & Dynes, 1972, 1979). Many of these observations apply just as well to disasters for which humans are responsible, such as mine cave-ins or the collapse of buildings and other structures.

Hurricane Andrew.   One of the most devastating natural disasters in U. S. history hit the coast of Florida in the summer of 1992. The storm, which generated winds of 150 miles an hour, hit land on August 24 and devastated south Dade County, creating a zone of destruction larger than the city of Chicago. More than 80,000 dwellings were demolished or rendered unlivable. Thirty billion dollars worth of property was destroyed. Due to the fact that many residents had obeyed evacuation orders, the death toll was only 43 in Florida; 15 more people were killed when the storm reached Louisiana (Gore, 1993).

After the storm, Dade County residents found themselves sweltering in the sun without food, electricity, or transportation. Thousands of cars were demolished, trees were down, and traffic lights were blown away. Almost as bad as the storm itself were the looters who suddenly appeared in large numbers. These predators made off with their neighbors' TVs, VCRs, and other valuables. Help was urgently needed but slow to arrive. Apparently, state and federal officials did not grasp the scope of the disaster until 2 days after the hurricane. Southern Baptist organizations were the first on the scene, setting up mobile kitchens and distributing thousands of meals a day. The Red Cross set up emergency shelters, and relief workers brought in medicine and other necessities. The most massive aid came from a joint military task force that directed traffic, restored order, and brought in supplies by means of truck convoys and helicopter (Gore, 1993).

Six months later, the region still looked like a war zone with emptied housing projects, roofless homes, boarded up shops, and thousands still living in tents. Many children showed signs of having been traumatized by the event. A dozen elementary school children had attempted suicide, one by hanging and another by jumping in front of the school bus. Many children, and some adults, became anxious and upset during storms after the hurricane, afraid that Andrew had come back. Counselors and school psychologists reassured parents that these responses were entirely to be expected under the conditions. In school, counselors watched for signs of despondency among the students. Not surprisingly, grades were falling and more students were being disruptive in class; others fell asleep during the day. In some instances, parents were contributing to the problem because they themselves were stressed out and short tempered with their children. One counselor hit upon the idea of giving out toys during therapy sessions and found that even older children could take comfort from stuffed animals. An 11-year-old boy clutched a pink bear and said, "A whole buncha houses come down and fall on mine" (Gelman & Katel, 1993, p. 65). It seems clear that the work of psychological counseling needs to go on for an extended period after a disaster.

Technological Disasters

Technological disasters differ in some respects from natural disasters. They are usually due to human error, carelessness, avarice, or in some instances, to a callous disregard for human values in the pursuit of profit (Rice, 1987). Since they are preventable, there is generally more rage and anger among victims following a technological disaster than after a natural disaster.

The nuclear accident at Three Mile Island, Pennsylvania, in 1979 was a major technological disaster. It began when a malfunction at one unit caused a release of radioactive gases into the atmosphere. During the immediate crisis, which lasted several days, there was massive disruption of life and evacuations from the surrounding area. The threat of radioactive leaks lasted for over 1 year. The victims exhibited increased psychological distress, increased physical complaints, and heightened levels of adrenaline, indicating high anxiety and tension. It was also reported that residents who had little or no social support showed more stress than those with good support (Fleming, Baum, Gisriel, & Gatchel, 1982).

An even more terrible disaster took place during 1986 at the Chernobyl nuclear power plant in the Soviet Union. Thirty-one people died in the initial explosion and fire at the Number 4 reactor of the plant, and about 300 have died subsequently. Initially, the plant managers delayed in informing the government of the extent of the damage, thereby slowing the evacuation of nearby residents. The Soviet government then misled the world and its own citizens about the seriousness of the problem; only later did the government admit to severe medical and environmental consequences (Barringer, 1990). Specifically, it was revealed that 4 million people in the Ukraine and western Russia are living on contaminated ground. Their exposure to radioactivity is resulting in high rates of thyroid cancer, leukemia, and premature death. The initial cover-up of the accident's scope prevented timely actions aimed at protecting people from radioactivity.

As a consequence of the incidents at Three Mile Island and Chernobyl, there is intense worldwide controversy about the safety of nuclear power. Although the workers in and around the plants are at greatest risk, nuclear accidents also pose a threat to people living far away from the scene. Radioactivity may be carried by wind currents and contaminate distant soil, plants, and animals as well as people.

The Needs of Emergency Services Workers. Although the victims of disaster are of immediate concern, the mental health needs of emergency workers must not be overlooked. In attempting to help victims under stressful and chaotic conditions, these workers may suffer extreme fatigue, stress reactions, and burnout. The National Institute of Mental Health (1985) has provided some suggestions that will help prevent and control stress among workers.

◆ Preventive efforts might include predisaster training in the mental health aspects of the work. Workers can learn to recognize the stresses inherent in their work and to develop strategies for dealing with those stresses. For example, the workers can learn about resources, such as debriefing and counseling, available to them for dealing with stress. The workers should also receive training in their particular role in the organization's overall plan and should participate in disaster drills.

◆ During the disaster, workers should be provided with as much factual information as possible about what they will find at the scene, and they should be informed about the well-being of their family members. Workers should be checked by supervisors for signs of stress and, perhaps, rotated between assignments of varying difficulty. Workers should be required to take breaks, especially if their capacity to help is diminishing.

♦ After the disaster, all who participated in the work should be debriefed. The debriefing may be one-to-one or it may be a group meeting in which the emotional aspects of the experience are discussed. The leader should be skilled in group dynamics and be trained to handle strong emotions. The debriefing is usually held between 24 and 48 hours after the incident, allowing time to overcome the initial fatigue and numbness. Two to four hours should be allowed for the debriefing, and both the positive and negative emotional responses should be reviewed. Finally, the organization should have some means of monitoring the worker's recovery from traumatic events and, if needed, the worker should be referred for counseling.

The victims of disasters are a small percentage of those who receive aid from human services. Most people who receive help are victims of social conditions such as poverty, discrimination, and technological change.

Poverty

Poverty was the norm among the successive waves of immigrants to this country during the previous century. Most immigrants regarded it as a temporary state that could be overcome by hard work and a bit of luck. During the 1800s, this optimism was justified by the dynamic growth of the nation and by the ample space for expansion westward. There were abundant opportunities for the enterprising individual, and it was expected that the second generation would surpass the immigrant parents in financial achievement.

In modern times, however, poverty tends to persist from one generation to the next. As Harrington (1968) pointed out, poverty may become a self-fulfilling prophecy, a kind of vicious cycle that robs the individual of the means to escape. The poverty cycle is perpetuated by the fact that the disadvantages of poverty hinder the next generation's chances to succeed. The high prevalence of broken homes and single-parent families sometimes results in insufficient supervision of and encouragement to children. Poor language skills and a lack of early environmental stimulation may make it difficult for children to take full advantage of educational resources. It becomes difficult for children to develop the skills and attitudes necessary to break out of the poverty cycle.

Of all social problems, poverty is the one that has received the largest share of attention from social planners. Poverty is a critical problem because so many other problems are linked to it; juvenile delinquency, criminality, drug abuse, and mental illness are disproportionately represented in poor communities. Serious health problems and high rates of infant mortality are also found in poor neighborhoods. Affluent persons are often appalled by the conditions existing in poverty areas and sometimes blame the victims for choosing to live so badly. The poor, on the other hand, think of themselves as having few options and as being trapped by the culture of poverty.

Poverty is a particular problem in the inner cities. Many of the big cities of this country contain decaying neighborhoods occupied mainly by poor households and devastated by arson, vandalism, high crime rates, and abandoned housing. Since World War II, thousands of relatively affluent households, especially those with school-age children, have moved to the suburbs (Bradbury, Downs, & Small, 1982). The result is that the cities are tending to concentrate poor residents who have a great need for services and limited ability to pay for them. In some big cities, one out of five residents is living on public assistance. There is controversy about what to do about this immense problem. Some social planners have thrown up their hands and suggested that it is futile to pour any more money into inner cities. They fear that increased services would only attract more poor people to the cities. Others have proposed that city governments should do everything possible to encourage middle-class people to return to the big cities. This would provide additional tax revenues, which could be used to benefit the poverty population. By and large, however, the inner cities still constitute an enormous reservoir of unmet needs.

Prejudice and Discrimination

The problems of poverty, racism, and prejudice are so deeply intertwined in this country that it is difficult to talk about one without referring to the others. Prejudice is based on preconceived attitudes and feelings about certain races, religions, or ethnic groups, and people of a certain gender. These attitudes reflect negative stereotypes that are often nothing more than simpleminded overgeneralizations about certain groups. Typically, these attitudes are not based on real experience with the group in question but are learned from prejudiced individuals. Prejudicial attitudes not only attack the self-esteem of victims but are often the basis for discrimination in employment, housing, and education. Patterns of discrimination aim to keep certain minorities at the bottom of the economic ladder and in a specific neighborhood or ghetto. Although the United States has made progress in reducing discrimination in recent decades, the lingering effects of mistrust are still with us.

Discrimination against African Americans, Latinos, and women is discussed in the following sections. These groups are highlighted because of their large numbers and because of their great importance to human services. There are, of course, many other groups that have been victims of discrimination, and you are invited to study these independently. Probably no other group has been treated with such consistent savagery as Native Americans. Brown's (1971) *Bury My Heart at Wounded Knee* provides a moving account of this shameful episode in American history. At times, Asian Americans have been victimized by the white majority. See the Additional Reading section at the end of the chapter for recommended books on this and related topics.

Discrimination Against African Americans.   For a number of historical reasons, African Americans for many years were denied access to the political and social life of the United States. They were segregated in regard to where they lived and went to school. They were relegated to low-level jobs that often provided little more than a marginal income. Family life was disrupted by many factors including the greater availability of jobs for African American females than for African American males. While successive waves of European immigrants were being assimilated into mainstream America, African Americans were held back by their obvious racial features. Even when they achieved wealth and fame, they were not readily accepted by affluent white communities. Discrimination tended to force African Americans into a circular pattern in which limited education barred them from higher education and career opportunities.

The African American people made slow but definite progress toward equality during the century following emancipation. This was followed by a period of accelerated progress beginning in the mid-1960s. The political initiatives of the 1960s and 1970s to be described in Chapter 3, were successful in achieving a higher level of opportunity for African Americans. These positive trends continue to the present day. African Americans are gaining in political power; their income is on the rise and more are now seeking higher education than ever before; a small but significant African American middle class has been established. But it is also clear that much remains to be done. Many African Americans are still deeply rooted in poverty and deprivation. Per capita unemployment is significantly higher among African Americans than whites, and African American teenagers have high rates of unemployment.

A Census Bureau report confirmed that more African Americans are getting a piece of the American dream—finishing their educations and finding good jobs. Specifically, 73% of African Americans aged 25 and older completed high school in 1994 compared to 51% in 1980. About 13% of African American adults had bachelor's degrees in 1994 compared to 8% in 1980. However, the income gaps between blacks and whites remained wide: Median family income for white families increased 9% over the past 20 years to $39,310, but the income of African American families remained stagnant at $21,550. The really bad news was that 46.1% of African American children lived in poverty in 1993 compared to 13.6% of white children. This was directly related to the high birthrate of unmarried teens in the black community ("More Blacks in Middle Class," 1995).

Discrimination Against Latinos.   Spanish-speaking Americans have also been victims of a pervasive pattern of discrimination that limits their opportunities for advancement. Virtually every indicator of well-being reflects the results of this discrimination: Their unemployment rates tend to be high; their health is not as good on the average as that of whites; and their educational achievement scores tend to be low, partly because of the language barrier (Freeman, Jones, & Zucker, 1979)

Although Latinos are a smaller group than African Americans in the United States, it is difficult to determine their precise number. Included in their ranks are a large but unknown number of illegal aliens. Migrant workers are another group not usually included in census surveys. In any case, Latinos cannot be considered a homogeneous group. Some can trace their ancestry back to the origins of this country and are well established in their communities. Many others are recent immigrants who came here looking for work. Those who came from Mexico tend to be concentrated in the Southwest, whereas Puerto Ricans tend to live along the East Coast. Many Cubans have settled in the greater Miami area. Other Spanish-speaking people have come here from Central and South America. The tendency of these various subgroups to retain their separate identities has frustrated efforts to join together to advance political and economic objectives.

One group in urgent need of help are the migrant workers who follow the harvest from south to north along the Pacific Coast. The plight of these workers, who are mostly of Mexican origin, has been publicized in books, movies, and magazine articles. However, they have not benefited greatly from this media attention. They work for low pay and are often provided with filthy, substandard housing. The state laws regarding living conditions are sometimes ignored because of official indifference and corruption (Garza, 1973). They are exploited not only by the growers, but also by recruiters who take a percentage of their wages. Perhaps the best hope of improving their living conditions comes from the increasing strength of agricultural unions.

Illegal immigrants are another group in need of assistance. Although illegal workers come from Ireland, India, the Caribbean, Asia, and poor countries all over the globe, the great majority are Spanish-speaking, with Mexicans making up the largest single subgroup. They may be employed in agriculture, the garment industry, factories, hotels, restaurants, gas stations, and many other settings. For the most part, they get the jobs that are dirty, demeaning, boring, and that offer little hope of advancement, and pay badly to boot (Crewdson, 1983). They typically lack union representation and do not usually receive sick leave, insurance benefits, or other fringe benefits. Their illegal status makes them easy prey for unscrupulous employers. To make matters worse, many American citizens resent their presence and blame them for taking away scarce jobs. Moreover, their position in this country has been made even more precarious by recent legislation.

The Immigration Reform and Control Act of 1986, the most important piece of legislation pertaining to immigration in decades, attempted to deal with the problem of illegal immigration by granting amnesty to illegal aliens living continuously in the United States since January 1, 1982 and to agricultural workers if they worked here for at least 3 months from May 1985 to May 1986. The Act also provides stiff penalties for employers who hire undocumented workers. In 1991, the federal government admitted that the 1986 law had not stopped the influx of illegal workers (Pear, 1991).

These workers are ineligible for welfare or other services sponsored by the government for the benefit of U. S. citizens, but they are periodically accused of taking advantage of these services anyway. The evidence reviewed by Crewdson (1983) suggests that they use social services far less than do American citizens. They tend to shy away from contact with authorities and sometimes even avoid services that are legally available to them. For example, they are sometimes reluctant to seek medical treatment except in emergency circumstances. This poses a serious public health problem in southern California and other areas of high concentration, because illegals suffer higher rates of infectious disease than do American citizens. Obviously, these workers are not examined for communicable diseases before entering the country. They may seek help from agricultural unions, immigrant fraternal organizations, and church-sponsored helping agencies. For the most part, however, these private agencies do not have the resources to provide more than temporary emergency help for some of those who need it.

During recent years, there were signs of increasingly negative attitudes toward the estimated 4 million illegal immigrants in this country (Verhovek, 1994). This trend was most pronounced in states with large illegal populations such as Florida and California. During 1994, Governor Lawton Chiles of Florida sued the federal government, asking for more than $1 billion in reimbursement for services it had been required to give illegal aliens. Governor Chiles, a Democrat, said the people of Florida were tired of spending huge amounts on services, education, medical care, and welfare for illegal aliens. In addition, there were the considerable additional expenses involved in jailing illegal aliens who committed crimes in the state. The governor estimated that there were 350,000 illegal aliens in Florida, a state of 13 million people. He argued that Florida was paying for the apparent inability of the U. S. government to protect its borders ("U. S. Is Sued over Aliens," 1994).

California voters passed Proposition 187 during the election of 1994. This initiative, strongly backed by Governor Pete Wilson, would have cut off most government services to illegal aliens. Specifically, the measure would deny welfare, nonemergency medical treatment, and public schooling to this group. There was no immediate impact of the law because federal and state judges blocked enforcement pending a review. Nevertheless, the passage of the measure illustrates the fact that Americans are becoming increasingly reluctant to provide services to these people. Although it is true that illegal immigrants contribute to the American economy, data provided by the Texas Office of Immigration suggest that on balance they cost more than they contribute in tax revenues. The greatest expense by far is associated with public schooling for the children of illegals. For example, the city of Houston pays $4683 a year for each student. Nationwide, $4.5 billion a year is expended on educating illegal immigrants and their U. S. born children (Verhovek, 1994).

The issue of illegal immigration raises important questions for class discussion:

Should we as a nation put a stop to further illegal immigration?

Governor Pete Wilson is in favor of a constitutional amendment that would deny citizenship to the children of illegal immigrants. What would be the consequences of such a step?

Women's Issues. We do not have definite knowledge of the status of women in prehistory (i.e., before the development of written records). During the late 1800s, a number of authors advanced the idea that women tended to be dominant in some early societies; goddesses were worshipped, and women controlled religion, property, and marriage. These authors then offered various explanations for the shift to male dominance that gradually took place. Feminist authors attempted to bolster their current agendas by asserting that male dominance was culturally imposed and should be ended. Others argued that the evidence for matriarchies, or female controlled societies, was not convincing and that males had always been dominant. Feminist historians Anderson and Zinsser (1988) reviewed these writings and concluded that we simply do not know very much about the relationships between men and women in early societies. There is no reason to believe that either male or female dominance was universal in prehistory. Nor can we conclude that women's traditional role in giving birth and nurturing children was viewed as secondary or unimportant by members of early societies.

What is certain is that women were clearly subordinate by the time written records began to appear. How did this happen? Based on a survey of many early cultures, anthropologist Peggy Sanday (1981) concluded that as the number of early societies grew, they began to compete with one another for scarce resources. As war and forced migration became the means of survival, women began to assume a subordinate role to men. Physically stronger on the average, males were expected to be more active and aggressive than women. Weapons skills were taught to male children. Once warfare is present, a woman needs protection from other warriors, especially if she is pregnant or caring for an infant or young child. In warrior cultures, men came to be viewed as more valuable and important than women (Anderson & Zinsser, 1988).

Female subordination was enshrined in the earliest and most sacred writings of the Greek, Roman, Hebrew, Germanic, and Celtic cultures. This idea passed intact to the emerging European culture and was later embodied in Christian beliefs (Anderson & Zinsser, 1988). Women were generally excluded from important activities such as warfare, politics, philosophy, and even the study of sacred books. By the fourth century B.C., Aristotle proclaimed that the male is naturally superior to the female. (He also believed that women had fewer teeth than men.). By the first century A.D., Jewish men in their morning prayers thanked God for not having been made women.

Although there had always been women who believed in equal rights for women, it wasn't until the 1800s that they developed effective organizations to achieve this goal. In part, the move to organize was a reaction against changes in law, government, and the economy that were limiting women's options still further. Significant progress was made by women's movements in both Europe and the United States. Most women in affluent Western nations now enjoy full rights of citizenship, including the right to vote, have access to higher education, and enjoy significantly widened employment opportunities.

In past generations, women in this country were discouraged from entering certain jobs or careers. For example, mechanical work, physical sciences, administration, engineering, and police work have traditionally been considered male provinces. Females have been regarded as more suited to clerical and secretarial jobs as well as certain nurturing professions such as nursing and social work. During the past three decades, many occupations, professions, clubs, associations, and government positions—once reserved for men—were opened to women. Although it is true that one in five of all working women holds a secretarial or clerical job, it is also evident that women now make up a majority in a wide range of professions that were once male dominated (Roberts, 1995). Here is a comparison of the percentages of all jobs in certain occupations held by women in 1970 and 1990:

Occupation	1970	1990
Bartender	27%	57%
Chemist	17%	29%
Doctor	11%	22%
Economist	14%	44%
Farmer	7%	17%
Industrial engineer	3%	27%
Librarian	84%	85%
Nurse	91%	94%
Police detective	5%	13%
Psychologist	43%	59%
Public official	24%	59%
Secretary	98%	98%
Teacher	74%	74%

SOURCE: From "Women's Work: What's New, What Isn't?" by S. Roberts, *New York Times,* April 27, 1995, p. B6. Copyright © 1995 by The New York Times Co. Reprinted by permission.

Although there has been an opening up in nontraditional areas, these data make it clear that many women are choosing nurturing professions. About 1 in 20 female workers is a schoolteacher, a proportion that hasn't changed much since 1940. Nursing continues to be a predominantly female profession, and the majority of psychologists are now women. Add to this

the increasing role of women in other medical professions and their continued dominance in social work and its becomes obvious that women are the
major providers of human services.

For a variety of reasons, women generally still earn less than men
within a given job category. One reason is that women tend to have shorter
job tenures than men because of their role as mothers and homemakers.
Women also tend to work more often at part-time jobs than men. The third
reason is sexism, a pattern of discrimination against women. Some women
activists have discerned a disturbing pattern: When women begin to dominate a field, the pay and prestige begin to go down (Roberts, 1995). There
may be some truth to this idea, but there are also other reasons why salary
levels have tended to stagnate in the human service field. We discuss these
reasons in more detail elsewhere in the book.

Perhaps even more significant than the movement of women into jobs
once held by males is the great increase in the number of women who work
outside the home. This has been called "one of the great transformations"
in American society (Peterson, 1994, p. 140). Today, close to 60% of all
American women aged 16 to 65 are in the labor force compared to 75% of
the men. Among younger workers, there are almost as many women in the
work force as men. The majority of women with young children were in the
labor force in 1993. Indeed, women now make up about 45% of the total
labor force (U. S. Bureau of the Census, 1994).

The Women's Movement, which did much to change attitudes about the
role of women, is one factor that helped create this great change in American life. Although only a small percentage of women belong to activist
groups such as the National Organization for Women (NOW), the basic
concepts of the movement have become part of the thinking of many American men and women (Mehr, 1995, p. 281). The final victory of the movement was supposed to be passage of the Equal Rights Amendment to the
constitution, which would have made a person's sex an irrelevant distinction under the law. Although the amendment passed both houses of Congress in 1972, it failed to win ratification from the required three-quarters
of state legislatures. A coalition of groups, composed overwhelmingly of
women, fought against ratification. Apparently, the women's movement did
not represent all women. Some continued to desire a traditional gender
role of homemaker and mother (Finsterbusch & McKenna, 1994, p. 43).

There is some reason to believe that a significant number of women are
not happy with the changes brought about, in part, by contemporary feminism. A Gallup Poll conducted in 1990 showed that 67% of the women sur-
veyed do not describe themselves as feminists, and many blame feminist
ideas for making life more difficult. A majority of women told Gallup in
1994 that the women's movement is hurting relations between the sexes.
When asked if the changes in women's lives has made life easier or harder
than they were 20 years ago, 48% responded that life was now harder. Gallup Polls also showed that large majorities believed that it is now harder for
marriages to be successful, and a whopping 82% believed it is now harder

for parents to raise children ("Has Feminism Made Lives Harder?" 1995). Another source of opposition directed at the feminist movement is based on the tendency of radical feminists to downgrade the traditional roles of women, viewing homemaking as mere drudgery.

Questions for Class Discussion or Special Assignment:

> What are the potential effects on human services of the changes in American society just discussed? Specifically, what sort of problems and challenges can be anticipated if a large majority of women continue to join the work force?
> What might be the effect on children in the family in which both parents work?

Social Change

Americans are gradually changing their attitudes toward the poor and minority groups. Actually, this change is only one aspect of what amounts to a revolution in customs and attitudes that has taken place in the last few decades. One major trend has been a liberalization of attitudes toward sexual behavior. Homosexuals are pressing for social acceptance of their sexual preference. Sex is more openly discussed than ever before, and premarital sexual relations are accepted by many teenagers. At the same time, women are challenging traditional roles, and there is much public discussion of alternative lifestyles. The rapid pace of social change, particularly during the late 1960s and early 1970s, has stimulated a conservative reaction that aims to preserve traditional social roles and customs. For example, members of the so-called Moral Majority championed a return to values based on fundamentalist religious beliefs. Without taking sides in these controversies, we can note that the rapid pace of these developments has created a sense of insecurity in many individuals. The contemporary American is faced with a bewildering range of options with regard to sexual behavior, role, and lifestyle.

The Changing American Family.   Family therapists have observed an important change in the American family during the past several decades: The family is no longer organized primarily around child-rearing (Carter & McGoldrick, 1989). The lower birthrate, the longer life expectancy, and increasing divorce and remarriage rates are some of the contributing factors. In the past, the lives of women were linked to their role in child-rearing activities. Now, as previously noted, more women are entering the labor market and are developing personal goals and an identity apart from the home.

Women who choose primary career goals may find themselves wrestling with a severe conflict. For men, the goals of family and career are parallel, but for women, the goals are more likely to conflict (Carter &

McGoldrick, 1989). This conflict is due to the perception that the primary responsibility for child care still rests with women. The traditional view that expects women to assume primary emotional responsibility for family relationships runs counter to the demands of a job or career. It is not surprising that more women than men seek counseling during the child-rearing years.

If it is true that child-rearing no longer occupies center state in family life, then what does? The new priorities have been identified by some writers as *individualism* (see Zastrow, 1988, p. 357). This is the belief that people should seek their own happiness, develop their capacities to the fullest, and fulfill their own needs and desires. In other words, the interests of the individual man and woman are taking precedence over the interests of the family. These personal goals are often centered around personal prestige, success, and the accumulation of material possessions. These values are by no means peculiar to the United States but may be found in many Western developed nations. In contrast, Eastern nations, such as India, are more likely to be organized around the family as the primary focus of daily life. An individual's identity is thus likely to be bound up with the family—usually the extended family.

Some social critics have expressed concern that children are becoming a liability to their parents. Once cherished, children are now more likely to be merely tolerated by adults. In the worst cases, as described in the next chapter, children may be seriously abused or neglected. Columnist William Raspberry (1991) stated that American children are in trouble: "too poor, too likely to grow up in a single parent household, too little supported by their government, and too low a priority for the society at large" (p. 12). He wondered if we can eliminate the career costs of parenthood and still do what we need to do for children.

Here is a brief listing of some of the changes in living arrangements and family structure that have taken place in recent years.

- Young women are more likely than their mothers were to live on their own rather than going right from school into marriage.
- An increasing percentage of the population of couples are living together, and sometimes having children, without marrying.
- An increasing percentage of women will never marry or have children.
- About half of marriages end in divorce.
- Whether by choice or necessity, in present-day marriages both husband and wife are working.
- There has been a large increase in single-parent households in recent years.
- There has also been an increase in the number of homosexual people openly living together.
- American children are increasingly products of broken or never-formed marriages.

Senator Moynihan (1993/1994) compared the changes that have taken place in the American family to an earthquake. Thirty years ago, one in every forty white children was born to an unmarried mother; today it is one in five. Among blacks, two of three children are now born to unmarried mothers. There is a wealth of data showing that intact biological families offer very large advantages compared to any other family structure. For example, the family background of students plays a much larger role in student achievement than standard measures of school quality. Furthermore, continued Moynihan, there is a mountain of evidence showing that children from disintegrating families end up with intellectual, physical, and emotional scars that persist for life. Many of the social problems that concern human services workers (e.g., the drug crisis, the education crisis, teenage pregnancy, and juvenile crime) can be traced to broken homes. Moynihan stated that a community that allows a large number of young men growing up in broken families dominated by women, never acquiring any stable relationship with male authority, and never acquiring any set of positive expectations about the future is asking for and getting chaos. Crime, violence, and unrest are nearly inevitable under these circumstances (Moynihan, 1993/1994).

Economic and Technological Changes

Dramatic changes have taken place since the 1970s in the way income is distributed in the United States. Until recent decades, most Americans were poor by contemporary standards. For example, the median income for a male worker in 1950 was $13,768 in 1994 dollars. The very rich were a small number of elite professionals, bankers, and business leaders. In 1950, fewer than 1 million American families earned as much as $60,000. But by 1980, 2.7 million households counted incomes of more than $100,000, and by 1993, this fortunate group doubled to 5.6 million households. At the same time, nearly 1 million households were enjoying incomes of over $200,000. "Nothing like this immense crowd of wealthy people has been seen in the history of the planet," commented a *New York Times* editorialist (Frum, 1995, p. A15). This is the first time in history that we have had a mass upper class.

Unfortunately, most Americans did not share in this great income surge. The proportion of American families earning less than $25,000, about 40%, has remained the same for 20 years (Frum, 1995). And the income of average families, adjusted for inflation, has remained about the same since the early 1970s.

Why were some able to do extremely well in the economic expansion of recent decades, whereas others are barely holding their own? It appears that highly educated, computer literate workers, skilled in the art of manipulating information, are doing well in the current economy. However, people with limited education find themselves placed in jeopardy by far-reaching developments in the global economy (Peterson, 1994). Secretary of Labor Robert Reich put it succinctly when he said, "If you are well prepared, technology is your friend; if you are not well prepared, technology is your enemy" (quoted in Simon, 1995, p. 959).

American workers are in essence competing against workers in other countries who are often paid less than they. Routine production work in manufacturing and in data processing can be done anywhere around the world. "So routine workers in advanced economies like the United States find themselves in competition with low-paid workers in Third World nations," explained Peterson (1994, p. 125). This competition is exerting downward pressure on the wages of unskilled workers. Along with these trends went a loss of power on the part of trade unions who formerly acted to protect the wages and working conditions of members. In a climate of global competition, an increase in pay for an American worker might place the company at a competitive disadvantage. In any case, the employer could hold out the threat of relocating overseas if wage demands were pressed.

Many skilled American workers can no longer find industrial employment at all, according to Luttwak (1993, p. 124), and are seeking "traditional underclass jobs" as janitors, warehouse loaders, cleaners, and security guards. This trend exerts downward pressure on unskilled workers who face a tighter job market or are being pushed out into the cold. They may then join a large group of discouraged workers who no longer seek regular employment. We elaborate on the unemployed or marginally employed in the next chapter.

What do these trends mean for America's working poor? The fact is that millions of families hold two or three jobs but still can't afford the necessities of life. Consider the situation of Terri Yates as she explained it to a *Time* magazine reporter. In 1994, Terri earned $10,000 as a full-time cab driver while her husband earned somewhat more driving a cab 7 days a week. The Yates can't afford a down payment on a house, are paying off a pickup truck, and are deferring repairs on a 10-year-old Pontiac. "I'm making less money than ever in my life, and I'm working more," Terri told reporter Gibbs (1995, p. 17). She added she can't send her daughter to the dentist because money is so tight. The parents feel they have "no life" and don't see things getting better. They are proud that they have never been on welfare but feel little respect for the politicians who applaud their struggle.

The prospect of joining the working poor is, in fact, not very attractive to those on welfare. An Urban Institute study considered the case of a hypothetical Pennsylvania woman with two children who received $4836 in Aid to Families with Dependent Children (AFDC), $2701 in food stamps, and $3000 in Medicaid benefits for a total of $10,537 in cash and benefits. If she took a full-time job at the minimum wage, her family would gain $9516 in earnings before taxes but lose Medicaid, AFDC, and one-third of her food stamps. In addition, she would have to pay for day care for her children (Gibbs, 1995). It seems obvious that she would be better off on welfare, particularly when you consider that welfare status might make her eligible for job training and education programs.

The Labor Department confirmed the perceptions of workers like the Yates that real wages are falling. For the lowest 10% of workers, the weekly paycheck averaged $225 in 1994, a 10% drop since the late 1970s after inflation is taken into account (Gibbs, 1995). Millions of people are just getting by, one crisis away from disaster. A crisis might be an illness to one person in the family, an unexpected loss or injury, or losing a job.

The estimated 10 million working poor in the country are victims of the global competition that we have discussed. They are also being replaced by automated, programmed machines that require little human supervision. For example, robots are now doing welding and assembly jobs once done by human beings. Many of the working poor are now stuck in service jobs that take up so much time and energy that resuming education seems like an impossible dream. They are not eligible for government sponsored training programs, do not receive free day care, and often do not have medical insurance or retirement benefits. They constitute a large group, vulnerable to destitution, that receives little or no help from human services. It is becoming more difficult for them to move up the economic ladder and easier to slip into homelessness or welfare dependence.

The implications of these data are disturbing to human service workers. The trend is clearly in the direction of a two-tier society with the very rich separated from the great mass of struggling poor people. The large number of very rich, coupled with the influence that their money assures, gives them increasing power in the political arena. The danger is that they may neglect the interests of their less affluent fellow citizens. We may slip into the situation that prevails in many poor developing countries: The poor simply do without the basic services that are considered essential in affluent nations.

Population Changes.   The 1990 census showed that more Americans live in suburbs than in any other social setting. There has been a vast exodus of people and jobs from both farm and city into the suburbs that ring the nation's cities. This shift in population carries with it a shift in political and economic power (Walters, 1992). It is well known that as voters age and move to the suburbs they tend to become more conservative in voting patterns. This may partly explain why politicians are addressing the concerns of middle-class home owners, while downplaying their sympathy for the urban underclass.

Walters (1992) described these changes in the state of California where population increased by an astonishing 6 million in the decade of the 1980s. Its increase alone was more than the total population of all but a dozen states. The growth came from two factors: immigration and high birthrates among non-Anglo groups, especially Asian and Latino immigrants. As the immigrants packed into the central urban areas, hundreds of thousands of Anglo-Californians, especially young workers looking for affordable homes, began moving into the new suburbs that sprouted 50 or more miles from the urban cores. This process was aided by the shift from an industrial to service-based economy in which job sites could be dispersed easily. These new suburbanites were seeking the American dream, a home in the suburbs to call one's own. "And . . . they were escaping from an urban environment that more each day was resembling Beirut—a fear dramatically underscored by the deadly . . . riots that erupted . . . after the verdict in the Rodney King police-brutality case," wrote Walters (1992, p. 88).

What does all this mean for human services? The white Anglo populations of the suburbs, although declining proportionately, are still politically dominant. As Walters (1992) put it, the voters of California don't like crime or property taxes and are only marginally supportive of schools, health, and welfare issues. This seems to reinforce the impression we have gained from other sources: A large increase in unmet human needs in the central cities exists in an increasingly hostile political environment. We have highlighted California not only because it is America's most populous state but because the trends apparent there are visible in other states with significant immigrant populations. Walters (1992) described California as the nation's social laboratory, testing whether a society of dozens of ethnic, linguistic, economic, and geographic subgroups can find any sense of common purpose. "To date, the drift is toward some kind of twenty-first century American tribalism, with suburbanites being the dominant tribe," Walters wrote (1992, p. 89).

A Crisis in Morals?

A number of authors have recently expressed alarm about the general decline in American morals that has taken place since the 1960s. Not only the United States but Great Britain and other affluent countries have undergone an immense increase in many kinds of deviant and antisocial behavior in recent decades. The increase in out-of-wedlock births has just been discussed, and in Chapter 2, we provide details about increased crime, drug abuse, child neglect, and other undesirable behavior. Daniel Moynihan (1994) warned that a disastrous social crisis is under way in America. Behaviors once regarded as wholly unacceptable are gradually being accepted as a normal part of American life. Crime, increasing teenage pregnancy and suicide, the breakup of families, murders by young school children, guns in schools, the spread of AIDS, the abuse of children, the battery of women, and drug abuse are some of the behaviors that concerned Moynihan. Part of the process involves changing the words we use to describe behavior. For example, when the term *illegitimate* birth becomes *out-of-wedlock* or *single parenting*, we imply acceptance of the behavior.

Himmelfarb (1995) pointed out how we have become very uncomfortable about making moral judgments, particularly about condemning certain behaviors. "Public officials in particular shy away from the word immoral, lest they be accused of racism, sexism, elitism, or simply a lack of compassion" (Himmelfarb, 1995, p. 240). When members of the president's cabinet were asked whether it is immoral to have children out of wedlock, they refused to put it in moral terms. The Secretary of Health and Human Services was quoted by Himmelfarb (1995), as saying, "I don't like to put this in moral terms, but I do believe that having children out of wedlock is just wrong" (pp. 240–241). It is not only our political and cultural leaders who are prone to this failure of moral nerve, but everyone is infected by it to some degree.

In an influential book, Magnet (1993) described the revolution that in the 1960s led to a strange alliance between the haves and have-nots. The intent of social planners was to liberate the poor from the political, economic, and racial oppression that held them in bondage. Along with this went a cultural revolution that liberated the poor from stodgy middle-class values and the Puritan ethic. Magnet argued that these new values had a disastrous effect: By putting down the attitudes that previously made for economic advance—sobriety, thrift, and hard work—they locked many of the poor into permanent poverty.

Noted black author Stanley Crouch made a similar point. During the 1960s, he stated, large numbers of gullible young people—black and white—were convinced that discipline, planning, and mastery of the English language were irrelevant. "Inferior preparation " was elevated to a "position of purity." Blacks who worked hard and educated themselves were referred to as "Oreos," that is, black on the outside but white on the inside (quoted in Brownfeld, 1993, p. 6).

The authors previously cited make the point that values and morals of a society powerfully influence human services. One example is the Supplemental Security Income Program, which was introduced in 1972 to provide a minimum income for the blind, the elderly , and the disabled poor. The program was subsequently extended to drug addicts and alcoholics. This involved redefining behavior pattens that were once considered vices as disabilities. As Himmelfarb (1995) pointed out, this redefinition has the effect of actually encouraging these disabilities. The program rewards those who try to overcome the addiction and cuts off benefits for those who succeed.

Drawing distinctions between good and bad behavior is implied in all of our thinking about social policy. We may disguise the underlying moral judgment when we speak of the *pathology* of crime, drugs, and welfare dependence. When we say workfare is better than welfare, we are again making a moral judgment. Equally, when we consider promoting sexual abstinence among young people, we are making another moral statement. Confusion about this point arises when we try to cover up morality by using scientific terminology.

Luttwak (1993) attributed the decline in U. S. culture to an unrestrained individualism that knows no balance. The United States has historically championed individual rights over the rights of the general public, but in the past, this emphasis on personal freedom was balanced by a strong sense of duty to family and community. However, in recent decades, the balance has shifted toward a drive for self-fulfillment that is pursued at the expense of the family. The interest of young children are often sacrificed by parents who wish to pursue personal happiness.

If the values of the liberal counterculture of the 1960s are increasingly being rejected, it does not follow that conservative values are morally up-lifting. There has been a shift in conservative values during recent years toward even greater emphasis on free markets and competition. This change is reflected in the transformation of the American corporation. What Luttwak (1993, p. 164) called the "old quiet-life corporation," which often provided lifetime jobs for its workers, became the "lean and mean" corporation. To increase profits and maintain a competitive edge, it became commonplace to fire large numbers of midlevel executives, a trend that continues to the present day. At the same time, there was no hesitancy to send assembly line jobs overseas to take advantage of cheaper labor. In other words, the corporation no longer experienced the previous sense of loyalty or obligation to its employees, many of whom have experienced a humiliating loss of self-respect along with a feeling of betrayal. The whole-sale firings and layoffs inevitably had a disruptive effect on family life. Con-servative economists defended these new policies as examples of creative destruction, meaning that the overall improvement in U. S. competitive-ness justifies the sacrifice of certain individuals (Cobb, Halstead, & Rowe, 1995). Luttwak (1993), himself a conservative, argued that workers and their families need stability more than they need new goods on the market. He suggested that conservative politicians do not feel free to talk about this issue because much of their funding comes from corporations.

Recent years have also witnessed a sharp decline in public confidence in our political institutions. According to pollster Stanley Greenberg (1995), beliefs that the government could be trusted to do what is right declined sharply after 1988. He went on to say,

> The lies, the perks, the bounced checks, the waste, the sweetheart deals, the privileges, the indifference to popular opinion—all stirred outrage when the country's leaders could no longer show ordinary Americans the way forward. And no amount . . . of ethics investigations, campaign re-form, or term limits will restore the public trust. (p. 19)

Psychological Stress

The large-scale problems just described have their final impact on individu-als. In our complex, rapidly changing culture, it is probable that an individ-ual will sometimes be frustrated in trying to meet the needs described at the beginning of this chapter. All kinds of obstacles including prejudice, poverty, and other factors just reviewed can stand in the way of fulfilling needs. Typically, disadvantaged people are preoccupied with basic survival needs, whereas the more affluent are concerned with higher needs relating to self-esteem and fulfillment of creative urges. To some extent, everyone experiences the pressure of these needs, and this is one important source of psychological stress.

Stress is sometimes defined as the strain imposed on an individual by threatening life events. However, it has been found that some desirable events, such as job promotion, may also impose strain on the individual. Bloom (1984) covered both possibilities by defining stressful life events as "those external events that make adaptive demands on a person" (p. 244). These events may be successfully handled or, in some instances, may lead to illness or psychological breakdown.

A team of researchers studied life events that occurred shortly before the onset of serious illness (Holmes & Rahe, 1967; Rahe, 1979; Rahe & Arthur, 1978). They developed a list of 43 life events and scaled them in terms of how much stress they evoke. The list is reprinted here as Table 1–1. It is not particularly surprising that death of a spouse ranks as the most stressful kind of event. But it is surprising that joyful life events such as marriage or marital reconciliation prove to be more stressful than financial catastrophes such as bankruptcy or mortgage foreclosure. All of the events listed in Table 1–1 have one feature in common: They require a person to adjust to a change in his or her life situation.

It is not only major life events that have an effect on physical health but also the ordinary hassles of daily life. Hassles are those apparently minor events that can make you tense, frustrated, and irritable. Losing your wallet, getting involved in a minor car accident, and waiting in long lines are just a few of the bothersome situations that interrupt the smooth flow of daily events. When hassles take place frequently over an extended period, they can have a negative impact on health and well-being. In fact, one team of researchers reported that hassles far outweigh major life events in predicating psychological and somatic symptoms (Lazarus & Folkman, 1984, p. 312).

Some people are better able to tolerate stress than others. It has already been pointed out that stress tolerance is partly dependent on the amount of emotional support one receives from other people. This is why divorce or death of a loved one is particularly stressful; it leaves the victim to face the situation without familiar supports.

Certain personality traits also play a role in how a person handles stress. Kobasa (1979), for example, studied how a person can remain healthy in the face of great stress. She reported that those who do so have a clear sense of their values, goals, and capabilities; a strong tendency toward active involvement with the environment; and a belief in their capacity to control and transform life experiences.

Developmental Crises

Psychological stress is intensified at certain phases of a person's development or maturation. This kind of stress is the unavoidable consequence of moving from one phase of development to the next. The stages of development include the prenatal period, infancy, childhood, puberty, adolescence, young adulthood, middle age, old age, and death. During each transition

TABLE 1–1   Social Readjustment Rating Scale

Life Event	Stress Value
Death of spouse	100
Divorce	73
Marital separation	65
Jail term	63
Death of close family member	63
Personal injury or illness	53
Marriage	50
Fired at work	47
Marital reconciliation	45
Retirement	45
Change in health of family member	44
Pregnancy	40
Sex difficulties	39
Gain of a new family member	39
Business adjustment	39
Change in financial state	38
Death of a close friend	37
Change to a different line of work	36
Change in number of arguments with spouse	35
Mortgage or loan for major purchase (home, etc.)	31
Foreclosure of mortgage or loan	30
Change in responsibilities at work	29
Son or daughter leaving home	29
Trouble with in-laws	29
Outstanding personal achievement	28
Wife begins or stops work	26
Begin or end school	26
Change in living conditions	25
Revision of personal habits	24
Trouble with boss	23
Change in work hours or conditions	20
Change in residence	20
Change in school	20
Change in recreation	19
Change in church activities	19
Change in social activities	18
Mortgage or loan for lesser purchase (car, TV, etc.)	17
Change in sleeping habits	16
Change in number of family get-togethers	15
Change in eating habits	15
Vacation	13
Christmas	12
Minor violations of the law	11

SOURCE: Reprinted by permission of the publisher from "The Social Readjustment Rating Scale" by T. H. Holmes and R. H. Rahe, 1967, *Journal of Psychosomatic Research, 11,* 213–218. Copyright © 1967 by Elsevier Science Inc.

from one stage to the next, a person is subjected to novel challenges and tasks that tend to increase anxiety. The changes might involve new responsibilities, bodily alterations, and new ways of relating to others. For example, the individual entering young adulthood has reached physical maturity and is expected to make serious plans for a career and to begin serious sexual relationships. The major thrust of a person's activities is toward the achievement of independent, self-supporting status. With support and nurturance from others, most are able to master the demands of the new phase successfully.

However, developmental stresses can overwhelm some individuals, particularly those whose needs for support and nurturance are not being met. There is a wide variation in how people react to developmental transitions. What is a crisis for one may be an interesting challenge for another. A crisis occurs when an individual feels overwhelmed by the demands of the next phase of development. If a person is completely unable to master the requirements of the next developmental stage, further growth is prevented. The consequences of this failure may range from temporary emotional disturbance to serious disorganization of personality.

During recent decades, there has been a marked change in attitudes of human services workers toward people in crisis. It is now accepted that people may become anxious or upset during transitions in development and that such reactions are not necessarily a sign of serious mental illness. Hoff (1978) pointed out that modern crisis theory has established a new approach to people with such problems. It is no longer assumed that they are completely irrational or that they cannot help themselves. Furthermore, it is becoming more accepted that it does not require a highly trained psychotherapist to help people get through a crisis. Counselors, police officers, nurses, laypersons with training in crisis intervention, and family members can be very helpful in getting someone through a difficult developmental phase.

The Crisis in Health Care

The health care system in the United States has become a major source of public concern in recent years. An editorial that appeared in the *American Journal of Public Health* charged that this country lacks a coherent national health policy and that the system has become indifferent to the real health needs of society (Sultz, 1991, p. 418). Sultz called for the creation of a network of health services that will care humanely for the poor, the sick, the elderly, and the most vulnerable Americans. We are falling far short of this goal. Although this country spends more on health on a per capita basis than does any other developed nation, millions of Americans do not have access to affordable health care. It has been estimated that about 34 million Americans do not have any health insurance at all (Matthiessen, 1990).

One of the major problems is that the costs of health care are running out of control. Today, health care consumes about 12% of our national wealth (about $500 billion!) compared to 4.4% (or $12.7 billion) in 1950. Why are costs so high? Here are some factors that play a role.

- ◆ The increasing costs of malpractice suits brought against providers are passed along to the consumer.

- The fear of malpractice leads to the practice of defensive medicine. In order to protect against being charged with malpractice, the doctor is likely to call for every test and diagnostic procedure that could possibly apply to a given case.
- Technological advances have led to the development of extremely costly medical equipment.
- Treatment is now available for some diseases (e.g., kidney failure) that were formerly untreatable and, possibly, terminal.
- The administrative costs of processing millions of insurance claims are considerable.
- Owing in part to the fact that Americans are living longer, there is a large and growing population of people with chronic diseases.
- The costs of treating patients with Acquired Immune Deficiency Syndrome (AIDS) have added greatly to the strain on the system.

Another difficulty is that our system, if it can be called that, has become very complex and unwieldy. Many other developed nations provide medical care through a unified system of government-operated clinics and hospitals. In contrast, we provide health care via a bewildering mix of public and private facilities funded by a large number of private and government insurance programs. The government insurance programs, chiefly Medicare for the elderly and Medicaid for the poor, provide limited coverage to millions of Americans but do not cover the majority of working people. Many workers receive medical coverage, usually through a private insurance company, as a fringe benefit of employment. The extent of coverage varies greatly, often with a single carrier offering a range of policies to choose from. Of course, the more limited the coverage, the more that must be paid out of pocket by the patient. The physician and patient are typically confronted with complex fee schedules detailing how much is to be paid for each medical procedure. Increasingly, the insurance companies are questioning the doctors' judgments, particularly with regard to costly procedures. There is a chorus of complaints about the forms to be filled out and the difficulties involved in trying to deal with the impersonal bureaucracies that administer the program.

Many people fall through the gaps in this network of coverage. When medical insurance is linked to employment, the worker may lose the insurance when he or she is laid off or fired from the job. Part-time workers, low-paid workers, and those employed by small firms are often without medical insurance at all. These people are in a serious dilemma; they can neither afford to buy their own insurance nor can they afford to pay for any extended medical treatment. Consequently, they put off doctor visits as long as possible and may end up in emergency rooms being treated for a condition that has become serious or life-threatening through neglect. All too often, the emergency room is replacing the family doctor's office.

Another criticism of our health care delivery system is that it tends to emphasize treatment rather than prevention. Most health care providers define successful treatment as the elimination of disease. Physicians understandably give precedence to a patient with existing symptoms rather than to a healthy patient who wants a program of diet and exercise. Many insurance companies do not reimburse subscribers for health maintenance visits, such as physical exams, but reimburse only for definable illness (Prokop, Bradley, Burish, Anderson, & Fox, 1991).

The reform of our health care system was one of the major goals of the Clinton administration. First Lady Hillary Rodham Clinton led a 500-person task force that was to accomplish three basic tasks: (a) extending medical benefits to the uninsured at reasonable cost, (b) guaranteeing continued coverage when workers change jobs or get sick, and (c) generally controlling the steadily rising costs of health care. Under the proposed Clinton plan, the President would establish government sponsored "health alliances" to bargain with insurers on our behalf, and a National Health Board would determine what medical services we may or may not have. Costs would be controlled by fines when health plans exceeded their budgets. States would be given standby power to regulate prices directly.

The Clinton plan was met with a torrent of criticism and failed to garner the support needed to get through Congress. Some of the criticisms were that it made the health care system even more complex and unwieldy than it already was and that it would create brand new bureaucracies entailing more government regulations. Paperwork would increase, and treatment decisions would be second-guessed by government officials (Butler, 1993).

The failure of the Clinton plan meant that the original problems were still there. Many alternative plans are being considered. One is the Canadian plan, which would allow the government simply to buy medical care for us with tax dollars. This would effectively sweep away the current insurance companies and employer provided insurance with its choice of services. It would be relatively simple and would reduce administrative costs. The disadvantages might be some rationing of care and less freedom to choose providers. Enactment of any such plan would be met by intense opposition from the nation's insurance companies, which profit from administering the present programs.

Another alternative is to model the system on the Federal Employees Health benefits system, which covers nearly 10 million employees, retirees, and their dependents (Butler, 1993). Under this plan, the workers decide for themselves what services they want. Once a year, they receive information on a menu of perhaps two dozen insurance plans available to them where they live. The cost of premiums, the services covered, the out-of-pocket expenses are all described in detail. The workers pay about one-third of the premium for whatever plan is selected with the government paying the rest. The government has nothing to do with setting the prices or determining the benefits package. One clear advantage is that costs are held down not by government regulation but by the competitive nature of this approach. Each insurer wants to attract clients to its program and tries to offer the

The Canadian National Health Plan:
A Model for the U. S.?

The citizens of Canada are beneficiaries of one of the most comprehensive health insurance programs in the world. The plan uses provincial (provinces are like our states) tax money, supplemented by federal funds, to provide medical care to everyone at no charge. All medical care is free, including long-term home care and nursing home care in many provinces. There are no bills, and no money is paid to patients to doctors; the doctors bill the government. By and large, the doctors are satisfied with the system, although there have been battles with the government over fees. Doctors' charges for services are lower than in the United States, but so are administrative expenses and malpractice premiums (Rosenthal, 1991). Incredibly, the system provides health care to all at less cost than the U. S. system.

It sounds good, but there are some disadvantages. The level of care is probably not as good as that received by wealthy people in this country. There are sometimes waits for tests and treatment, and the system is slow to buy expensive new machines and procedures. Advanced diagnostic equipment is in short supply, and patients may have to travel in order to benefit from this equipment. Also, Canadians do not enjoy the same ready access to specialists as do wealthy Americans. The ratio of specialists to general practitioners is 1:1 in the United States compared to 1:4 in Canada.

The basic advantage of the Canadian system is that everyone is covered; the patient's financial status is never an issue. In this country, there is much greater variation in the level of care, depending on a person's income and resources. As we have seen, millions of people in the United States have no medical coverage at all, whereas the wealthy have available the latest in advanced medical technology. ◆

most benefits for the least expense. The problem comes in with persons who have no employer to pick up the premium. In the case of a worker who was recently laid off, for example, government would have to pay the entire tab. The costs would be considerable and added to the expenses already incurred by Medicaid and Medicare.

Defining Managed Care

Managed care is an umbrella term for health care insurance systems that contract with a network of hospitals, clinics, and doctors who agree to accept set fees for each service or flat payments per patient. The advantage to providers is that they are given a ready source of referrals. There are several different kinds of managed care plans:

• **HMO: The health maintenance organization** is the most highly structured, providing comprehensive health services for a fixed prepaid rate. Some HMOs have their own clinics, whereas others have a "panel" or network of independent doctors. Care is coordinated by a primary-care doctor or "gatekeeper." The main advantage is that costs are relatively low. The owners of small or medium sized businesses may find that this is the least expensive way of providing workers with medical coverage. The disadvantage is that patients are limited to the HMOs clinics and providers. If they go out of network, they must pay the costs out of pocket.

◆ **PPO: Preferred provider organizations** are groups of doctors and hospitals that agree to provide health services at a fixed rate. The prospective patient is usually given a list of providers and may go directly to any of them. There is no gatekeeper or individual to coordinate care. Typically, the patient must pay a modest copayment fee for the service.

◆ **POS: Point-of-service** plans also have networks of providers, but patients may seek treatment outside of the network if they are willing to pay a greater share of the cost. This is becoming increasingly popular because patients need not forfeit their freedom to choose their doctors and hospitals. Some traditional HMOs, like Kaiser Permanente, have started to offer a point-of-service option. Coverage for out-of-network benefits varies from plan to plan; for example, some pay 70% of what the HMO considers a "reasonable and customary" fee, which is generally less than the actual charge (Durkin, 1995).

The recent growth of managed care plans is due to the fact that they provide a means of controlling the escalating costs of medical care. They are sometimes criticized on the grounds of providing limited or assembly line service and for intruding into the doctor-patient relationship.

Interaction Among Problems

For purposes of description, contemporary problems have been treated here as separate and distinct from one another. In real life, there is a dynamic interplay among these factors. Close examination shows that certain individuals or groups may have to struggle against the cumulative impact of many stressful factors. For example, a technological change that puts a poor southern agricultural worker out of work immediately places the family under stress. The need for money may force the older children to quit school and seek work, which reduces their chances of escaping the poverty cycle. If the family relocates to a northern ghetto in search of work, they may be disappointed to find many others like themselves also out of work. The hopelessness of the situation may promote attempts to temporarily escape by means of drugs or alcohol. High levels of violence, crime, and gang activity may also threaten family cohesion. Medical care may be poor or completely inadequate in the community. These negative influences tend to accumulate to the point that cause and effect act in a circular fashion. For example, the mental breakdown and hospitalization of a mother may be traced to poverty and other factors; in turn, her breakdown becomes a major obstacle to the adjustment of her children, who may be shunted from one person or institution to another. The cycle goes on.

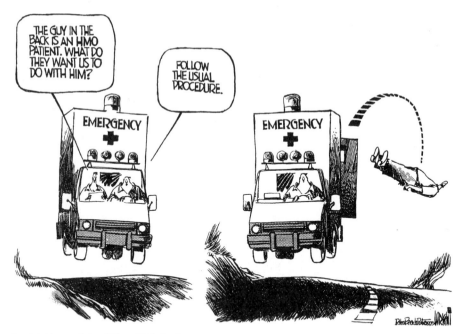

Reprinted by permission: Tribune Media Services.

SUMMARY

The United States monitors its economic health by means of a sophisticated system of indicators that provide a basis for informed discussion
about economic activity. In contrast, we do a relatively poor job of monitoring our social health. As Miringoff (1995) pointed out, social indicators appear less often and are assessed in isolation with no context or connection.
Poverty, for example, is reported once a year and teenage suicide every 2
years. There are no national measures of homelessness and illiteracy. The
Fordham Institute for Innovation in Social Policy has published an annual
Index of Social Health for the United States. Although not as precise as our
measures of economic health, it certainly represents a significant advance
in social monitoring. The Index consists of 16 social indicators including
infant mortality, child abuse, poverty, teenage suicide, drug abuse, unemployment, homicide rates, and others (Miringoff, 1995).

The results reveal a sharp decline in America's social health. Since
1970, the Index showed a drop of about 45%. The decline was due to increased numbers of children in poverty, increased child abuse and teenage
suicide, lower average weekly wages, increased homicide rates, a widening
gap between rich and poor, and other factors. The findings generally support the picture we have presented in this chapter: a decline in social
health in the context of general affluence. As social indicators have gone
down since 1970, most measures of economic activity have shown robust

growth. The Dow Jones stock average, for example, reflected steady advances in corporate profits, and other measures showed yearly advances in economic productivity.

More vivid than statistics is an eyewitness account provided by Mario Cuomo (1994). When governor of New York, he visited the neighborhood in Queens where he grew up and found himself unprepared for so many dramatic changes:

> Instead of the faint hope of the 1930s . . . I saw the despair of the 1990s. Instead of people of diverse backgrounds working . . . to get ahead, I saw people in desperation, unemployed, without any purpose or prospects. The houses were crumbling; children loitered when they should have been in school . . . Pimps and prostitutes patrolled the streets. I even saw a couple fornicating in the street. My part of South Jamaica, once a pocket of modest dreams . . . had become . . . ravaged by neglect, a vivid example of societal failure (Cuomo, 1994, p. 158).

These conditions, he continued, are not unique to this neighborhood but may be found in cities all across the country.

In this context, it is clear that an increasing number of people need help from human services. It is therefore ironic, and troubling, that several trends are acting to reduce support for human services at this time. The huge deficits run up by the federal government are partly responsible for this predicament. The federal government spends more paying interest on the national debt than it does on all state and local governments combined. This payment does not build a single building, create a single job, or feed a single person (Cuomo, 1994, p. 5). In the 1996 fiscal year, we spent 12 times as much on repaying interest than on education and twice as much as on poverty programs. The impact on human services is enormous because the debt robs us of our ability to fund services adequately and, at the same time, makes our social problems worse. Many agencies at both federal and state levels are under pressure to cut back services.

Another trend is the belief on the part of some policymakers that human service programs are adding to our problems. For example, William J. Bennett (1993, p. ii), noted conservative commentator, stated that "over the years the government has often done unintended harm to many of the people it was trying to help." This was particularly true, he continued, of programs designed to help poor people. Bennett suggested that we need to ask some tough questions when we design programs. What kind of behavior will the program encourage or discourage? Will the program undermine families? Will it encourage self-responsibility or long-term dependence? Will the money appropriated go to recipients or will it be diverted to massive bureaucracies?

This may indeed be a time for honest self-examination by service providers. The criticisms of human services need to be taken seriously. Some agencies may in fact be bloated with political appointees and administrators who provide no useful services to anybody. Although we recognize the need for greater accountability and cost effectiveness on the part of agencies, we are greatly concerned about the potential dangers of undisciplined cutting of essential services. As people fall through the safety net, they are more likely to become dysfunctional, unstable, and possibly, violent. Human services are essential to a civil, well-ordered society. A failure to provide important services in a timely fashion is often counterproductive because more serious problems may be created. In the chapters that follow, many specific examples of this process will be provided.

ADDITIONAL READING

Adam, B. D. (1987). *The rise of a gay and lesbian movement.* Boston: Twayne Publishers.

Azarnoff, R. S., & Seliger, J. S. (1982). *Delivering human services.* Englewood Cliffs, NJ: Prentice Hall.

Brown, D. (1971). *Bury my heart at Wounded Knee: An Indian history of the American West.* New York: Holt, Rinehart & Winston.

Button, J. W. (1978). *Black violence.* Princeton, NJ: Princeton University Press.

Crewdson, J. (1983). *The tarnished door: The new immigrants and the transformation of America.* New York: Times Books.

Ehrenreich, B. (1989). *Fear of falling: The inner life of the middle class.* New York: Pantheon.

Gilder, G. (1981). *Wealth and poverty.* New York: Basic Books.

Hacker, A. (1992). *Two nations: Black and white, separate, hostile, unequal.* New York: Charles Scribner's Sons.

Himmelfarb, G. (1995). *The de-moralization of society: From Victorian virtues to modern values.* New York: Knopf.

Lott, B. (1994). *Women's lives: Themes and variations in gender learning* (2nd ed.). Pacific Grove, CA: Brooks/Cole.

Luttwak, E. (1993). *The endangered American dream.* New York: Simon & Schuster.

Magnet, M. (1993). *The dream and the nightmare: The sixties' legacy to the underclass.* New York: Morrow.

Moore, J. W. (1977). *Mexican-Americans.* Englewood Cliffs, NJ: Prentice Hall.

Oates, S. B. (1982). *Let the trumpet sound: The life of Martin Luther King, Jr.* New York: Harper & Row.

Petersen, W. (1971). *Japanese Americans: Oppression and success.* New York: Random House.

Peterson, W. C. (1994). *Silent depression: The fate of the American dream.* New York: Norton.

Pettigrew, T. F. (1980). *The sociology of race relations: Reflection and reform.* New York: Free Press.

Rose, P. I., & Smith, S. (1990). *They and we: Racial and ethnic relations in the United States* (4th ed.). New York: McGraw-Hill.

Ryan, M. P. (1983). *Womanhood in America: From colonial times to the present.* New York: Franklin Watts.

Schaefer, R. T. (1995). *Race and ethnicity in the United States.* New York: Harper Collins.

Sowell, T. (1981). *Ethnic America.* New York: Basic Books.

Steinberg, S. (1981). *The ethnic myth: Race, ethnicity, and class in America.* New York: Atheneum.

Toffler, A. (1980). *The third wave.* New York: Morrow.

Tsongas, P. (1981). *The road from here: Liberalism and the realities in the 1980s.* New York: Knopf.

Unger, R., & Crawford, M. (1992). *Women and gender: A feminist psychology.* New York: McGraw-Hill.

West, G. (1981). *The national welfare rights movement: The social protest of poor women.* New York: Praeger.

Wilson, W. J. (1987). *The truly disadvantaged.* Chicago: University of Chicago Press.

Zastrow, C. (1990). *Introduction to social welfare: Social problems, services, and current issues* (4th ed.). Belmont, CA: Wadsworth.

REFERENCES

AAFRC (American Association of Fund-Raising Counsel). (1990). *Giving U.S.A.* (1990 ed.). New York: AAFRC Trust for Philanthropy.

Anderson, B. S., & Zinsser, J. P. (1988). *A history of their own: Women in Europe from prehistory to the present* (Vol. 1). New York: Harper & Row.

Barkan, J. (1991, June 24). Saved from the fate of the Swedes. *New York Teacher,* p. 19.

Barringer, F. (1990, April 28). Four years later, Soviets reveal wider scope to Chernobyl horror. *The New York Times,* pp. 1, 4.

Bennett, W. J. (1993, March). *The index of leading cultural indicators* (Vol. 1). Washington, DC: The Heritage Foundation.

Bloch, S., Croch, E., & Reibstein, J. (1982). Therapeutic factors in group psychotherapy: A review. *Archives of General Psychiatry, 27,* 216–224.

Bloom, B. L. (1984). *Community mental health: A general introduction* (2nd ed.). Pacific Grove, CA: Brooks/Cole.

Bradbury, K. L., Downs, A., & Small, K. A. (1982). *Urban decline and the future of American cities.* Washington, DC: The Brookings Institution.

Brill, N. (1990). *Working with people: The helping process* (4th ed.). New York: Longman.

Brown, D. (1971). *Bury my heart at Wounded Knee: An Indian history of the American West.* New York: Holt, Rinehart & Winston.

Brownfeld. A. C. (1993, November). Stanley Crouch: Courageous voice across racial divide. *The Washington Inquirer,* pp. 5, 6.

Butler, S., & Kondratas, A. (1987). *Out of the poverty trap: A conservative strategy for welfare reform.* New York: Free Press.

Butler, S. M. (1993, September 28). Rube Goldberg, call your office. *The New York Times,* p. 25.

Caplow, T. (1976). *How to run any organization.* New York: Holt, Rinehart & Winston.

Carter, B., & McGoldrick, M. (1989). *The changing family life cycle: A framework for family therapy* (2nd ed.). Needham Heights, MA: Allyn & Bacon.

Cassel, J. (1990). The contribution of the social environment to host resistance. In M. R. Ornstein & C. Swencionis (Eds.), *The healing brain: A scientific reader* (pp. 31–42). New York: Guilford Press.

Clymer, A. (1994, November 10). G.O.P. celebrates its sweep to power; Clinton vows to find common ground. *The New York Times,* pp. A1, B5.

Cobb, C., Halstead, T., & Rowe, J. (1995, October). If the GDP is up, why is America down? *Atlantic Monthly,* pp. 59–60, 62–68, 70, 72–73, 76, 78.

Comer, R. J. (1996). *Fundamentals of abnormal psychology.* New York: W. H. Freeman.

Crewdson, J. (1983). *The tarnished door: The new immigrants and the transformation of America.* New York: Times Books.

Cuomo, M. (1994). *The New York idea: An experiment in democracy.* New York: Crown.

DeParle, J. (1991, May 29). "Thousand Points" as a cottage industry. *The New York Times,* pp. A1, A18.

Durkin, B. J. (1995, March 14). New choice on the road to managed care. *The Standard Star, Gannett Suburban Newspapers,* pp. 1A, 2A.

Ebenstein, W., Pritchett, C. H., Turner, H. A., & Mann, D. (1970). *American democracy in world perspective* (2nd ed.). New York: Harper & Row.

Ehrenreich, B. (1989). *Fear of falling: The inner life of the middle class.* New York: Pantheon.

Finsterbusch, K., & McKenna, G. (1994). Is feminism a harmful ideology? In K. Finsterbusch & G. McKenna (Eds.), *Taking sides: Clashing views on controversial social issues* (8th ed., pp. 42–43). Guilford, CT: Dushkin.

Fleming, R., Baum, A., Gisriel, M. M., & Gatchel, R. J. (1982). Mediating influences of social support on stress at Three Mile Island. *Journal of Human Stress, 8,* 116–125.

Frazier, K. (1979). *The violent face of nature: Severe phenomena and natural disasters.* New York: Morrow.

Freeman, H. E., Jones, W. C., & Zucker, L. G. (1979). *Social problems: A policy perspective* (3rd ed.) Chicago: Rand McNally College Publishing.

Frum, D. (1995, August 14). Welcome, nouveaux riches. *The New York Times,* p. 15.

Garza, H. A. (1973, Spring). Administration of justice: Chicanos in Monterey County. *Aztlan, 1,*137–146.

Geen, R. G., Beatty, W., & Arkin, R. (1984). *Human motivation: Physiological, behavioral and social approaches.* Boston: Allyn & Bacon.

Gelman, D., & Katel, P. (1993, April 5). The trauma after the storm. *Newsweek,* p. 65.

Gibbs, N. (1995, July 3). Working harder, getting nowhere. *Time Magazine,* pp. 16–20.

Glazer, N. (1988). *The limits of social policy.* Cambridge, MA: Harvard University Press.

Goldwater, B. (1978). *The conscience of a majority.* Englewood Cliffs, NJ: Prentice Hall.

Gore, A. (1993, April). Andrew aftermath. *National Geographic,* pp. 2–37.

Greenberg, S. B. (1995). *Middle class dreams.* New York: Random House.

Harrington, M. (1968). Preface. In L. A. Fenman & J. L. Kornbluh (Eds.), *Poverty in America.* Ann Arbor: University of Michigan Press.

Has feminism made lives harder? (1995, May/June). *The American Enterprise,* p. 19.

Hasenfeld, Y. (1983). *Human service organizations.* Englewood Cliffs, NJ: Prentice Hall.

Himmelfarb, G. (1995). *The de-moralization of society: From Victorian virtues to modern values.* New York: Knopf.

Hoff, L. A. (1978). *People in crisis: Understanding and helping.* Menlo Park, CA: Addison-Wesley.

Holmes, T. H., & Rahe, R. H. (1967). The social readjustment rating scale. *Journal of Psychosomatic Research, 11,* 213–218.

Kobasa, S. C. (1979). Personality and resistance to illness. *American Journal of Community Psychology, 7,* 413–423.

Lazarus, R. S., & Folkman, S. (1984). *Stress, appraisal and coping.* New York: Springer.

Lin, N., Simeone, R. S., Ensel, W. M., & Kuo, W. (1979). Social support, stressful life events, and illness: A model and an empirical test. *Journal of Health and Social Behavior, 20,* 108–119.

Linowes, D. (1995, November 15). The rationale for privatization. *Vital Speeches of the Day,* pp. 86–88.

Luttwak, E. (1993). *The endangered American dream.* New York: Simon & Schuster.

Lynch, J. J. (1977). *The broken heart.* New York: Basic Books.

Macht, M. W., & Ashford, J. B. (1990). *Introduction to social work and social welfare.* New York: Macmillan.

Magnet, M. (1993). *The dream and the nightmare: The sixties' legacy to the underclass.* New York: Morrow.

Maslow, A. H. (1968). *Toward a psychology of being* (2nd ed.). New York: Van Nostrand Reinhold.

Maslow, A. H. (1970). *Motivation and personality* (2nd ed.). New York: Harper & Row.

Maslow, A. H. (1987). *Motivation and personality* (3rd ed.). New York: Harper & Row.

Matthiessen, C. (1990, October/November). Bordering on collapse. *Modern Maturity, 33,* pp. 30, 32, 38, 39, 82, 83.

Mehr, J. (1995). *Human services: Concepts and intervention strategies.* Boston: Allyn & Bacon.

Miringoff, M. L. (1995). Toward a national standard of social health. *American Journal of Orthopsychiatry, 65,* 462–467.

More blacks in middle class. (1995, February 23). *The Standard Star, Gannett Suburban Newspapers,* p. 1B.

Moynihan, D. P. (1993/1994). Defining defiancy down: How we've become accustomed to alarming levels of crime and destructive behavior. *American Education, 17,* 10–18.

Murray, C. (1984). *Losing ground: American social policy, 1950–1980.* New York: Basic Books.

National Institute of Mental Health. (1985). *Disaster work and mental health: Prevention and control of stress among workers* (DHHS Publications No. ADM 87–1422). Rockville, MD: Author.

Neher, A. (1991). Maslow's theory of motivation: A critique. *Journal of Humanistic Psychology, 31,* 89–112.

Neukrug, E. (1994). *Theory, practice, and trends in human services: A overview of an emerging profession.* Pacific Grove, CA: Brooks/Cole.

Pear, R. (1987, October 3). U. S. moves to fine hotel for employing illegal aliens. *The New York Times,* p. 16.

Pear, R (1991, August 7). U. S. intensifies campaign against employers of illegal aliens. *The New York Times,* p. A10.

Peterson, W. C. (1994). *Silent depression: The fate of the American dream.* New York: Norton.

Prokop, C. K., Bradley, L. A., Burish, T. G., Anderson, K. O., & Fox, J. E. (1991). *Health psychology.* New York: Macmillan.

Quarantelli, E. L., & Dynes, R. R. (1972, February). When disaster strikes (It isn't much like what you've heard and read about). *Psychology Today,* pp. 66–70.

Quarantelli, E. L., & Dynes, R. R. (1979). Response to social crisis and disaster. *Annual Review of Sociology, 3,* 23–49.

Rahe, R H. (1979). Life change events and mental illness: An overview. *Journal of Human Stress, 5,* 2–10.

Rahe, R. H., & Arthur, R. J. (1978). Life change and illness studies: Past history and future directions. *Human Stress, 4,* 3–15.

Raspberry, W. (1991, July 30). When few aim for the "family track." *The Standard Star, Gannett Suburban Newspapers,* p. 12.

Rice, P. L. (1987). *Stress and health.* Pacific Grove, CA: Brooks/Cole.

Roberts, S. (1995, April 27). Women's work: What's new, what isn't? *The New York Times,* p. B6.

Rosenthal, E. (1991, April 30). Canada's national health plan gives care to all, with limits. *The New York Times,* pp. A1, A16.

Ryan, M. P. (1983). *Womankind in America: From colonial times to the present.* New York: Franklin Watts.

Sanday, P. R. (1981). *Female power and male dominance: On the origins of sexual inequality.* Cambridge: Cambridge University Press.

Sarason, I. G. (1980). Life stress, self-preoccupation and social supports. In I. G. Sarason & C. D. Spielberger (Eds.), *Stress and anxiety* (Vol. 7). Washington, DC: Halsted.

Schlesinger, A. (1962). *The vital center.* Boston: Houghton Mifflin.

Scham, M. (1973). *Blacks and American medical care.* Minneapolis: University of Minnesota Press.

Schindler, R., & Brawley, E. A. (1993). Community college programs for the human services: A continuing challenge for social work education and practice. *Journal of Social Work Education, 29,* 253–262.

Schmolling, P. (1995). Human services. In A. E. Dell Orto & R. P. Marinelli (Eds.). (1995). *Encyclopedia of disability and rehabilitation* (pp. 395–397). New York: Macmillan.

Simon, P. (1995, October 18). Throw out the pollsters: An interview with Paul Simon. *The Christian Century,* pp. 958–960.

Social Security Administration. (1994). *Annual statistical supplement to the Social Security Bulletin.* Washington, DC: U. S. Department of Health and Human Services.

Southern Regional Education Board. (1966). *The community college in mental health training: Report of a conference.* Atlanta, GA: Southern Regional Education Board.

Sullivan, J., & Purdy, M. (1995, July 23). Parlaying the detention business into profit. *The New York Times,* pp. 1, 28.

Sultz, H. (1991). Health policy: If you don't know where you are going, any road will take you. *American Journal of Public Health, 81,* 418–420.

Toner, R. (1995, April 9). G.O.P. blitz of first 100 days now brings pivotal second 100. *The New York Times,* pp. 1, 18.

Uchitelle, L. (1987, December 27). Hiring is up—to serve the middle class. *The New York Times*, p. E5.

U. S. Bureau of the Census (1994). *Statistical abstract of the United States* (115th ed.). Washington, DC: U. S. Government Printing Office.

U. S. is sued over aliens. (1994, April 12). *The New York Times*, p. A13.

Verhovek, S.H. (1994, June 8). Stop benefits for aliens? It wouldn't be that easy. *The New York Times*, pp. A1, B10.

Wahba, M., & Bridwell, L. (1976). Maslow reconsidered: A review of research on the response hierarchy. *Organizational Behavior and Human Performance, 15*, 212–240.

Walters, D. (1992). Isolationism. *Metropolis*, pp. 69, 88–89.

Wilson, D. (1995, July 19). Privatizing public services. *The Standard Star, Gannett Suburban Newspapers*, pp. 1A, 2A.

Women make slight gain in closing the wage gap. (1987, July 31). *Gannett Westchester Newspapers*, p. D1.

Zastrow, C. (1988). *Social problems: Issues and solutions*. Chicago: Nelson-Hall.

Groups in Need

INTRODUCTION

This chapter is devoted to groups of people selected for help by human services. They are sometimes called **target populations** or consumers of human services. The poor, the elderly, mental patients, abused children, and teenage runaways are examples of groups that have been targeted by specific programs and agencies. There is nothing permanent about target populations. Current public opinion, availability of funding, and political climate determine which groups may be relatively favored at a particular time. Populations that have always existed may suddenly be chosen for benefits. For example, victims of crime have only recently been targeted for benefits in a systematic way. The critical question of who determines which groups will receive aid is discussed in Chapter 7.

There are literally hundreds of target groups of varying sizes, and we can't cover all of them here. We limit our discussion to some of the larger groups that are being helped in an organized way. For each group, we give a rough estimate of the number of people included, along with a brief account of some of the programs and services provided. In regard to kinds of help provided, we place emphasis on large-scale federal programs, because these have become the vital bedrock of support for millions of Americans. You are encouraged to investigate some of the smaller target populations, as well as some of the local and private helping agencies, on your own.

AMERICA'S POOR

The United States is one of the wealthiest nations in the world: Its gross national product (the value of all goods produced and services provided) is higher than that of any other country. Although this country enjoys a high level of affluence, the data presented in Chapter 1 showed that millions of Americans are not sharing in the general wealth. Their relative deprivation affects the style and quality of their lives; it extends beyond mere distribution of income and includes inequality in education, health care, police protection, job opportunity, legal justice, and other areas (Julian & Kornblum, 1986, p. 202).

There is continuing debate about the degree of hardship faced by the nation's poor people. Conservatives point out that many poor people receive noncash benefits such as food stamps, public housing subsidies, and health insurance that help provide the necessities of life. Others charge that millions of Americans are so poor that they cannot make ends meet and that many are actually going hungry. For example, the Physician Task Force on Hunger in America (1985) reported that hunger had become an epidemic in some parts of America.

Measuring Poverty

Exactly how many Americans are living in poverty? There is no definite answer to this question because the number depends on the standard used to define poverty. Perhaps the most widely used measure is the threshold, or poverty line, provided by the Social Security Administration. This figure is based on the fact that an average low-income family spends one-third of its total income for food. The poverty line, then, is the food budget for a family of a given size multiplied by 3. Adjustments are made for changes in the cost of living for a given year. Another consideration is whether or not the family lives on a farm. Farm families supply some of their own food and are therefore assigned a lower figure. The poverty line should be taken as a general measure of economic well-being. It is *not* necessarily the income level used to determine eligibility for government assistance, a figure which varies by locality.

In 1994, a nonfarm family of four was considered poor if it had an income below $15,141 (Frum, 1995). This meant that roughly 38 million Americans (14.5% of the population) were poor by this standard. Although varying with the state of the economy, the poverty rate has been stuck in a range between 13–15% since the early 1980s.

The official poverty threshold allows convenient comparisons of poverty levels from year to year. It is not implied that the family could actually live on that amount. Schwarz and Volgy (1992) proposed a more realistic alternative measure. Their *self-sufficiency threshold* is defined as an economic budget that would allow a family of four to purchase minimum but essential items for food, housing, clothing, transportation, medical and personal expenses, and to pay taxes. Their self-sufficiency threshold for 1990 was $20,658 compared to $13,359 for the official poverty line. In other words, a family of four actually needs about 150% of the poverty line to get by. Schwarz and Volgy (1992) estimated that there are about 24 million persons among the working poor, that is, those who are employed full time, receive no welfare benefits, and live below the self-sufficiency threshold.

Who Are the Poor?

Obviously, poor people are those with a relative lack of money, resources, and possessions. Beyond this shared characteristic, America's poor may have little else in common. One important subgroup of poor people consists of those who have suffered a temporary setback that has reduced their ability to be self-supporting. These groups include workers who have been laid off, women who have been deserted by a spouse, and persons needed at home in a family crisis. Most of these people would be considered *able-bodied poor* because they are potentially employable.

A quite different subgroup of poor, sometimes called the *deserving poor,* is made up of people who are not able to be self-supporting. Included are the aged poor, young children of poor families, some discharged mental patients, and people who are permanently disabled.

According to Brieland, Costin, and Atherton (1980), this diversity among subgroups of poor has been an obstacle in developing satisfactory programs to help the poor; programs that suit one group may be inadequate for another. To encourage able-bodied poor to enter the job market, an aid program should pay only low benefits. However, low benefits would be an undeserved penalty to a person who could not work in any case.

We pointed out in Chapter 1 that a disproportionate number of poor can be found among minority groups. The poverty rate for African Americans and Latinos is considerably higher than that of whites. Women and children were also overrepresented among the ranks of the poor. In fact, the great majority of those living in poverty consist of women and children; they are the major recipients of welfare benefits, food stamps, and other programs for the poor.

Welfare and AFDC

At present, the single most important weapon in the war on poverty is public welfare. It is difficult to provide a clear picture of welfare because it is not one but many programs. Local, state, and federal governments are all involved in a complex, interlocking fashion. The basic responsibility rests with local (i.e., county or city) governments, which determine who is eligible for welfare and what benefits will be given. There is great variation in benefits paid by the various states, even when differences in cost of living are taken into account. Southeastern states, for example, tend to pay much less than California or some northern industrial states.

Aid to Families with Dependent Children (AFDC) is the program most people mean when they refer to welfare. Before this program was enacted, there were few acceptable options available to a parent with no means of supporting young children. One alternative was to turn the children over to an orphanage; another was to seek work outside the home, leaving the children unsupervised. Neither alternative was satisfactory to the family or to the community. Considerations such as these led to the birth of the AFDC program in 1935. This program provides benefits to the mother and child. Although there is also some provision for husbands with limited income, over 80% of those receiving aid are members of female-headed households.

The federal government pays 50–80% of AFDC benefits, whereas state and local governments administer the program. The federal government also pays half the administrative costs, but there is variation in the proportion paid by state and local governments. Some states take on the entire nonfederal portion, whereas other states require local communities to pay some portion of the nonfederal share. The lack of uniformity has contributed to the creation of a monstrous bureaucratic maze with agencies having different regulations and eligibility requirements.

AFDC has probably generated more political controversy than any other social program. Part of the difficulty centers around the great increase in the size of the program. In 1960, AFDC served only 745,000 families at a cost of $1 billion a year. The expansion of the program that began under Presidents Kennedy and Johnson continued during subsequent administrations. Between 1965 and 1972, antipoverty programs lifted half of the poor over the poverty line, but the costs were enormous. Presently, AFDC reaches 14 million households at the cost of $23 billion a year (Wines, 1995). What caused the surge in welfare rolls? Part of the answer is that the civil rights movement of the 1960s and 1970s encouraged poor people to think of welfare as a right rather than a privilege. Previously, many poor people who were eligible had not applied. Some actually did not know about their entitlements; others were too ashamed to apply. Increasingly, poor people rejected the idea that they were to blame for their destitution. At the same time, the liberal political climate caused welfare agencies to be more receptive toward applicants than they had been.

Aside from growing costs of the program, criticisms about other aspects of AFDC were raised by conservative and some liberal commentators. Perhaps the most serious is that AFDC works against keeping the family together. The assumption underlying this criticism is that the program promotes family nonformation or breakup of existing families. The fathers are usually men without technical skills whose income is low and who may not be able to work on a steady basis. In contrast, the welfare income is regular, and the system provides other benefits that the father may not be able to supply. For example. welfare status usually assures eligibility for health insurance—an important consideration in these days of rising health costs. The net effect is that the poor father may help the family by leaving it. If he elects to stay with the family, he cannot earn more than a limited amount without jeopardizing the welfare benefits.

As discussed in Chapter 1, some commentators blame welfare for the great increase in out-of-wedlock births to teenage girls. In fact, more than half a million teenage girls gave birth in 1991. Many of these girls are not ready to deal with a pregnancy or to raise a child. A teenage mother is much less likely to complete high school and is more likely to be poor in later life than is a mature mother. Babies born to teenage mothers are at relatively high risk of illness, low birth weight, and developmental delays (Ventura, 1994). Clearly, they are at risk to perpetuate the cycle of poverty and end up as welfare recipients themselves.

It is adult males, 20 and older, who are responsible for the majority of babies born to teenagers aged 15–17. What has changed in recent decades is that pregnant teenage girls no longer marry the father. Although some girls choose older boyfriends whom they regard as mature, a sizable amount of teenage sex is not consensual. In some poor areas, teenage girls report high rates of rape and sexual abuse. Many of the fathers in depressed areas are not able to provide support for a family. In one study, 32% of the adult male partners of teenage girls were neither working nor in school at the time of the child's birth (Shapiro, 1995). Under these circumstances, it is not surprising that the girls seek welfare support.

The Future of Welfare

During 1995, there was a growing political consensus that the welfare system needed a complete overhaul. As we have seen, the welfare state was criticized for breaking up families, rewarding irresponsible behavior, and minimizing work incentives for the poor. Democrats conceded that their party had failed to strongly support the federal safety net for poor people (Toner, 1995). Some Democrats stated that they had failed to keep vigil over welfare programs with the result that the programs did not change with the times. Mario Cuomo said, "We blew it. We were in power for a long time. We didn't correct ourselves . . . We didn't stay up to date and we paid the price" (quoted in Wines, 1995, p. E1). The result was that 87 of 100 senators, included 3 of 4 Democrats, voted to abandon the federal welfare system that had been in place for three decades. Plans were underway to restructure the system.

Although the details are not known, it seems certain that the states of the union will play an increasing role in managing welfare programs during the next decade. Increased money in the form of block grants will be sent from federal to state levels. In fact, many states have already seized the initiative in reorganizing welfare programs. The names of some of the new state programs provide clues to the direction of the changes. Consider the Virginia Independence Program, Wisconsin's Work Not Welfare Program, and Colorado's Personal Responsibility and Employment Program. In Massachusetts, the Department of Public Welfare became the Department of Transitional Assistance (Verhovek, 1995). It seems obvious that recipients are being told to assume more self-responsibility, prepare to work, and not to expect benefits for an extended period.

Other state reforms center around teenage girls who produce out-of-wedlock children. California now requires that grants to teenage mothers be given only if the teen is living with a parent or guardian with the money going to the adult. The basic idea is that the girl's parents are primarily responsible for supervising her and taking care of her children. Under the old system, girls were rewarded with a benefits package and, sometimes, an apartment when they gave birth. They were treated as though they had become mature women overnight. In reality, they were often children themselves, lacking the skills needed to earn a living or to socialize a child (Schmolling, 1994).

Another reform is the imposition of a time limit on welfare benefits. Wisconsin is experimenting with a 2-year limit on benefits in two counties. The idea is to prevent welfare from becoming a permanent lifestyle. Under the old system, fully 25% of the recipients received assistance for 10 years or more. Vermont and Florida were also developing time-limit plans. Other proposals were aimed at promoting socially desirable behavior. In Maryland, for example, there is a 30% reduction in welfare payments unless parents prove they have paid rent, kept children in school, and obtained preventive health care (e.g., vaccinations). Other ideas are aimed at keeping the family together. For instance, some states have a "wedfare" component that allows the woman to retain a portion of grants after marriage (Schmolling, 1994).

In summary, it appears that the states of the union will have greater freedom in designing their own welfare programs. Ideally, they will use this freedom to develop innovative programs that successfully move recipients into productive lifestyles. There are, of course, various dangers in turning welfare over to the states. One is the possibility of negative competition between states to see who can offer the lowest benefits, the object being to discourage welfare migration into the home state. Advocates for the poor have expressed concern about the fact that only one state, New York, has a constitutional provision that guarantees aid to its poorest citizens. A state court ruled that Connecticut has no such responsibility, paving the way for cutbacks in benefits and the imposition of time limits on how long benefits may be received (Rabinovitz, 1995). The idea that poor people are entitled to a guarantee of at least minimal subsistence seems out of favor at both federal and state levels.

Liberal commentator Mark Rank argued that welfare reform does not address the basic problem—poverty. Although no one doubts that individuals abuse the welfare system, it is important to remember that the majority who receive welfare do want to work. The real problem, he suggests, is that viable opportunities are not available to everyone because low-paying and part-time jobs simply do not pay enough money to provide for a family. Minimum wage jobs such as fast-food, clerical, and cleaning positions do not pay enough to keep a family above the poverty level (cited by Popple & Leighninger, 1990, pp. 243–244).

One of the major obstacles to employment for poor people is a lack of basic educational literacy. Presently, about 20 million adults are functionally illiterate. More than one-third of adult illiterates had incomes below the poverty line. The federal government, which plays an important role in education and job-training programs for unskilled adults, reduced funding for those "second chance" programs during the 1980s (Caputo, 1989).

Home Relief

Presently, only a minority of states choose to provide Home Relief (or General Assistance) to unemployed adults who are under 65 and not disabled, and the number is declining. Unlike AFDC, this program is financed without federal assistance and hence is vulnerable to political attack on the local level. Monthly benefits for a destitute person range from nothing to New York's high of $352 a month. Even this maximum grant is not nearly enough to elevate the recipient above the poverty line or even to guarantee shelter. The reason for the reluctant giving is obvious; the beneficiaries are able-bodied and capable of working; therefore, some citizens suspect them of being lazy and unwilling to work (Sack, 1991). This stereotype ignores the fact that jobs may not be available in some areas or during economically depressed times. It is also possible that the worker does not have the skills demanded by the jobs that are available. The vulnerability of Home Relief was demonstrated during the recession of 1989–1991 when benefits were cut back just when high unemployment rates made them more necessary.

Other Programs for the Poor

The federal government supports a number of other programs for people with limited income. These include food stamps, free or reduced-price school lunches, housing subsidies, and Medicaid benefits. We'll take a closer look at some of these programs here.

Some low-income families are eligible for food stamps, which can only be used for the purpose of buying food in an authorized food market. They cannot be used for buying liquor, beer, cigarettes, soap, paper products, or other nonfood items. The stamps cannot be redeemed for cash. At present about 27 million Americans receive food stamps, that is, one out of every ten Americans (Pear, 1995).

Poor people may also be eligible for various kinds of help with housing. Some communities provide low-cost housing, often called "projects," for poor people. In some cases, welfare provides a rent subsidy for those unable to pay the full amount of their rent. Homeless people are put up in low-cost hotels until a permanent place is found. Regardless of the form of housing, poor people tend to be placed together in ghettolike environments where crime, addiction, and substandard conditions are common.

The federal government provides health care to those of limited income through Medicaid, a system that offers an array of inpatient and outpatient medical services. Although it has helped poor people gain access to improved medical care, the program is riddled with abuses, especially in poor areas. Some unscrupulous people set up "Medicaid mills" in poor neighborhoods where the patient is routinely run through a lengthy series of tests and procedures, many of which are unnecessary. Another limitation of the Medicaid system is that many doctors simply refuse to accept Medicaid patients because the level of reimbursement is too low.

Not all programs for the poor are concerned with basic survival needs. For example, many city and state governments provide low-cost or free college education for low-income students. Many of these colleges have an open enrollment policy and make some provision for the underprepared student in the form of remediation courses.

Most of the programs just mentioned are means-tested, which means that a recipient's total financial support must fall below a certain level before he or she is eligible. Although these and other programs have improved the quality of life for many poor persons, life for the poor is far from easy. There continues to be a strong undercurrent of hostility toward the poor in this country. Many hardworking Americans, convinced that welfare recipients are lazy and/or immoral people, bitterly resent paying tax money to support them. The poor themselves sometimes have incorporated these negative attitudes into their own thinking. They feel ashamed of not being independent and self-reliant, important values to Americans. These attitudes may be shared by the politicians who establish budgets and eligibility requirements, as well as by the workers who administer the programs. It is not surprising that welfare recipients often band together into informal groups where they may find not only understanding and support but more practical kinds of help.

This section can best be closed by recalling Will Rogers's remark, "It's no crime to be poor but it might as well be."

A Suggested Class Assignment:

> Report on the welfare system in your state, answering the following items:
> What are the eligibility requirements for entering the program?
> Describe the benefits including cash awards, housing subsidies, and other allowances.
> Describe the recipient population in terms of age, gender, race, and education.
> What arrangements are made regarding employment, job training, or education?
> What changes, if any, have been made in the system in recent years?
> How does this program compare to that of neighboring states?
> How do recipients feel about the program?
> How does the program deal with unmarried teenage mothers?

THE UNEMPLOYED

Let's begin our discussion of unemployment with some of the obvious benefits that typically come from having a steady job.

- It provides income needed for the necessities of life.
- It helps one to be independent and self-supporting.
- It helps one feel like a useful member of society.
- It structures time in a useful way.
- It provides social contacts with others.
- It may place one in a stimulating environment.
- It provides an opportunity to use and develop talents.

The Consequences of Joblessness

These benefits vanish when a worker is laid off or fired. Instead, there is often a sense of absence of control over one's life, coupled with a fear of having to depend on others. The unemployed person begins to feel cut off from the mainstream of life, a feeling that deepens as time goes on. Julian and Kornblum (1986, p. 417) reviewed some data that support the idea that work is necessary if one is to be, in any full sense, "among the living."

The devastating consequences of unemployment were highlighted by a study of white-collar men who had lost their jobs in the recession of the mid-1970s; they showed signs of severe psychological stress (Braginsky & Braginsky, 1975). Although many were college graduates and had held prestigious managerial positions, their self-esteem was sharply lowered by the experience. Most suffered deep shame, avoided friends, and felt isolated from society. They felt insignificant and suffered from the feeling that they had lost value in the eyes of family members. Another consequence of their prolonged unemployment was a deep cynicism toward established institutions.

Unemployment Rates

Each month, the U. S. Bureau of Labor Statistics reports the official rate of unemployment in the labor force. The labor force is defined as people 16 years of age or over who worked 1 hour for pay during 1 survey week or who did not have a job and were actively seeking work. The nation's official unemployment rate in recent years has ranged from 7.1% during the 1991 recession to 5.5% during the recovery of 1995 (Hershey, 1995). This means that the average number of unemployed has ranged between 8–9 million workers during this period. This does *not* include the estimated 1 million discouraged workers who are no longer even trying to find jobs. Nor does it include the more than 6 million underemployed persons who are working part-time because they could not find full-time jobs (Tumulty, 1992). In all, there are 15–16 million workers who were either underemployed or unemployed.

The jobless rate for whites is usually much less than that for African Americans, with the Latino rate falling between these groups (Hershey, 1988). It is suspected that a disproportionate number of minorities are involved in the *underground economy,* a term that refers to exchange of goods and services—both legal and illegal—that are not regulated or taxed by government (Julian & Kornblum, 1986). This economy includes income from drugs, prostitution, flea markets, and gambling, as well as employment with wages that are paid "under the table" or "off the books." By and large, those involved in these unrecorded activities are not eligible for social services or pension plans.

Unemployment Insurance

The unemployment compensation system is our way of helping people who have been laid off from their jobs. The states regulate unemployment insurance programs, and they vary in rules and eligibility requirements. In most states, workers and employers contribute to the program. Often the amount and duration of payments are based on the individual's earnings history and length of employment. Most states pay benefits for up to 26 weeks and usually require some evidence that the person is actually looking for work. In addition, a federal-state extended benefit program is sometimes activated when unemployment rates become relatively high in a particular state; it provides up to 13 additional weeks of regular benefits (Hope & Young, 1986). A further increase in the number of weeks of coverage has been provided by Congress during times of high unemployment. Even when maximum supplements are available, an unemployed worker runs out of benefits in 65 weeks.

The Impact of Unemployment on Human Services

Increases in unemployment have a number of direct and indirect effects on human services. Certainly, there are increased numbers applying for unemployment insurance and public assistance. Less obvious are the indirect consequences of unemployment on human services. Brenner's (1973) study clearly showed that economic reverses result in increases in certain physical illnesses, elevated crime rates, and increased first admissions to both state prisons and mental hospitals. These and other negative effects of economic downturns may take several years to fully develop. It appears that the stress associated with loss of livelihood may have a long-term, insidious effect. It is equally clear that people react to this stress in very different ways. Some lash out with antisocial behavior, and others may suffer physical or mental breakdowns. The shock waves of unemployment ultimately reach mental hospitals, general hospitals, prisons, and a variety of other agencies.

CHILDREN IN NEED

Children are endangered not only by poverty but by illness, rejection, lack of understanding, the inability of parents to socialize them properly, and many other factors. Human services workers realize that children are a high-risk group for developing all sorts of physical and emotional problems. Children often haven't fully developed the skills and defenses needed to deal with the stresses of life. Although some remarkable children do well in spite of grave hardships, most require some minimal care, love, and guidance. If these are not adequately supplied, the risk of developing a serious disorder increases.

According to the Joint Commission on Mental Health of Children (1970), 8–10% of all children are suffering from a childhood problem serious enough to require professional help. Another 2–3% are severely disturbed. These problems range from serious disorders such as childhood psychoses, retardation, and physical abuse to milder disorders such as school phobia, bed-wetting, and extreme shyness. These and other dysfunctions, fully described in abnormal psychology courses, will not be detailed here. Instead, we will examine the vulnerability of children in terms of the changing American family. There has been a great deal of recent public discussion about how these sweeping changes have affected children.

Children and the Changing American Family

In Chapter 1, we noted the dramatic changes that have taken place in the American family in recent decades. It seems clear that, on average, American children are now worse off in some respects than children of the recent past. More children are growing up with fewer parental resources: less time, only one parent, stress due to separations (Wolfe, 1991). In addition, many children—about one in five—are living below the poverty line (Gannett, 1991). Today's youngsters perform worse at school, are twice as likely to commit suicide, use much more alcohol and drugs, and are twice as likely to be obese as children of the previous generation (Fuchs, 1991).

Children of Single-Parent Families

In 1960, 9.1% of America's children lived in single-parent families; the percentage increased steadily during the following decades reaching 28.6% in 1991 (U. S. Bureau of the Census, 1991). About 17 million children currently live in such families. The Census Bureau also revealed that the percentage of children in these homes is disproportionately high in our central cities, for example 55% in Detroit, 53% in Washington, DC, and 49% in Atlanta. The great majority of these homes are without a father. In Chapter 1, we discussed some of the disadvantages of single-parent families including the fact that there is a greater likelihood of living in poverty. Children from these families also have above average levels of youth suicide, mental illness, violence, and drug use. When you add poor school performance to the list of problems, it becomes obvious that this population is likely to be in need of help from a range of human service agencies.

Perhaps the greatest disadvantage of single parenthood is the negative effect on the income and employment of the head of the family. Mother-only families have very high rates of poverty. After a divorce or separation, the mother's earnings become the major source of family income, accounting for 60–70% of the total income (Garfinkel & McLanahan, 1986, pp. 18–22). Usually, the postdivorce income of men is higher than that of divorced women. For single parents of both sexes, there are likely to be problems associated with combining work with child-rearing. Job mobility, earning power, freedom to work late, and job performance are all likely to be negatively affected (Grief, 1985, p. 181).

The psychological aspects of single parenthood tend to compound the difficulties. In a sense, the single parent must play all the roles once shared by mother and father. In addition to providing love and nurturance, the single parent "must represent the family interests to society at large, interpret society to the children, and be a figure of authority and discipline for them" (Costin, Bell, & Downs, 1991, p. 137). For many single parents, the pressures of playing these roles, along with the need to make a living, create considerable stress.

The single-parent situation may present serious problems to the children. Helping efforts have been centered in the schools. One approach that has enjoyed some success is peer counseling in the form of "rap groups" for children. Whether sponsored by the school or a local counseling agency, these groups help the youngster to ventilate strong feelings about the disrupted home life and also to reduce the sense of isolation that some feel. In the group setting, children realize that their feelings are shared by many others in similar situations.

In some cases, the child may be so disturbed that professional help is sought. Some community agencies, such as child guidance centers, offer individual or family therapy with a social worker, psychologist, or psychiatrist. Some of these agencies maintain a reference library of books, pamphlets, and films on death and divorce for use by clients and families of clients.

In addition to psychotherapeutic intervention, a great many other kinds of services may be available to these children and their families. There are so many, in fact, that we can only provide a brief listing.

- Daytime care programs for young children aim to foster optimal intellectual development and to help overcome some of the emotional effects of early deprivation.
- Parent assistance programs are designed to help the inexperienced or overburdened parent to deal with some of the practical problems of child and home care.
- Socially supportive organizations like Big Brothers/Sisters may help fill the gap in a child's life that was left by a departing parent.
- Family crisis intervention may combine the skills of police and human services workers to help resolve intense domestic disputes that require police intervention.
- Teenage mothers may be provided with programs to help them continue their education and also to instruct them about parenting, sexuality, and social services for which they may be eligible.
- Community centers may offer an array of useful services, including social and recreational programs for children at different ages.

Abused and Neglected Children

It is not known how much the recent changes in American family life have contributed to the apparent increase in child abuse. It is certain only that there has been a huge increase in the number of reports of abuse during recent decades. Some experts attribute part of the increase to intensive case finding and reporting, implying that similar cases existed in the past but were not reported. During recent decades, the media have reported many sensational stories, which have increased public awareness of the suffering of young victims of abuse. As we shall see, it is even possible that our concern for these youngsters have ushered in a phase of overreporting of doubtful or unfounded cases of abuse.

Exactly how do we define child abuse or maltreatment? Abuse and neglect cases are so varied that they defy any simple or uniform definition. A preliminary definition would encompass maltreatment of a child in physical, emotional, or sexual areas. And of course, in each area, there are degrees of severity of maltreatment. In a given case, experts might disagree on whether or not a given treatment constituted abuse.

The following list offers an idea of the various types of maltreatment that have come to the attention of human services workers.

- Children have been physically assaulted—that is, beaten, kicked, slapped, punched, or shoved. In some cases, an implement such as a knife, whip, or strap has been used, and in still others, the child has been burned with a cigarette or scalded with a hot liquid.
- Sexual abuse of a child has involved a variety of acts ranging from fondling of genitals to penile penetration. The atrocious crimes of incest and child rape are included in this category.
- The abuse has taken the form of emotional assaults, such as threatening, belittling, or disparaging the child.
- In some cases, the child has been confined by being tied up, chained, or locked in a closet or room.
- Neglect of the child's needs may also be viewed as abusive. Examples have included outright abandonment of the child, failure to provide needed medical care, inadequate supervision, poor nutrition, inadequate clothing, neglect of the child's education, and disregard of the child's safety.

A distinction is usually made between abuse and neglect of a child. Abuse is usually an act of *commission* on the part of the caregiver, meaning a voluntary act, whereas neglect is an act of *omission*, in which some ingredient important to the child's welfare is not provided. Many instances of neglect are involuntary on the part of the parent or caregiver. Sometimes, the caregiver may be unable to provide for the child because of illness, incarceration, loss of income, or some other unforeseen event.

The number of cases of child abuse and neglect cannot be stated with certainty because estimates come from so many different sources. The U. S. Department of Health and Human Services (1988) found that in one recent year, 1,584,700 cases of maltreatment were reported to community professionals in schools, hospitals, police departments, juvenile probation departments, day care centers, mental health agencies, and welfare departments. About 63% of the cases involved neglect and fewer than 50% involved abuse. About 19% of the children involved were considered to be endangered by the treatment they received, and many had suffered serious injuries. Although these data are the most comprehensive available, it should be kept in mind that they include only those cases that actually come to the attention of community agencies. There are probably many cases that go unreported. Some people who suspect that a child is being abused may decide not to get involved, may be afraid of retaliation on the part of the abuser, or perhaps, doubt that the authorities will take any effective action.

Estimates of the actual as opposed to the reported number of cases have ranged between 2.5 million to over 6 million(!), with most studies showing a dramatic increase in recent years (Popple & Leighninger, 1990, p. 260). The American Humane Association reported that the total number of reported cases jumped to nearly 2 million in 1985 from 669,000 in 1976 (Miller, 1987). The American Humane Association studies are produced annually and have the advantage of including cases reported by neighbors and other nonprofessionals. The great increase in the number of reported cases in recent years has raised doubts about the validity of some. One possible source of invalid cases comes from divorced parents who wish to gain custody of their children by denigrating the care provided by the former spouse. It is also possible that the intense emotions aroused by child abuse has led to overzealous and unfounded prosecutions. The fact is that at least half of all reports of alleged child abuse cases are unfounded in the sense that they lack credible evidence (Waller, 1991). It seems clear that false reporting of child abuse cases is a disservice to the children who are involved. They are forced to undergo the pressures of public hearings and are generally placed under great stress. Another problem is that the unfounded cases necessitate the waste of professional time, which could be put to better use in valid cases.

The Causes of Child Abuse

There are many factors that play a role in child abuse. Some have to do with environmental stress, whereas others involve the personality traits of the abusing caregiver. Abusive parents tend to be young, of lower-class status, frustrated, unemployed, alcohol abusers, and often suffer from marital discontent (Egeland, Clochetti, & Taraldson, 1976). Child abuse also takes place in middle- and upper-class homes, but the affluence of the parents is often used to prevent incidents from becoming known. Regardless of class, the abusing parents often take out their frustrations on their helpless children.

Very often, abusing parents lacked effective role models in childhood and were themselves abused or neglected. However, it would be a mistake to

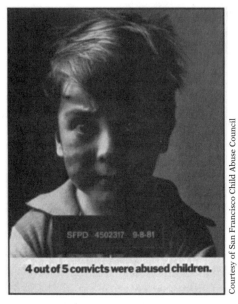

4 out of 5 convicts were abused children.

This poster makes a powerful appeal on
behalf of abused children.

conclude that child abuse inexorably repeats itself in successive generations.
Kaufman and Zigler (1987) warn against repeatedly telling adults who were
maltreated as youngsters that they will abuse their own children, because for
some it may become a self-fulfilling prophecy. These authors reviewed the
child abuse literature and concluded that about 30% of those who were
abused as children complete the cycle with their own offspring. This rate is
six times higher than the rate in the general population, but it is important to
note that the vicious cycle is the exception, not the rule. The cycle is less
likely to be repeated in adults who have a loving, supportive relationship
with a spouse or a lover and who have relatively few stressful events in their
lives. It also helps if the adult consciously resolves not to repeat the cycle of
abuse and seeks counseling to discuss effective parenting.

Although abusing parents may come from any background, there is a
very strong relationship between poverty and abuse. In fact, family income is
probably the most powerful single indicator of child abuse and neglect (U. S.
Department of Health and Human Services, 1988). As shown in Table 2–1,
maltreatment was about seven times more likely to occur in families with an
annual income under $15,000 than in families with income above this figure.
There is nothing very surprising about this finding, because poverty is likely
to bring with it frustration, insecurity, and stress. People with low incomes
tend to have more children than those from upper income levels while having
fewer resources to take care of them. Substance abuse, criminal behavior,
and high rates of mental illness are just a few of the other negative factors
that tend to be prevalent in poor families and that contribute to abuse.

TABLE 2-1   Maltreatment Rates Based on Family Income
(per 1000 Children from Families in That Income Category in the
Population)

Category	Less Than $15,000	$15,000 or More
All maltreatment	54.0	7.9
All abuse	19.9	4.4
Physical abuse	10.2	2.5
Sexual abuse	4.8	1.1
Emotional abuse	6.1	1.2
All neglect	36.8	4.1
Physical neglect	22.6	1.9
Educational neglect	10.1	1.3
Emotional neglect	6.9	1.5
Fatal injury/impairment	0.03	0.01
Serious injury/impairment	6.0	0.9
Moderate injury/impairment	30.9	5.5
Probable injury/impairment	5.4	0.9
Severity-endangered	11.7	0.6

SOURCE: U. S. Department of Health and Human Services. National Center on Child Abuse and Neglect. (1988). *Study Findings, Study of National Incidence and Prevalence of Child Abuse and Neglect.* Washington, DC: U. S. Government Printing Office.

Helping the Abused or Neglected Child

Child protective services are offered by many private and government agencies. Some of the most important are state social service agencies, which may be designated as the department of social services, the department of human resources, or the department of human services. These agencies process most of the cases of abuse and are responsible for making a determination of whether or not to accept the case for services. If the case is accepted, the agency must decide what services are needed. In some cases, the parents will be helped to improve their level of care by means of counseling. However, if the abusing parents are not cooperative, the case may be referred to court, which may in turn assign legal custody to the agency (Popple & Leighninger, 1990). The parents may sometimes be granted physical custody of the children, provided they accept monitoring and services by the agency. The worker may supervise the home to make sure there is no further maltreatment of the child. Various community services, such as tutoring or recreation, may be provided to the children while the parents are taught the skills needed to be successful caregivers. In a minority of cases, the court and the agency may decide that the child would be seriously endangered by remaining in the home. Foster placement then becomes the option of choice.

Nationwide, federal, state, and local agencies spend more than $10 billion a year caring for an estimated 460,000 children in foster care (Kramer, 1994). An increased demand for placements, due to the spread of crack use among women, has come at a time when fewer foster homes are available because more women have joined the work force. This situation has prompted many state and local agencies to cut corners on foster home investigations. Children are sometimes placed in overcrowded homes with unsuitable guardians. Consequently, there have been many reports of children being raped, beaten, and neglected in their foster homes. For example, a suit filed on behalf of 2800 foster children in Baltimore charged that children as young as 3 have been raped and that many were medically neglected and otherwise mistreated (Miller, 1987). There have also been disturbing reports of abuse of children entrusted to state mental health and retardation facilities (McFadden, 1987). These are children who could not be placed in foster homes.

It should be pointed out that most foster parents are decent people who raise children for little monetary reward. States and localities are generally raising the amount paid to foster parents. Some pay between $250–$400 a month per child. Other steps taken to deal with the crisis in foster care are the recruitment of more (and better) foster parents, training of foster parents, increasing the number of caseworkers, and when feasible, helping the abusive biological parents to keep their children at home.

The preferred approach is to hold the family together if that is at all possible and to give the parents the support they need to become adequate parents. Rather than to punish the parents, the goal is to help them break the cycle of abuse. One approach is to use groups to teach effective parenting to those whose own parents were usually disastrous role models. The abusing parents are encouraged to call staff of the mental health agency when they feel the impulse to hurt their children. It must be understood by all concerned that effective parenting does not come naturally but must be learned in a step-by-step fashion. The study of child abuse makes it quite obvious that maternal and paternal "instincts" cannot be relied upon to produce love and care for a child. Parenting involves a wide range of skills, attitudes, and knowledge that are normally acquired from one's own parents. Child abusers often fall into the pattern of imitating the abusive parents that raised them.

Another approach to treatment is Parents Anonymous (PA), a group founded in 1970. Being a self-help group, it avoids the angry feelings that are often generated by an outside authority intruding into a home. Often, the abusing parents feel guilty about their maltreatment of their children. They are very sensitive to being shamed and belittled by authorities, however much they may "deserve" it. In the PA meetings, modeled after Alcoholics Anonymous, the abusing parents voluntarily admit their tendencies to others like themselves. With the support of the group, they struggle to control themselves and to find other ways of dealing with their children. Although it is too early for a definitive assessment of the effectiveness of this approach, it can be said that PA is growing in popularity. There are now more than 100 chapters in the United States.

Children are members of many target populations. Additional references to children may be found in subsequent sections on people with disabilities, mental illness, and retardation.

THE ELDERLY

During the 1980s, there was a dramatic rise in the number of Americans aged 65 and older; the 1990 census counted 31.2 million Americans in this age group, a 22% increase since 1980 (Crispell & Frey, 1993). Elderly people now accounted for 13% of the entire U. S. adult population. It is expected that both the percentage and absolute number of elderly will continue to increase. By 2030, there will be about 65 million older persons in the country.

This huge increase in the elderly population will have a profound influence on human services, because the chances of needing outside help increase sharply with age. The percentage needing the help of another person to perform personal care or home management is 14% for those aged 65–74, 26% for those aged 75–84, and 48% for those 85 and older. Older persons account for a relatively high percentage of hospital stays, have longer hospital stays, and average more visits to the doctor than people under 65. In 1984, the 65-and-over group accounted for 31% of total personal health care expenditure (AARP, 1986). Also to be considered is the fact that the elderly suffer higher rates of depression and suicide than the general population.

Older people inevitably undergo physical changes that increase susceptibility to diseases such as cancer, heart disease, arthritis, and diabetes. As the body declines in vitality, it becomes less able to deal with stress and malfunction. The physical problems are compounded by social and psychological difficulties. For example, the elderly person has to face up to the loss of loved ones as well as to the possibility of feeling less useful and more of a burden to others. Financial problems are also likely to come with old age. The majority of elderly people leave the work force, sometimes pressured to do so by rules and regulations of their employers. With retirement, income drops sharply. This explains why social security benefits are of such vital concern to many elderly Americans.

Social Security

The federal government plays a major role in providing for the needs of the elderly. The Old-age, Survivors, and Disability Insurance (OASDI) program, popularly known as social security, is the largest social welfare program in the United States. During 1994, 42.6 million individuals were receiving OASDI benefits. The majority of the beneficiaries were retired workers and their spouses; a smaller number were disabled workers. The amount of money received is adjusted yearly and is pegged to the Consumer Price Index. The idea is to help beneficiaries keep up with the rising costs of living. For example, benefits in 1992 were increased 3.7% over the previous year, bringing the average benefit to $629 a month for an individual retiree and to $1067 for an elderly couple (Pear, 1991). Continued yearly increases have raised the average monthly benefit to $698 for a single retired worker, and to $1178 for a retired couple in 1995.

Headlines have sometimes conveyed the impression that social security may be going broke. There is, in fact, no immediate problem. The retirement and disability trust funds are currently running a surplus with 1994 income exceeding expenses by over $58 billion. The excess is loaned to the U. S. government in the form of special issue, interest-bearing bonds (AARP, 1995). It *is* true that the funds will be exhausted by 2030 unless Congress takes action, and there are several reasons for the projected shortfall. The looming retirement of 70 million baby boomers (persons born during the late 1940s and early 1950s) is one factor. Another is that people are living longer and, consequently, collecting benefits for a longer time. Even more important is the fact there will be fewer workers in the future to support more beneficiaries. In 1950, there were 16 workers for every person receiving benefits; today the ratio is 3:1, and by 2030 it will be 2:1. These figures again reflect the fact that the proportion of elderly in the U. S. population is increasing steadily (Carlson, 1995).

How is social security financed? Employers and employees each pay 6.2% of a worker's salary through payroll taxes up to the 1995 taxable minimum of $61,200. Self-employed persons must pay the entire 12.4% of their earnings into a special fund. The maximum taxable wage has been raised periodically and may go up again in the near future.

Some young people are dismayed by the fact that they are being asked to bear the brunt of expenses for the system even though their eventual benefits are being delayed and may be reduced. Starting in the year 2000, for people born in 1938 or later, the age for receiving full retirement benefits will increase in gradual steps from 65 to 67. For example, anyone born in 1960 or later will be eligible for full retirement benefits at 67.

How Are Benefits Determined?   The amount received is based on a formula that uses average earnings over an individual's entire working life. The worker receives credits based on the amount earned each year. The amount it takes to earn 1 credit changes annually. In 1995, an individual received 1 credit for each $630 of annual wages up to a maximum of 4 credits a year. At this rate, it would take 10 years to earn the 40 credits needed to qualify for benefits.

There is no doubt that social security has transformed the way older Americans live. By helping them to be independent, it has also changed the lives of many of their children (Rovner, 1995). It is by far the nation's largest and most successful antipoverty program. In 1992, social security lifted the incomes of 9.6 million Americans over 65 above the poverty threshold. In effect, without social security, the elderly poverty rate would have been almost 50% instead of only 11.8%. Few people realize that 6 of 10 workers in private industry have no pension other than social security (Rovner, 1995).

Those who want to earn money in addition to their benefits by continuing to work are penalized by the system. Between age 65 through 69, a recipient cannot earn more than $12,500 without losing some benefits; for each $3 earned above this amount, $1 in benefits is deducted. Nonwage income such as interest on savings may be earned in any amount without loss of benefits. These regulations appear to favor affluent people who are likely to enjoy this significant nonwage income and penalize poorer individuals who need to work to supplement meager incomes.

Supplemental Security Income (SSI) is a federal program that pays monthly cash benefits to people who are 65 or older, *or* are blind, *or* who have a disability *and* who have limited resources and income. As of 1991, a person with unearned income of less than $4884 is eligible (unearned income includes social security benefits, pensions, rent, and interest). A person may have a somewhat larger amount in wages, classified by the government as earned income, and still be eligible. A person is considered disabled if he or she is unable to work because of a physical or mental impairment, but of course, the disability must be medically certified. The maximum monthly payment in 1991 was $407 payable to an individual and $610 a month for a couple. However, states may add to the federal SSI payments if they wish. Another benefit provided by SSI is a small payment of $30 a month to people living in institutions such as mental hospitals (Social Security Administration, 1991).

We cannot go further in explaining the eligibility rules and benefits because they are quite complex. The interested student is urged to visit a social security office to obtain further information. Several pamphlets containing useful information are usually available for the taking. For example, "A Guide to SSI for Groups and Organizations," put out by the Social Security Administration, gives a clear, brief description of the program.

Health Care for the Aged

"No longer will older Americans be denied the healing miracle of modern medicine. No longer will illness crush and destroy the savings they have so carefully put away over a lifetime." These words were spoken by President Lyndon Johnson in 1965 when Medicare was created as an amendment to the Social Security Act (Connell, 1995, p. 3B).

At that time, only half of the American elderly had any health insurance. Thirty years later, 97% of seniors (about 37 million) held Medicare cards. Medicare provides hospital benefits, operating room charges, regular nursing care, and medical supplies. It also covers some services at home such as part-time skilled nursing care for convalescents who no longer need to be in a hospital. However, the program does not cover routine physical exams, eyeglasses, hearing aids, or immunizations. Some critics believe that these limitations effectively deny some older people access to preventive medical services. Whether the government saves money in the long run by curtailing preventive services is open to question.

Medicare does not by any means pay all of the costs of medical treatment. There are significant deductibles and limitations of coverage. The deductible, now $100, is the amount the person must pay out of pocket per year before the insurance goes into effect. Once the deductible is met, Medicare pays a set fee for covered doctor and hospital services and procedures. When all is said and done, Medicare ends up paying about 45% of the actual expenses incurred (Connell, 1995). This is why many elderly buy private Medigap insurance to help cover the costs not covered by Medicare.

Providers complain about the complexity of the system and about the need to hire clerical staff to process the paperwork. Huge manuals, listing each procedure along with a designated fee and code number, must be consulted. There may be frustrating delays when a provider tries to get through to a representative to correct errors or resolve complaints. Some doctors do not "accept assignment," meaning to accept what Medicare pays as full payment. The patient must then pay the difference between the fee and the Medicare payment. In fairness, it must be said that many of the same kind of complaints by providers are made about private medical insurers.

In spite of its limitations, Medicare is a very popular program with the elderly. Changes in the program are considered with caution by politicians who fear the wrath of the elderly at election time. However, it is widely accepted in Washington that changes are necessary. Policymakers with all shades of political opinion agree that Medicare cannot be sustained in its present form because the costs are out of control (Toner & Pear, 1995). In 1994, nearly $160 billion was spent by Medicare, and the costs are rising at an annual rate of 10%. At this rate, the trust funds would be depleted by the year 2002. During the year 2010, the great wave of baby boomers will begin their senior years, placing a severe strain on the system.

Medicare is financed, in part, by a payroll tax that has been increased frequently since its inception. Some policymakers now feel that tinkering with the existing system will not solve the problem. They favor a complete redesign of Medicare along the lines of a voucher system. Presently, the government acts as insurer, paying doctors and hospitals for covered services. Under a proposed plan, the government would contribute a fixed amount of money to each Medicare beneficiary who would then go into the marketplace to purchase his or her own insurance plan. The elderly person would be able to pick and choose among health plans offering different benefit packages and, of course, different premiums. The beneficiary would receive cash rebates if selecting a plan charging less than the standard federal payment (Toner & Pear, 1995).

Medicaid for the Elderly.   Medicaid was created as part of the social security system at the same time as Medicare. It was intended primarily to provide health insurance for persons with low incomes or serious disabilities. In practice, the elderly and persons with disabilities consume two-thirds of Medicaid's dollars with poor, able-bodied individuals taking up the rest. A major expense is caring for the elderly in nursing homes, which now cost about $38,000 a year on average for each resident. Two of three nursing home residents have their bills paid by Medicaid (Connell, 1995). The remainder must "spend down" their savings until they have become paupers, at which point Medicaid kicks in.

Medicare facts

- One in ten Medicare beneficiaries is over 85.
- The average 65-year-old can expect to live past 82, 3 years longer than before.
- Medicare spends about $4000 a year per recipient, but the sickest 10% average over $28,000 per year.
- Medicare fueled the growth of the health care sector of the economy in this country. Hospitals now routinely provide services and surgical procedures (e.g., hip replacements), which were uncommon in 1965.
- The U. S. spent $204 per person on health care in 1965 (5.9% of the gross national product) compared to $3685 per person (14% of the gross national product) in 1995.
- Medicare was enacted over the strenuous objections of the American Medical Association. In order to secure its passage, the Johnson administration set only the loosest limits on doctors' fees. The result was that some physicians were charging Medicare four times what they charged private insurers for the same procedure.
- It wasn't until the 1980s that Medicare got around to setting limits on hospital and physicians' fees (Connell, 1995; Toner & Pear, 1995).

The Dementias

Dementia is not one but a group of disorders caused by damage of brain tissue. Regardless of the specific type of damage, individuals suffering from any of these disorders tend to show similar deficits, such as short-term memory loss, reduced ability to learn new material, and difficulties in understanding abstract or symbolic ideas. Problems in concentration, judgment, and emotional control are likely to become more noticeable as the disease progresses. Eventually, the person may have difficulty in recalling words or the labels of common objects, or may begin repeating the same phrases over and over again. Finally, the victim may be unable to recognize friends and family.

Until recently, it was assumed that these dysfunctions were due to arteriosclerosis, popularly known as hardening of the arteries. In this form of dementia, certain areas of the brain show infarcts, or small strokes, that damage blood vessels feeding the brain. Those with multi-infarct dementia, as it is called, often have a history of strokes and high blood pressure. We now know that this type of dementia represents only about 15–20% of dementia cases (Hooyman & Kiyak, 1991).

The most common dementia of later life is Alzheimer's disease, which accounts for over 50% of all cases of dementia. The diagnosis of Alzheimer's disease can be absolutely confirmed only after a patient has died and the brain tissue is examined: The typical features are neurofibrillary tangles (distorted nerve fibers) and senile plaques (nerve fiber lesions) in the brain tissue. However, early diagnosis can now be made with a high degree of accuracy, based on an extensive series of physical and psychological tests. The prevalence rates of this disorder tend to increase sharply with age. Although less than 2% of the general population under age 60 are afflicted, rates climb to 20% for those over the age of 80. Even higher rates have been reported for those over age 85 (Hooyman & Kiyak, 1991, p. 269).

Unfortunately, there are no completely successful treatments for dementia. However, many victims can benefit from changes in the environment aimed at helping them find their way around. Simplified routes from room to room can be indicated with tape or markers. Written schedules of activities and written directions for cooking, bathing, and taking medications can serve to support the victim's memory. It is also important to maintain a regular schedule and to keep the patient active (Hooyman & Kiyak, 1991). Victims of dementia are generally aware that something is wrong with them, so depression is a real possibility. Everything feasible should be done to help engage the person in recreational activities. Ideally, these kinds of therapeutic steps will help slow the rate of deterioration.

The dementias may have devastating consequences for the victims and their loved ones. It is estimated that some form of dementia, or senility, is involved in over 50% of admissions to nursing homes (Weiler, 1987). For every American who suffers dementia, there are three more close family members who are affected by the emotional, physical, social, and financial burdens of caring for the primary patient. Family caregivers often face the prospect of witnessing the gradual deterioration of a loved one's intellect and personal relationships. To make matters worse, health, social, and personal care services in the community are often unresponsive to the needs of patients and families, and institutional care is often characterized by a lack of thorough assessment, heavy reliance on convenient drug therapies, and little attention to psychological interventions that may help families to cope (Weiler, 1987).

The economic costs of the dementias are huge and steadily increasing. The net annual costs per patient, most from direct medical and social services, are $18,517 in the first year and slightly less in subsequent years (Hay & Ernst, 1987). The total cost of caring for the disease per patient ranges from about $49,000–500,000 depending on the patient's age at the onset of the disease. These figures do not include lost productivity of afflicted people. Unfortunately, there are no means of fully insuring against the economic costs of these disorders. The families of victims must often pay thousands of dollars out of pocket. Insurers and government programs have been reluctant to make chronic diseases eligible for coverage.

Community Programs for the Elderly

Aside from social security, there are an array of programs that help maintain the elderly in the community. Elderly Americans with low income may be eligible for food stamps and low-cost housing. In addition, many communities have senior centers that offer a range of services, including social clubs, counseling, leisure-time skills training, and inexpensive meals. The general thrust of these programs is to reduce the isolation that many elderly persons experience, especially after the loss of a spouse. An attempt is made to connect the person with a lively social group and to enhance the sense of commitment to the community. For those seniors with problems in getting around, some agencies provide visitors to homebound seniors or offer escorts to those who need help getting to the doctor, bank, or market. Meals on Wheels provides hot meals to seniors who can't get out of the house.

These programs provide the link between the person and the community, sometimes delaying or preventing institutionalization. However, not all seniors avail themselves of these programs. Some see themselves as extremely capable, not "old" at all, and resent any implication that they need help.

Nursing Homes

Although the great majority of elderly people are able to live in the community, about 5% are presently living in institutions, including hospitals for the chronically ill, mental hospitals, prisons, and nursing homes (Beaver, 1983). By far the greatest number of institutionalized elderly persons, about 1 million, are living in nursing homes. Nursing homes vary in the amount of skilled nursing care that they provide. Some care for relatively disabled individuals, whereas others cater to those with less severe limitations. It should be made clear that nursing homes are not hospitals in that they do not provide service for the acutely ill. Rather, they maintain those with a chronic condition who do not require active medical intervention. These may be people with mild brain damage or physical handicaps that limit mobility.

What factors determine the need to place an elderly person in a nursing home? Tobin and Lieberman (1976) identified the following: physical deterioration, lack of support services in the community, and the inability of the family to provide the level of care needed by the older person. There is little evidence to support the belief that large numbers of elderly people are "dumped" into institutions. Usually, American families try to keep their older members in the community if at all possible. In fact, many elderly members with mild limitations do live with their relatives. However, sometimes the elderly person deteriorates to the point where round-the-clock care is required. As suggested before, the changing patterns of the family, especially the increase in working mothers, make it increasingly difficult to care for an infirm elderly person at home.

There has been an increase in recent years in the number of elderly living in nursing homes. This may be in part owing to changing family patterns, but it is also related to the increased availability of nursing homes. This increase was spurred by federal funding for this purpose in the 1960s when it became clear that there was a shortage of facilities for elderly Americans. The availability of Medicaid in the mid-1960s also stimulated

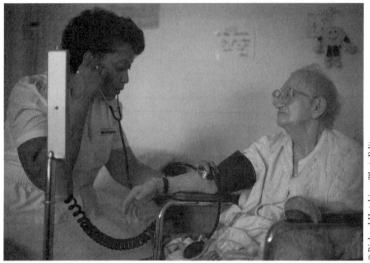

A nurse providing care to a nursing home resident

the growth of nursing homes. Most residents pay for their care through Medicaid. The costs are so high that relatively few individuals could afford to pay out of their own resources.

The idea of putting an older person in a nursing home arouses strongly negative feelings on the part of all concerned. Some of this revulsion is due to horror stories about nursing homes that neglect or even abuse patients in their care. Some critics believe that many nursing homes are chiefly concerned with the profit and convenience of management. It is true that the nursing home industry is composed largely of private, profit-making concerns, many of which are part of larger chains. There is no doubt that abuses do occur and that some nursing homes seem to be places where patients wait to die. The general trend, however, is that most homes provide adequate custodial care along with token recreation and rehabilitation programs. Even in places where physical care is beyond reproach, the patients seem to spend inordinate amounts of time just sitting around. They are often babied to an unnecessary degree because it is faster and easier for staff to feed, bathe, and dress them than to wait for patients to do it themselves. The lack of therapeutic programs is due simply to the fact that it costs money to provide them. Many nursing home administrators are unaware that improvements can be made with no increase in cost by training existing staff to encourage patients to function maximally.

Working with the Elderly

Kahn and Antonucci (1982) reported that older people who are active and in control of life are less likely to be depressed and are more successful in coping with problems. Although encouraging older people to be active is desirable, it must be kept in mind that older people may have some realistic limitations on their activities. These limitations might be due to irreversible physical deterioration or to loss of loved ones. Older people often need help in accepting their realistic losses before they can go on to develop new activities and new social relationships.

These realistic limitations only partly explain why some human services workers do not seek to work with the aged. This trend has been observed in social work, psychology, medicine, and other helping professions. The Group for the Advancement of Psychiatry (1971) studied reasons for negative staff attitudes toward older clients and came up with these: The elderly stimulate the workers' fears of their own old age and also arouse the workers' conflicts with parental figures. Some helpers believe that old people are too rigid to change their ways, and others are concerned about devoting a lot of time and energy to a patient who might soon die.

Those workers who put their fears and prejudices aside find that working with the aged can be very rewarding and enjoyable. The prognosis is not usually as negative as feared, and there are pleasures and delights to be derived from contact with old persons. In our experience, student workers often begin fieldwork training with the aged with distaste but come away from the experience with positive feelings. Often, students are deeply touched by their contacts with elderly shut-ins and nursing home residents. More important is the sense of really making a difference in a client's life.

PEOPLE WITH DISABILITIES

Included in this category are people with a physical or mental impairment that limits one or more major life activities such as seeing, hearing, speaking, or moving. The disabled include not only those who are blind, deaf, physically impaired, mentally retarded, or mentally ill, but also those with hidden impairments such as arthritis, diabetes, heart and back problems, and cancer (Asch, 1984a). Some authors make a distinction between the terms *handicap* and *disability. Disability* refers to a diagnosed condition, such as blindness or deafness, whereas *handicap* refers to the consequences of the disability. The implication is that the consequences can be greater or lesser depending on various factors, such as society's attitude toward the disability in question.

There are no exact estimates of the number of people with disabilities, partly because of the uncertainty about including people with mild impairments. Bowe (1980) estimated that the total number of disabled in the U. S. is about 36 million, or about 15% of the entire population. Estimates of the disabled population of working age vary from 8.5% to a high of 17% (Asch, 1984a). It has also been estimated that 10% of the children under 21 are disabled (Gliedman & Roth, 1980), and that 46% of those 65 and over report a health impairment (DeJong & Lifchez, 1983). By any estimate, the number of people with serious disabilities is awesome.

Mainstreaming People with Disabilities

The history of society's treatment of the disabled can be summed up in two words: segregation and inequality (Burgdorf, 1980). People with disabilities have often been denied their rights and have not been readily admitted into the mainstream of American life. It is only in recent years that this country has witnessed a wave of activism and accomplishment for these people. Senator Lowell Weicker (1984) documented some of the social and legal steps that have been taken to help people with disabilities. For example, federal courts have issued landmark decisions that state that physical handicap is not a legitimate excuse for denying a person's constitutional rights. Congress passed the Rehabilitation Act of 1973, which prohibits discrimination against qualified handicapped people in regard to federal programs, services, and benefits. Perhaps even more important is the Education for All Handicapped Children Act of 1975, which calls for a free, appropriate education for handicapped children in the least restrictive setting. Despite these positive steps, the struggle to admit the handicapped into the mainstream of social and economic life has just begun.

The person with a disability who wishes to participate more fully in community life is often faced with a wide array of barriers. Some of these are physical or architectural. For example, a person in a wheelchair cannot climb stairs or may not be able to open a door without help. A person on crutches may not be able to use certain kinds of public transportation. Governments on all levels have taken steps to eliminate these architectural barriers. To an increasing extent, the handicapped are being provided with ready access to public buildings. Ramps enable the wheelchair-bound person to enter buildings with relative ease. Sidewalks are being modified to allow passage of wheelchairs, and doors and elevators are being changed to permit easier operation by the handicapped. The considerable costs of these alterations have kept them from being instituted in some settings.

Despite legislation calling for the inclusion of handicapped children in regular classrooms, some school systems have not fully complied with the law. In fairness, it must be stated that the special needs of disabled children do impose extra expenses on a school budget that may be tight in the first place. Aside from the costs of physical renovations, there may be additional expenses of providing special equipment and transportation. For example, visually impaired youngsters might need learning materials on tape or in Braille. Turnbill (1982) pointed out that court cases that establish the right of some handicapped children to attend school 12 months a year, of deaf children to obtain interpreters during all aspects of their training, and of handicapped children to obtain psychotherapy at school expense are costly not only in terms of money but also in terms of political capital. What Turnbill implied is that activists who fight for the rights of handicapped children must show some reasonableness in the demands they make. If demands seem excessive to the citizens in a community, there is danger of a loss of public support for services to the handicapped.

The right of individuals with disabilities to equal opportunity in employment is clearly established. However, an important unsolved problem centers around the fact that social security and Medicare regulations tend to discourage disabled people from looking for work. Their support payments and medical benefits often exceed what they could earn after taxes, particularly if their jobs were not steady. If a person with a disability earns more than $3000 a year, he or she risks losing government support. There isn't much incentive to work under these conditions.

Psychological Barriers Against People with Disabilities

Negative societal attitudes are another obstacle that limits the acceptance of people with disabilities into the mainstream. American culture prizes competence, autonomy, and physical attractiveness. Americans are daily subjected to a media barrage of sexy, youthful, healthy people who entertain, sell products, and provide role models. In this atmosphere, it is inevitable that disability, particularly obvious disability, would have a negative impact on a person's sense of self-worth. Some handicapped people have incorporated these negative cultural attitudes and made them the basis for self-defeating behaviors (Fenderson, 1984). In other words, some people with disabilities behave in such a way as to unnecessarily limit their participation in life roles and functions. Some may feel that there is no use in trying because they will not be accepted anyway.

There is abundant evidence, reviewed by Asch (1984a), that people with disabilities arouse strong negative emotions in able-bodied people. In particular, handicapped people arouse anxieties about loss, vulnerability, and weakness. The able-bodied person may be repulsed or embarrassed by anything awkward or unusual about the disabled person. It is not surprising, then, that some nonhandicapped people prefer to avoid social contact with the disabled. When forced to interact, they may behave in unnatural ways. For example, the able-bodied person is apt to go to one of two extremes: either pretending that the disability doesn't exist and doesn't matter or feeling sorry for the disabled person and being excessively helpful. Richardson (1976) and Goffman (1963) have both written about the rarity of meaningful social interaction between those with disabilities and those without. It is difficult for the able-bodied person to get beyond another's disability and relate on the basis of shared human feelings and desires.

◆ CASE STUDY ◆

Personal Reflections of a Blind Psychologist

Adrienne Asch (1984b) contributed the following reflections about her experiences as a person with a disability:

> Once, in a group dynamics program, I had to decide under which sign I would stand for an exercise in difference and group identification—white, straight, young, Jewish, woman, or disabled. Because many of the participants had focused on my disability in their dealings with me during the two-week program, because I had already revealed many aspects of myself, including my similarities with others (whether or not they had been seen), and because no other person with a disability was there to convey what it meant to be disabled, I stood under the disability sign.
>
> An acquaintance overhead me say that it had been hard to decide whether to stand under the sign for disabled or that for woman. "If you hadn't identified as disabled," she said, "I would have said you were denying." With more honesty and irritation than tact, I replied, "It's for people like you that I have to stand under that sign. You and your attitudes have put me there, not my blindness itself."
>
> Were it not a social problem, disability would require no discussion. In a more just world, disability might not be a social, economic, or political problem. It would not be a topic for meetings and discussions, I write out of conscience, anger, and disappointment—that to live with myself, to better myself and others like me, I have no choice but to speak about what could have and should have been a rather inconsequential part of myself and my life. I write in neither pride nor shame, but simply because I have no other choice.
>
> I long for the day when I, other disabled psychologists, and other disabled people will go into any room in any convention, any meeting, or gathering or job in the world and be greeted, evaluated, rejected, or accepted for who we are as total human beings. We need such a forum not because disabled people are so special, separate, or unique but because we must let people know of our desire and right to be part of the world from which we should never have been excluded. (pp. 551–552) ◆

The Rehabilitation Process

The process of helping people with disabilities to achieve the highest possible level of productivity and independent functioning is a team effort in which many different professionals play a role. Clearly, the task of physicians, nurses, and other medical specialists is to help the person with a disability attain maximum use of self. This is one step in the process of rehabilitation. Psychological aspects of the process are of equal importance. In some cases, the person with a disability may become so discouraged as to be unresponsive to counseling. Some patients refuse to accept the seriousness of the disability or any limits that it may impose. The rehabilitation counselor helps the patient to deal with psychological obstacles, oversees the patient's progress, and is usually available to the client from the beginning to the end of the process.

In the rehabilitation agency, the patient's school and job history are reviewed in light of future job or training possibilities. A counseling psychologist may be asked to administer a battery of tests to the patient. The results often provide valuable information about the person's abilities, interests, and aptitudes. Using all of the available information, a plan is developed that involves either training or actual placement on a job. Some large rehabilitation centers are equipped with workshops where patients can try various activities such as carpentry, clerical work, machine operation, and so on. Here, the client is able to gain confidence by achieving success at various tasks. An occupational therapist may be assigned to help the client increase skills and to build up tolerance for sustained work. Even after the client is placed on a job or begins school in the community, follow-up interviews are arranged to resolve any problems that come up in the placement.

The disabled are often perceived by others in a somewhat distorted way. The disability tends to generalize in the minds of others to the whole person—that is, to induce others to see the handicapped as more limited than they really are. In counseling, the person with a disability is helped to come to grips with these unrealistic perceptions and the effect of these perceptions on self-image. The effective counselor recognizes that the disabled are more like the able-bodied than otherwise and works with their real strengths and assets.

PERSONS WITH MENTAL ILLNESS

Physical illness is easier to define than mental illness because it involves bodily disorders that can be observed and measured in precise ways. Mental illness, on the other hand, involves feeling states, perceptions, and behaviors that sometimes depart only slightly from the normal range. To make matters worse, *mental illness* is sort of a catchall term that includes everything from temporary emotional upsets to long-lasting psychological breakdowns. An account of the heated controversies about the nature of mental illness will be reserved for Chapter 4. For the present, the mentally ill will be regarded as people with emotional and psychological problems who seek help from psychiatric and mental-health facilities.

Prevalance of Mental Illness

In any given year, about 30% of the adults and 17% of the children and adolescents in the United States display serious emotional disturbances and are in need of treatment. More specifically, it is estimated that out of every 100 adults:

13 have a significant anxiety disorder

6 suffer from a serious depression

5 display a personality disorder involving maladaptive tendencies that cause distress or impaired functioning

1 is schizophrenic, that is, shows disorganized thinking and is out of touch with reality

1 suffers from the brain disorder of Alzheimer's disease

10 abuse drugs or alcohol

These data strongly suggest that psychological and behavioral disorders are a major problem in our society (Comer, 1995; Regier et al., 1993). Nationwide surveys of adults showed that between 16–22 million people in this country receive therapy for psychological problems in the course of a year (Narrow, Regier, Rae, Manderscheid, & Locke, 1993; Regier et al., 1993). This represents about 12% of the entire adult population. Most of those who seek psychotherapy on an outpatient basis suffer from anxiety or depression. One recent trend is that people with serious disorders such as schizophrenia are increasingly seeking psychotherapy as are those with substance abuse disorders. Another recent trend is that therapy is no longer a privilege of the wealthy. Due in part to the expansion of medical insurance coverage, people at all economic levels, including minorities, are seeking treatment (Comer, 1995). The current cost of outpatient psychotherapy ranges from $50–160 per session (Jaegerman, 1993). In Chapter 4, we review the various theoretical models that guide treatment for psychological disorders.

◆ CASE STUDY ◆

The Crisis of Mental Illness

Joan Houghton is a young woman who provided the world with a moving account of her mental illness. She recalled that mental illness, in the form of a psychotic episode, struck her with the force of a nuclear explosion.

> All that I had known and enjoyed previously was suddenly transformed like some strange reverse process of nature, from a butterfly's beauty into a pupa's cocoon. There was a binding, confining quality to my life, in part chosen, in part imposed. Repeated rejections, the awkwardness of others around me, and my own discomfort and self-consciousness propelled me into solitary confinement. (Houghton, 1980, p. 8)

Joan remembered sitting with her mother in the waiting room of a mental hospital while her father investigated admission procedures. A young man was seated nearby. Perspiration dripped across his brow and down his cheeks. Joan took a tissue from her purse and gently wiped the moisture from his face. She tried to reassure him that everything would be fine. Presently, Joan was ushered into a small room where she met a social worker and a psychiatrist. After a brief conversation, they presented her with a piece of paper and instructed her to sign. She signed "Saint Joan," without realizing that she had thereby admitted herself to a mental hospital. "My first psychotic episode appeared as a private mental exorcism, ending with the honor of sainthood and the gifts of hope and faith" (Houghton, 1982, p. 547–552).

Joan was hospitalized for 5 weeks. Her recovery involved a struggle against her own body, which seemed to be drained of energy, and against a society that seemed to reject her. "It seemed that my greatest needs—to be wanted, needed, valued—were the very needs which others could not fulfill" (Houghton, 1980, p. 8).

Joan eventually recovered and was able to hold a job at the National Institute of Mental Health. An articulate young woman, she wrote eloquent accounts of her struggle with mental illness. It appeared that important unmet needs played a major role in precipitating her breakdown. ◆

Trends in Mental-Health Care

There have been dramatic changes in recent decades in *where* Americans are treated for serious mental illness. These changes center around a basic reform in psychiatric care started in the 1950s. The basic idea is to get mental patients out of institutions and to treat them in community-based facilities. In 1955, there were 560,000 patients in state and county mental hospitals. The numbers living in mental hospitals had steadily declined to 160,000 in 1978 (Coleman, Butcher, & Carson, 1984). This decline in occupancy reflects increasing awareness among mental health experts that long-term hospitalization is not the best choice of treatment for many patients. For one thing, lengthy hospitalization tends to create a dependence on the institution that hampers the patient's reentry into the community. Another contributory factor has been the introduction of powerful tranquilizing medications. These new drugs help suppress the disturbed and agitated behaviors of some patients, thereby making it possible to treat them on an outpatient basis.

Patients admitted to mental hospitals do not stay nearly as long on the average as in the decades prior to the 1950s. However, it soon became obvious that many briefly treated patients are not able to live in the community without recurring episodes of acute disturbance. Their symptoms flare up periodically, and they have to be readmitted to the hospital. It is not unusual for some mental patients to have 10, 15, or even 20 brief stays at mental hospitals. Critics began to talk about the "revolving door" effect. They also charged that many mental patients were simply being "dumped" into communities that often had not made adequate provisions for their aftercare.

It might be useful at this point to take a closer look at the two parts of the intended reform of mental-health care: The first is deinstitutionalization, which means simply getting patients out of long-stay hospitals; and the second is community-based treatment.

Deinstitutionalizing Mental Patients.   The 1960s were years of rapid social change. Old ways of doing things were challenged in every area of life,
including the mental-health field. Social activists charged that large numbers of mental patients were being detained, often against their will, in
huge, outmoded psychiatric hospitals. They further alleged that many of
these patients were simply being warehoused in custodial wards and not
getting much in the way of treatment. Very often, patients were not even
asked how they felt about being in the hospital. There was a great deal of
merit to these criticisms, especially in regard to the state hospitals. Many of
these were located far from the communities they served, making it difficult to reconnect patients with their former community.

Meanwhile, civil rights attorneys were active in championing the rights
of mental patients. They argued that mental patients were entitled to due
process of law before being committed against their will. If hospitalized,
the patients were to receive treatment in the least restrictive environment.
These legal efforts finally culminated in the landmark Supreme Court decision *O'Connor* v. *Donaldson,* which held that it is unconstitutional to con-
fine a nondangerous person in a mental hospital against his or her will
unless adequate treatment is provided.

Community Care for Mental Patients.   Of course, it was not enough simply to condemn the old approach to mental illness. In response to the pressures of social reformers, mental-health experts began to implement a
community-based approach to the problem that was designed to achieve
certain important goals. One was to prevent mental disability whenever
possible by fostering constructive social change. Another was to seek out
people in need of help and treat them in the community. Still another goal
was to facilitate the reentry of institutionalized people into the community.

The Community Mental Health Centers Act of 1963 was to provide the
means of achieving these and other goals. This federal legislation provided
for the establishment of a network of mental-health centers throughout the
nation. Each center was to provide an array of services to the community.
Five basic services were to be offered:

1. *Inpatient care.* Each community mental-health center was to have a
   hospital for seriously disordered mental patients. The plan was that
   patients would be treated as quickly as possible and returned to the
   community. Only patients who did not respond to treatment would
   be referred to long-stay institutions.
2. *Outpatient care.* The center was to provide psychological services
   through an outpatient clinic.
3. *Partial hospitalization.* A facility was to be provided to treat patients
   during the day but allow them to return home evenings and week-
   ends. The intent was to prevent patients from becoming dependent
   on the treatment facility as they might do if confined on a 24-hour
   basis.

4. *Emergency care.* The center was to maintain a 24-hour crisis center to deal with psychiatric emergencies.
5. *Consultation, education, and information.* The center was to offer consultation, education, and information to others vitally concerned with mental-health issues such as teachers, police, city officials, and probation officers. The idea was to facilitate social changes that might help prevent emotional disorders.

The act was subsequently amended to add several other desirable goals in addition to these mandated programs. These included rehabilitation in the form of vocational and physical training for patients as well as research and evaluation. For example, the center was to do research to evaluate its own effectiveness to explore the causes of psychological disorder.

The plan was a good one, but the community mental health centers have not been able to fully attain their goals. The original plan called for the establishment of 2000 centers, each serving a specific catchment or health service area. Only about 600 centers are currently in full operation, which means that only about 30% of the population in need is being served.

Current Problems in Mental-Health Care

Bassuk and Gerson (1978) wondered how the well-intentioned reform of deinstitutionalization could have created so many problems. These authors asserted that the discharged mental patient was to be supported by a full spectrum of aftercare services but that communities rarely provided such services. The living arrangements were often very poor. Many patients drifted to substandard inner-city housing that was unsafe, dirty, and over-crowded. There was a lack of vocational training, job referrals, transportation, and recreational facilities. Aftercare agencies complained that they were not given sufficient funds to provide services needed by expatients.

By the mid-1980s, it was generally accepted by mental-health professionals that deinstitutionalization had been a massive failure (Lyons, 1984). In retrospect, policymakers place the blame on three major factors. One was a tendency to view state mental hospitals as prisons that violated the civil rights of mental patients. As long ago as 1975, one of us wrote an article entitled "Civil Rights for Mental Patients: The Road to Neglect?" that argued

> while some of the early actions of the civil rights movement helped to publicize and correct long-standing abuses, the movement increasingly seems to be in pursuit of goals that are ultimately detrimental to patient welfare. . . . To an excessive degree, civil libertarians are operating under the influence of an analogy that equates mental patients with persecuted minority groups. (Schmolling, 1975, p. 168)

The author suggested that this analogy lends itself to rescue fantasies. Patients were, in fact, "rescued" and discharged from hospitals on a wholesale basis. Unfortunately, the extent of their social disability was not taken into account.

The second factor that led to the ultimate failure of this policy was the overselling of tranquilizing medicine. Scientific researchers had given us antibiotics and effective vaccines against certain diseases. It did not seem too much to expect that researchers would give us a pill that would revolutionize the treatment of the mentally ill. Tranquilizers were sold (by the carload) as a panacea for mental illness. Regretfully, the drugged patients did not do as well in the community as was hoped. Although drugs may help a patient return to the community, they do not meet the same needs as friends, family, a job, and continued support services.

The third factor was that deinstitutionalization was supported as a way to reduce the enormous costs of caring for patients on a round-the-clock basis. Ironically, the anticipated savings did not occur. The state hospitals tended to spend more and more as they cared for fewer and fewer patients. Johnson (1990, p. 103) presented data showing that the annual cost per mental patient nearly quadrupled between 1969 and 1977 and that some hospital systems showed large increases in overall costs as the inpatient population shriveled. One reason for this is that the political power of the state employee unions enabled them to maintain high levels of staffing even though the patients were disappearing from the wards. Politicians went along with this because they anticipated the support of these employees at election time.

What Services Are Needed?

Based on the commonsense ideas advanced by Johnson (1990), here is a partial list of the needs of mental patients living in the community.

♦ *Housing.* The mentally ill need a place to live where their sometimes eccentric behavior will be tolerated. In other words, they need a safe haven where they will not be subject to hostile criticism by intolerant persons.

♦ *Outreach.* Mental patients often lack a clear sense of time and place and are likely to miss their appointments. It is very often useful for staff members to go visit patients in their residences and engage them in their own environment.

♦ *Hospitalization readmission.* The chronic mental patient requires occasional readmission to the mental hospital. Once patients become openly bizarre, delusional, or dangerous to themselves and others, it should be possible to readmit them without a lot of bureaucratic red tape. The readmission need not be viewed as a failure of the aftercare program because these disorders are defined, in part, by a need for occasional removal to a safe inpatient setting. Sometimes, staff members delay too long in arranging the hospitalization because of their own sense of personal failure.

♦ *Skills of living.* The chronic mental patient often needs help with the skills of daily living and interpersonal relations. Such tasks as personal hygiene, grooming, shopping, budgeting, traveling, and everyday conversation need to be practiced. As Johnson (1990) suggested, many therapists do not find this kind of educational activity very interesting and would prefer a deeper, more verbal kind of therapy. Again, the helper must decide if the patient's needs are best served with deep analysis or with instruction in the skills of daily life.

The New Chronic Patient. Since the early 1970s when the policy to deinstitutionalize became dominant, the trend has been to provide acute hospital care for a few weeks to people with psychotic disorders and outpatient clinic treatment following discharge. The integration between hospital and clinic has often been inadequate. A number of younger Americans have become acutely, then chronically, ill during this era of limited care. They have gone from their 20s to their 30s while living in the community. Pepper (1987) described them like this:

> They do not carry shopping bags or wear three sweaters in the summertime. Most dress like their age-mates, aspire to hold a job, be in love, have children, take vacations, and in every other way fulfill the American dream. . . . But living in the community also offers them the opportunity to drink alcohol, smoke pot, do cocaine, heroin, LSD, PCP—just like everybody else. Unfortunately, most of them respond to even small doses of drugs with psychosis, depression, or a worsening of their personality disorders. Most regrettably, public policy and practice in the last decade have further tended to separate drug and alcohol treatment services from mental health treatment. It is a rare community today that offers integrated treatment for such individuals, who now constitute a majority of the younger seriously disturbed population. (p. 454)*

Is Reinstitutionalization the Answer? A backlash has resulted from the failure of deinstitutionalization to solve the problems of the mentally disabled. Some professionals have called for a halt to deinstitutionalization and a return to large-scale institutions. They point out that institutionalization is more humane than homelessness, hunger, and victimization. Plum (1987) argued that this is a shortsighted "solution" to the problem and that it would be preferable to develop better support systems in the community. She also suggested that we explore combinations of institutionalization and noninstitutional forms of mental-health services. Further discussion of these issues is presented in later chapters.

*From "A Public Policy for the Long-Term Mentally Ill: A Positive Alternative to Reinstitutionalization," by B. Pepper, *American Journal of Orthopsychiatry*, July, 1987, p. 454. Copyright © 1987 the American Orthopsychiatric Association, Inc. Reproduced by permission.

SUBSTANCE ABUSERS

The term *substance abusers* refers to people who misuse certain substances for the purpose of altering mood or psychological state. The substances used for this purpose range from foods like sugar and carbohydrates to alcohol and hard drugs such as heroin, amphetamines, and barbiturates. Virtually the entire adult population uses some of these substances at one time or another. What is the distinction between using and abusing a substance?

One important criterion is that the abuser employs the substance to avoid facing up to problems. When under stress, he or she "turns on" to the stuff in question in order to feel better without doing anything about the troublesome situation. The abuser runs the risk of becoming addicted; this means that he or she may become both psychologically and physiologically dependent on the substance. Certain drugs, including alcohol, alter body chemistry if taken to excess. Once addicted, the individual must continue to use the substance if unpleasant withdrawal symptoms are to be avoided. It is not practical to review all possible addictions in this section. Attention focuses on two addictions that have received the most attention from human services: alcoholism and heroin abuse. In addition, cocaine abuse is given extended coverage because it has become so prevalent in our society.

Alcoholics

Some experts believe that alcoholism is the number one public health problem in the United States today. The number of people who are psychologically dependent on alcohol has been estimated at anywhere from 8 to 20 million. The lack of precision in the count is due to difficulty in distinguishing between heavy drinkers and alcoholics, as well as the fact that many people abuse alcohol in secret. The majority of known alcoholics are adult men, but the number of adult women who drink to excess has increased in recent years. There is also significant alcohol abuse among teenagers and even among preteens.

Why are so many Americans dependent on alcohol? One important property of alcohol is that it helps the drinker to feel relaxed and uninhibited. Continued use, however, reduces motor coordination and causes a number of deficiencies such as blurred vision, thick speech, and the suspension of normal judgment. This combination of properties explains why the majority of serious auto accidents are alcohol related. Most individuals are able to use alcohol in moderation to feel at ease in social situations. However, the alcoholic comes to rely on alcohol to help deal with stressful and difficult situations. At some point on the path to addiction, the alcoholic becomes unable to face difficulties without using alcohol as a crutch. Prolonged excessive drinking can lead to a variety of health problems, including serious damage to the brain or liver. On a social level, the alcoholic may jeopardize both employment and family life.

Treatment for the alcoholic has changed dramatically in this century. Throughout most of our history, alcoholism was seen as a kind of moral weakness. Drunks were either ignored or treated as criminals. During the first half of this century, it was common practice to jail alcoholics, particularly those of low social status. It became obvious that this punishment had no long-range effect on the alcoholic, who never seemed to learn the "lesson."

Alcoholics Anonymous (AA), founded in 1934, called for an end to punitive, moralistic approaches to the problem. Instead, alcoholism was to be regarded as an illness and treated as such. AA bases its program for helping alcoholics on group meetings during which members confess their dependence on alcohol. One basic tenet of AA is that the alcoholic is not to think of himself or herself as cured at any time. The alcoholic is simply trying to live one day at a time without alcohol. At the same time, the alcoholic gains strength from meeting people who are controlling their desire for alcohol. Added to this is the spiritual emphasis that is one of the pillars of the AA approach. The alcoholic calls upon a higher power to help control the problem. It should be stressed that the organization was founded by and is run by alcoholics. As such, it is a self-help group and a model for similar groups such as Narcotics Anonymous and Cocaine Anonymous established by drug addicts. AA is certainly the most popular of the self-help groups: It has more than 2 million members in 89,000 groups across the United States and nearly 100 countries (Comer, 1995).

Al-Anon is a related self-help group that provides support for people who live with alcoholics. Members share their experiences and learn how to cope with the effects of drinking on their lives. They may also learn how to stop reinforcing the drinking and related behavior of loved ones (Comer, 1995).

For various reasons, discussed by Comer (1995, p. 477), it is difficult to determine the success of self-help groups. Some keep no records of members who drop out of the program. Others may be distrustful of professional researchers and don't cooperate with them, although this attitude is beginning to change. Most of the evidence of success comes from testimonials of many thousands who believe they have been helped.

Psychotherapy by itself has not proved to be of great value in treating alcoholics, nor have strictly medical approaches been of lasting value. For many years, hospitals—both general and psychiatric—were reluctant to undertake treatment of alcoholics. It seemed futile merely to provide the alcoholic with a place to "dry out" when the benefits usually were temporary. Most mental health professionals now believe that treatment must be multifaceted. The first step is primarily medical because it involves detoxification—that is, removing the toxic substances from the body and restoring the body chemistry to normal. Medication is used to control withdrawal symptoms. This may be followed by family and occupational counseling aimed at helping the patient to function better in the community without resorting to alcohol. Follow-up counseling in the community might subsequently be coupled with continued membership in AA. Gradually, hospitals are beginning to establish special units for the treatment of alcoholism along the lines just suggested. Concurrently, there has been a trend to train human services workers in counseling alcoholics.

Heroin Addicts

It is even more difficult to determine the number of heroin addicts than the number of alcoholics in the country because of the illegal nature of heroin use. Understandably, addicts are not eager to stand up and be counted. During the 1960s, there was such a great increase in heroin use that the media began talking about the "heroin epidemic" (Bazell, 1973). Recent surveys show that heroin use continues at a high rate (Carson, Butcher, & Coleman, 1988). Although it is difficult to gather precise data, the considered opinion among experts is that there are more than a million heroin addicts in the United States (Davison & Neale, 1996).

Whereas alcoholics are widely distributed throughout the range of social classes, heroin addicts tend to be concentrated in the lower socioeconomic classes, particularly among minority group members. Initially, narcotics addiction was seen primarily as a problem of the inner cities. However, during the last two decades, there has been a spread of heroin addiction to white suburban areas as well as to small towns and cities across America. Regardless of area, heroin addiction is most common in people in their late teens to early 20s. One other group with a high rate of addiction are physicians who have easy access to pure morphine and other narcotics; they typically become involved in drugs at a later age than street addicts and also seem better able to function on the job than street addicts.

A number of factors account for the appeal of narcotics, a class of drugs derived from opium, including heroin, morphine, and codeine. The immediate effect is a sense of euphoria, followed by a state of deep relaxation and contentment. This blissful state, which may last 4 to 6 hours, is followed by the unpleasant return to reality called "coming down." Frequent use of the drug for a month or so is sufficient to addict most people. Addiction is both physiological and psychological in nature. Once addicted, the user feels physically ill if he or she cannot get the drug. Unfortunately, larger and larger doses are needed to achieve the same effect. Drug addiction is then likely to become a way of life, with much time spent getting the money to feed the habit. The addict often turns to illegal means of raising the money, but reports of addicts turning to violence are greatly exaggerated. They are more likely to get involved in theft, burglary, and shoplifting because the income is more reliable. Another major source of income is selling drugs to others, thus perpetuating the problem. Female addicts often turn to prostitution to get money (Rorvik, 1979).

Aside from imprisonment, treatment for narcotics addicts has taken three basic forms: hospitalization, methadone maintenance programs, and self-help groups. Until the 1960s, hospitalization under supervision was usually the only practical alternative. As might be expected, this approach is most successful in helping the addict to "detox"—that is, to overcome the ill effects of withdrawal from heroin. However, the relapse rate is very high once addicts leave the hospital.

Methadone maintenance is probably the most frequently used approach at this time. Methadone is a synthetic narcotic chemically similar to morphine that is itself highly addictive. The presumed usefulness of this drug is derived from its capacity to satisfy or reduce the craving for heroin. Methadone does not produce the stupor associated with heroin, nor does it require ever-increasing doses to be effective. It frees the addict of the necessity of raising money for heroin and opens the door to normal job and social routines. Unfortunately, most addicts cannot be tapered off to the point where they can go drug-free. In effect, they substitute one addiction for another, but from society's point of view an addiction to methadone is preferable to an addiction to heroin because it decriminalizes the addiction.

The third major approach is based on intense group pressure brought to bear on addicts by their peers—reformed addicts. Synanon is perhaps the best known of these self-help groups for addicts. Founded in the 1960s, it grew to the point where it was able to maintain several residences for addicts in a number of cities. Similar groups began to mushroom in the late 1960s and early 1970s. The general approach is drug-free and stresses a tough-minded attitude toward the addict, who is seen as a dependent child with few redeeming qualities. In some programs, the group assault appears designed to break down the defenses of the addict so completely that new behaviors become a necessity. Drug addicts point out that middle-class professionals are too soft to work effectively with addicts. Whereas this may or may not be true, there is little solid evidence that these self-help groups have found the formula for success. One unsolved problem of such programs is the high dropout rate; the most difficult cases often simply leave the group.

Treatment with Drug Antagonists.   This refers to using drugs to change the effects of an addictive drug. The best known of these is Disulfiram, usually known by its trade name of Antabuse. It is used to treat chronic alcoholic patients who need special help to remain sober. Taken by itself the drug has few negative effects, but if the patient drinks alcohol after taking Antabuse, he or she will experience nausea, vomiting, and other ill effects. The idea is that persons on Antabuse will avoid alcohol knowing the consequences. The obvious disadvantage of this treatment is that patients can forget to take the drug if they plan to resume drinking.

A relatively new type of treatment is based on the use of narcotic antagonists such as naloxone, cyclazocine, and naltrexone. These drugs do not have an aversive effect but deprive the narcotic addict of the euphoria usually produced by opiates such as heroin. Without the high, there would seem to be little point in continuing the use of the narcotic. It has been reported that these drugs may also block the high that alcohol creates. Comer (1995) cited some studies that suggest the possibility of promising results with drugs of this type. However, these drugs may cause negative side effects in some persons, including severe withdrawal reactions (Goldstein, 1994).

Cocaine Abusers

Although there was a reduction in the number of cocaine users during the 1980s, there were still 1.6 million users in 1990 (Davison & Neale, 1996). Once a fashionable drug among affluent people, it is now widely used by young people in the inner cities (Weiss & Mirin, 1987). One reason for the spread of cocaine is that the supply has increased, resulting in lower prices.

Cocaine, a derivative of the coca plant, is sometimes called coke, snow, blow, toot, flake, nose candy, and other names. It is usually snorted into the nasal passages where it is readily absorbed. Some users melt the impurities, leaving pure cocaine or freebase, which is smoked for an intense high. Intravenous injection is the most hazardous way of administering cocaine; not only are the chances of addiction increased, but there also is an additional danger that comes from nonsterile needles.

In 1986, a new form of cocaine called crack became prevalent; it is a pea-sized crystallized form of the drug that is sold in small units for a relatively low price. Crack produces an intense high very quickly. It is this factor plus its low price that accounts for its attractiveness to teenagers and people with limited income.

Cocaine increases alertness and brings about a heightened sense of well-being verging on euphoria. In heavy users, this cocaine high is followed by a rapid descent into pain, anxiety, and depression, which in turn compels the user to find and use more. Some end up using cocaine almost continuously until the supply is exhausted. This pattern, called a "run," may go on for a number of days. Repetitive use is a clear sign of addiction or physical dependence on the drug.

Large doses of cocaine, or prolonged use, may produce a state of paranoia. Heavy users may feel under threat of attack and may arm themselves accordingly. In some people, cocaine abuse may lead to hallucinations of touch, taste, and smell. One strange consequence of abuse is cocaine psychosis—the belief that bugs or snakes are crawling under the skin. Gallagher (1987) noted that one Hollywood actress required plastic surgery after she clawed her face open to kill imaginary bugs.

There are as yet no widely accepted, specific treatments for cocaine abuse. Most treatment of cocaine abuse takes place in general drug and alcohol treatment programs that use the same methods in treating cocaine addicts as other substance abusers. The percentage of cocaine-related admissions to drug abuse facilities rose from 1.2% in 1976 to 9% in 1983 (Weiss & Mirin, 1987). It should be kept in mind that the classification of abusers into discrete categories (i.e., alcoholic, cocaine addict, etc.) may sometimes be misleading, because many individuals abuse more than one substance.

Cocaine Anonymous is a self-help group that began as an adjunct to Alcoholics Anonymous and now has about a thousand chapters nationwide. Like AA, it helps the user to achieve sobriety on a day-to-day basis. Coke-anon (or Cocanon) is a companion organization for relatives of the addict.

Some clinicians believe that cocaine abusers do not become motivated to stop their drug use until they "hit bottom" and lose everything. However, other experts in the field believe that this scenario can be avoided by means of a confrontation of the abuser by family and/or employer (Weiss & Mirin, 1987). At an intervention meeting, family members and friends may gather together with the abuser and a professional, typically a physician, psychologist, or social worker experienced in such work. They present the abuser with clear documentation of the results of the abuse, treatment options, and a statement of the family's response if he or she refuses treatment or continues the abuse. These meetings are emotionally charged and may cause the abuser to defend against what seems like a general attack. But when it goes well, the impact may be great enough to convince the addict to enter treatment immediately. If the user continues to deny the seriousness of the habit, the family may resolve to stop *enabling* the addiction by covering it up, taking over the responsibilities of the addict, supporting the addict, and so on. The family may go so far as to refuse to live in the same house with the addict. Instead, they focus on getting their own lives together.

Conflicting Approaches to the Drug Problem

What to do about drug addicts has been the subject of intense controversies during recent years. At least three different approaches can be identified, each of which has strong supporters. These are (a) legalization or decriminalization of drugs, (b) law enforcement, and (c) treatment for addicts.

Some Americans are so frustrated by the failure of our attempts to control narcotic abuse that they are ready to raise the white flag: Legalize narcotics, they say, and be done with it (Kupfer, 1988). They are willing to risk greater drug use in order to reduce the crime associated with illegal drug traffic. The underlying idea is to take the profit out of the drug business. Law enforcement efforts tend to drive up the prices of illegal substances, making the business more profitable. If we eliminate the laws against the possession, sale, and use of drugs, according to this view, we will reduce the violence, corruption, and medical problems associated with their use. Lazare (1990) argued that instead of spending vast sums for police, prosecutors, judges, prison guards, and so on, we should tax the sale of previously forbidden drugs and use the money for drug treatment.

A case against legalization was made by Schmolling (1993) who reviewed evidence showing that unregulated access to narcotics has led to disastrous results in the past. In fact, the Harrison Act of 1914, which outlawed self-administration of narcotics, was enacted because of the realization that cocaine and opiate addiction was causing crime and family instability (Musto, 1987). There is also reason to believe that legalization of narcotics would result in huge increases in the number of addicts (Wilson, 1990). Cocaine, for example, is intensely addictive and may produce a state in which other considerations such as job, family, children, sleep, food, and even sex go out the window. A policy of making cocaine freely available would undoubtedly increase the number of crack babies. Wilson (1990) stated that the only way to be certain of the effect of easy availability of cocaine would be to try it and see; he quickly added that this is one social experiment we dare not make because the consequences would be devastating.

The second approach, law enforcement, is the chief weapon that the government employs in the war on drugs. This approach is based on a moral (or punitive) model which holds that individuals must be held responsible for violating the law. In this view, violators are capable of choice and must face the consequences if they break the law. During the 1980s, adherents of this model argued that we were losing the drug war because we were too soft on users and dealers. This lead to more arrests, mandatory (and sometimes severe) sentences for dealers, and increased surveillance and interception of drugs smuggled into the country. The increased use of legal sanctions during the 1980s apparently had the effect of reducing drug use among casual users but had little effect on frequent users, defined as those who use drugs at least once a week (The White House, 1989). Other consequences of the "get tough" approach are overcrowded court dockets, increased expenses associated with enforcement efforts, and as we document in the next section, a huge increase in the prison population.

The third approach, treatment, is based on the medical model to be described in detail in Chapter 4. The general idea is that addicts are suffering from an illness and should be treated rather than punished. In this view, abusers are victims of compulsive, self-destructive cravings and are in need of medical and psychological treatments. Although governments spend more on law enforcement than on treatment, drug treatment is nevertheless a major industry in this country. There are 5000 drug agencies nationwide, including the following:

 detoxification units that have the short-range goal of ending physical dependence on drugs
 inpatient units that offer de-tox with a beginning of counseling to be continued on an outpatient basis
 outpatient clinics providing support and therapy
 methadone units designed to maintain heroin addicts in the community
 residential, drug-free, therapeutic communities that help the addict develop a new lifestyle

Private nonprofit facilities enroll about 60% of those in treatment; state and local governments enroll about 25%. Profit-making programs treat 11%, and a small number are in federal facilities (The White House, 1989).

Interactions Between Legal and Therapeutic Approaches

In debates about drug policies, conservatives tend to argue in favor of intensified law enforcement, whereas liberals are more inclined to favor treatment approaches. The two approaches are often presented as though they are opposed to one another. In reality, there is an intimate connection between the two that is often overlooked. Legal pressures account for 40–70% of all referrals to community alcohol and drug treatment programs (Schottenfeld, 1989). Agency statistics probably do not reflect the true magnitude of coerced referrals. Many seemingly self-referred individuals are responding to outside pressures but were not referred directly by the courts. Some are pressured by child welfare agencies, and others by a spouse or employer. Every intake worker at drug treatment agencies has listened to earnest pleas for treatment followed by a request beginning with the words, "By the way, I could use a letter showing I'm in treatment." The letter would be brought to court, to probation offices, or to an employer or a welfare agency providing benefits. The proportion of genuinely voluntary referrals to drug treatment agencies is probably quite low. Despite abundant evidence to the contrary, many heavy users believe they can "handle" their drugs of choice and perceive themselves to be recreational users rather than addicts. If it weren't for law enforcement and other forms of coercion, there would be little spontaneous demand for treatment aimed at a drug-free lifestyle.

Schmolling (1993) argued in favor of a more cooperative, rather than competitive, relationship between law enforcement and treatment agencies. Some existing programs involve what might be called a therapeutic use of law enforcement. The basic idea is to give addicts a clear choice; that is, personal freedom is made contingent on drug-free, responsible behavior. One model based on this concept is California's Civil Addict Program (CAP). As described by Anglin (1988), an addict convicted of property crimes or drug dealing could be committed to the program. The two-phase program consisted of an incarceration period followed by monitored release in the community. A crucial feature of the program was that addicts could be reincarcerated for infractions including drug use as determined by urine testing. The message of this program was clear: If you want your freedom, stay clean. Treatments that enhance social and vocational competence help the addict move toward a more productive way of life. Relatively few addicts choose conventional criminal processing over participating in this sort of program.

CRIMINALS

The United States has a relatively high rate of criminal activity compared to other affluent nations. Our homicide rate leads the industrialized world due, in part, to the drug problem and ready availability of handguns. How do we know how much criminal activity is taking place? There are two main sources of information: police reports and victim surveys. The FBI's Uniform Crime Reports, issued annually, are based on crime reports contributed by more than 16,000 law enforcement agencies. These reports tell us what crimes have actually been reported by citizens to the police. A victim survey is quite different because it is derived from a household poll in which people are asked whether they have been a victim of a crime during a given time period. The best known of these is the National Crime Survey, which is a poll of about 160,000 people in 84,000 households. This survey has been issued annually since its inception in 1973. The victim surveys reveal much higher rates of crime than do the police reports. The reason is obvious: Many crime victims do not file a complaint with the police. Why not? It may be that the perpetrator is a close friend or family member. Other victims do not want the nature of the crime to be made public, and still others may feel that "nothing will be done about it anyway, so why bother?" There is also the possibility of reprisals against the person bringing charges.

The data on crime must be viewed against the background of a major shift in the political environment that began in the 1980s, bringing with it changing policies related to crime and imprisonment. The previous emphasis on rehabilitation gave way to a more punitive approach. The public wanted more effective crime control and rewarded politicians who promised to get tough on criminals. Another reason for the change in policy was that a series of experimental studies raised serious doubts about the effectiveness of rehabilitation (Blumstein, 1995, p. 395). The dominant finding was that no particular approach consistently works in reducing postrelease criminal behavior. It appeared that the characteristics of offenders and the environment to which they return have more influence on recidivism than any special program. The major impact of the new policies was a huge increase in prison population. From 1980 to 1991, the average annual increase in the jail and prison population was an incredible 8.5% (Freeman, 1995). There are now about 1 million prisoners in state and federal institutions; this does not include another 445,000 in local jails (Holmes, 1994). The United States is second in the world, behind Russia, in rate of incarceration and has a rate 4 times that of Canada and 14 times that of Japan. Our high rates are due largely to violent crimes as opposed to property crimes. According to Holmes (1994), surveys of state prisoners have found that 94% had previous convictions or are in prison for violent crime; the data showed that when they were free they committed violent and repeated crimes. The public is concerned about the recycling of these violent offenders back into the community.

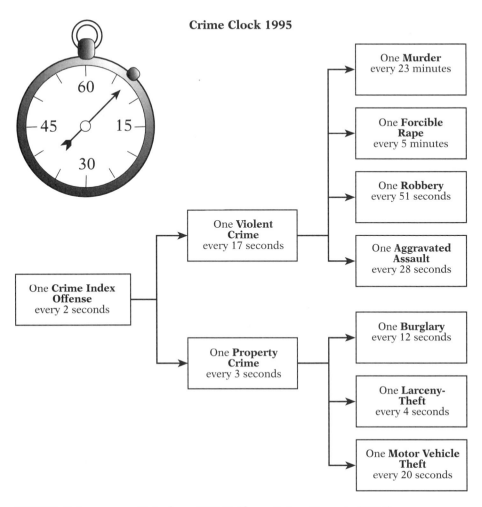

Crime Clock 1995

One **Murder** every 23 minutes

One **Forcible Rape** every 5 minutes

One **Robbery** every 51 seconds

One **Aggravated Assault** every 28 seconds

One **Violent Crime** every 17 seconds

One **Crime Index Offense** every 2 seconds

One **Property Crime** every 3 seconds

One **Burglary** every 12 seconds

One **Larceny-Theft** every 4 seconds

One **Motor Vehicle Theft** every 20 seconds

FIGURE 2–1   SOURCE: Data from FBI Uniform Crime Reports (1996)

Considering that an increasing number of people with criminal tendencies were in prison, it seems logical to expect the crime rate to go down. Actually, the Uniform Crime Reports showed a stabilization in reported crime rates but not a significant decline. An analysis of the data by Freeman (1995, p. 175) resulted in the chilling conclusion that the "propensity for crime among noninstitutionalized men increased immensely during the 1980s." In other words, the fact that massive incarceration did not reduce crime rates means that there are more criminals out there. In fact, the number of men "under supervision of the criminal justice system" was 6.6% of the entire male work force (Freeman, 1995, p. 172). To understand some of the causes of this increased propensity to crime in the United States, it would help to look at the youngsters—the juveniles—who are just beginning their criminal careers. Most criminal careers begin in the juvenile years.

Juvenile Offenders

The general public does not fully realize that juveniles, defined by most states as persons younger than 18, commit a large percentage of serious crimes. During the mid-1980s, persons under 18 accounted for about one out of every three arrests for robbery, about half of all arrests for property crimes, and about one of six arrests for rape. Each year, more than a million juveniles are arrested by the police in the United States (Inciardi, 1987). This alarmingly high rate of criminal activity among youngsters is by no means confined to inner cities. Similarly high rates have been reported for youngsters from suburban and rural areas (National Institute of Mental Health, 1974).

One repeated finding of studies both here and abroad is that 6% of the boys of a given age will commit half or more of all serious crimes in that age group. According to Wilson (1995), here are some of the characteristics of these young chronic offenders:

- They tend to have criminal parents.
- They tend to be low in verbal IQ and do poorly in school.
- They tend to live in cold, discordant families.
- They are emotionally cold and inclined to be impulsive.
- They typically reside in poor, disorderly communities.
- They begin their misconduct at an early age.
- They use drugs and alcohol.

These findings are in line with a number of other factors that have been identified as contributing to delinquency. Perhaps most basic is a home life characterized by insecurity and rejection of the youngster. Delinquent youths are likely to come from homes disrupted by divorce rather than by the death of a parent. Inconsistent discipline is another contributing factor. Parents are likely to alternate harsh punishment with periods of neglect or disinterest. The delinquent generalizes contempt for the parents to other authority figures, including teachers and police. Frequently, delinquents do not receive the kind of parental help and encouragement that is needed for success in school. One study demonstrated quite clearly that inner-city delinquents have little confidence that they can achieve success in our society (Institute for Social Research, 1979). They anticipate dropping out of high school and, at best, being stuck in a low-level job. Delinquents sometimes feel justified in breaking the rules because the system is so much against them.

The courts have generally treated juveniles differently than adult offenders. The juvenile court system was designed not so much to punish but to protect the best interests of the child. However, this approach is now under attack by citizens who feel the courts are too lenient with dangerous juveniles. The argument is that teenagers who commit adult crimes (e.g., rape, assault, and murder) should be treated as adults and dealt with severely. The courts are caught between the interests of an outraged community and the rights of the youngster.

Juvenile Correction Programs. A variety of programs are used to treat juvenile offenders. For juveniles whose crimes are not very serious, and who have supportive families, the court may recommend some form of in-home supervision. Informal probation, intensive supervision, mentoring programs, and after-school programs are some of the programs that may be considered.

For youngsters who pose greater risk but are not considered extremely dangerous, placement in group homes, foster care, and other community living situations are the programs of choice. For those who represent the highest risk to the community, most states provide a continuum of increasingly restrictive settings ranging from isolated wilderness camps to high-security locked facilities. According to Greenwood (1995), recent decades have seen a trend away from the large, traditional training schools where most serious juvenile offenders were once placed. These institutions were criticized for offering sterile and unimaginative programs and for allowing abuse and mistreatment of the weaker juveniles. In place of these institutions, many states are substituting smaller, often privately run, community-based settings. These community programs at least present the hope of offering a wider range of rehabilitative programs. An exception to the general trend toward community-based facilities is California, which continues to rely on large, secure training schools. These institutions house from 700 to 1500 youthful offenders. One reason for this preference is that California is inundated with juvenile offenders, accounting for 20% of the youth locked up in the entire nation (Greenwood, 1995). Many other state systems are struggling with reduced budgets to handle an increasingly difficult and dangerous population. This sometimes results in the provision of custodial care with little money left over for therapeutic programs.

We are indebted to Yoshikawa (1994) for identifying some programs that reduce delinquent misconduct and improve behavior at school. They include the Perry Preschool Project in Ypsilanti, Michigan; the Parent-Child Development Center in Houston, Texas; the Family Development Research Project in Syracuse, New York; and the Yale Child Welfare Project in New Haven, Connecticut. All dealt with low-income families, and all intervened during the first 5 years of a child's life and continued for up to an additional 5 years. The programs offered parent training along with preschool education for the child. Extensive home visits were included. Follow-up studies showed that these programs produced less aggressive, impulsive, and delinquent behavior. We cannot go into further detail, but students interested in effective delinquency programs should follow up on their own.

Adult Offenders

What should we do with those who violate the law? This is an intensely controversial issue that generates widely divergent answers from liberal and conservative commentators. Some believe that we are too soft on criminals and that many criminals escape prosecution on legal technicalities. Others argue that the entire system is heavily biased against poor people and minorities. For prosecutors, the central questions are how to allocate limited resources in regard to a bewildering variety of cases involving street crime, domestic violence, drug violations, child abuse, white-collar offenses, and repeat offenders (Forst, 1995).

There is intense conflict about imposing mandatory minimum sentences in drug cases. Indeed, some judges are now refusing to try minor drug cases. Judge Jack Weinstein (1993) is one of these; he argued that our justice system is in crisis largely because of drug prosecutions. He pointed out that nationwide, over one-third of all new inmates are drug offenders. Due to mandated sentences, he continued, drug smugglers and dealers are serving longer prison terms, sometimes 10-year minimums, than was previously the case. The resulting overcrowding in our prisons is wasteful and self-defeating because it deters no one from dealing in drugs.

Senator Phil Gramm (1993), on the other hand, is in favor of tough sentencing for drug dealers. He believes that most criminals are rational men and women who commit crime because they think it pays. And in America, they are right; crime does pay because there is a low expectancy of actually being arrested, convicted, and imprisoned. "When a potential criminal knows that if he is convicted he is *certain* to be sentenced, and his sentence is *certain* to be stiff, his cost-benefit calculus changes dramatically and his willingness to engage in criminal activity takes a nose dive," argued Senator Gramm (1993, p. A19). We have witnessed a dramatic increase in crime since the 1960s, he continued, because we have treated criminals as victims of dysfunctional families, of capitalism, and of society at large. Instead, we must keep criminals off the streets and keep them from harming our children.

Probation.   Some offenders receive suspended sentences and are placed under the supervision of a probation officer. Many of those on probation are nonviolent offenders with no prior convictions. About 80% of probationers complete their terms without a new arrest (Clear & Braga, 1995). However, the public is rightly concerned about a subgroup of offenders who have high rates of criminal activity.

An important recent trend in probation is the push toward better classification of probationers so that those who pose the greatest risk to the community receive more supervision. In the past, too little time was devoted to serious offenders. Now, cases are assigned "work units" in accordance with need, and each probation officer is responsible for a certain number of work units (Clear & Braga, 1995).

Prison and Correctional Programs. The finding that prisoners are not being rehabilitated in significant numbers is not surprising in view of the fact that most prisons provide little more than custodial care. Relatively little effort is devoted to treatment and job training. Life in prison is routinized, time is structured, and the social system is completely authoritarian. It is not the kind of place in which one can learn to function adaptively in a free society. Although incarceration undoubtedly has the effect of deterring some prisoners from future crime, it is also true that others become hardened by their total immersion in a society of criminals.

An influential early survey by Martinson (1974) suggested that various programs designed to reduce recidivism were not generally successful. Individual therapy, education, skill development, group therapy, and variations in sentencing and probation all proved to be of little avail. There was some evidence that the personal characteristics of offenders, such as age and type of offense, were more important than the form of treatment in determining future recidivism. Youthful offenders had the best chance of being rehabilitated. There is an urgent need for pilot studies on the kinds of prisoners that can best be integrated into the community and the kinds of programs that would serve this purpose.

Inciardi (1987, p. 580) suggested that each of the present correctional strategies—vocational training, education, penitence through prayer, recreation, group therapy—seems to work for somebody. The difficulty is that we do not know which approach is most effective for whom. Perhaps the greatest problem is in the selection of offenders for participation in a particular rehabilitative program. Inciardi suggested that we need to do a better job in the screening of offenders and that we should admit that some offenders cannot be helped by any known program. Improvement is also needed in determining when an offender has received maximum benefits from any given technique. All of this means that correctional programs should learn to be more efficient and cost effective.

Alternatives to Incarceration. Although some Americans believe that incarceration is the only adequate moral response to the suffering imposed upon innocent victims by criminals, various alternatives are being put into practice in many parts of the country. The high costs of incarceration, the overcrowding in prisons, and the lobbying of penal reformers are some of the factors that account for increasing the number of offenders who are assigned to some form of nonincarceration program (DeIulio, 1991). Here are brief descriptions of some approaches that are now being tried.

◆ *House arrest with electronic monitoring.* The offender, usually an adult who has committed property crimes, is required to stay in or around home except to participate in court-approved activities. He or she is required to wear an electronic monitoring device, usually in the form of an ankle bracelet, that enables corrections officers to know where the offender is at any time. The offender is incarcerated if there are any violations.

Early returns showed that these programs were plagued with equipment problems that resulted in erroneous reports that the offender was home and equally false reports that the offender was not home. There were many reports of noncompliance with the monitoring. Despite these problems, new arrests were relatively uncommon with offenders on house arrest (Petersilia, 1987). There is some hope that these programs will prove to be cost effective, especially if confined to nonviolent offenders.

 ◆ *Community service sentences.* This alternative to incarceration involves placing offenders in the community under close supervision and requiring them to perform any one of a number of socially useful tasks (e.g., painting buildings or cleaning vacant lots) to help pay part of the costs of their supervision. Usually, the offenders work in small groups supervised by a corrections officer.

 ◆ *Intensive supervision programs.* These programs differ from conventional probation and parole in that the supervision is much tighter. For example, the participants must either work or go to school, submit to random drug and alcohol tests, and reside in a community center having strict rules about chores, curfews, and social interactions. In addition, the offender may be required to make restitution to victims.

 ◆ Early results showed high rates of failure for these programs. These offenders did not seem to do better in terms of arrests and other measures than those on routine supervision (Clear & Braga, 1995).

 ◆ *Boot camps.* The idea of immersing offenders in a military style experience similar to basic training is popular with some politicians. It is hoped that this will instill some pride and self-discipline in the offender. The results of limited assessments done so far provide no basis for optimism (Clear & Braga, 1995). There is no evidence that these programs either deter or rehabilitate prisoners.

More assessments of these innovative approaches are needed before any final conclusions can be drawn. Certainly, there is an urgent need to find cost-effective alternatives to standard imprisonment. On average, it costs $75,000 to build a prison cell and $20,000 to maintain a prisoner for 1 year in a state prison (Blumstein, 1995).

PERSONS WITH MENTAL RETARDATION

It is apparent that some children are not able to learn as quickly as their age-mates. In fact, the first intelligence tests were designed to identify children who could not accomplish age-appropriate tasks. These tests measure the child's ability to memorize, concentrate, grasp verbal abstractions, do arithmetic, and other skills. By definition, the child who is average in ability for a particular age has an intelligence quotient (IQ) of 100. Those who score significantly below average in ability are classified as persons with retardation. The precise cutoff score is arbitrarily selected, and there is variation among scaling systems. However, most authorities consider individuals with IQs below 70 to be mentally retarded.

Causes of Retardation

Environmental factors account for the majority of cases of mental retardation. Few people realize that most individuals in this group show no evidence of brain injury or defect. These factors include a destructive or abusive home life, parents who are dysfunctional and poor role models, and limited learning opportunities during infancy and early childhood. The myth that learners with retardation are brain injured has been an obstacle to setting higher expectations for these individuals (Borich & Tombari, 1995, p. 525).

Certain genetic disorders may cause below average functioning in learning and achievement. Phenylketonuria (PKU) is an example of a single-gene disorder that may cause severe retardation. Babies with PKU appear normal at birth but are unable to metabolize an amino acid called phenylalanine, which then accumulates and converts to toxic substances. Fortunately, infants can now be screened for PKU. If diagnosed early and started on a low-phenylalanine diet, they may develop normally.

Chromosomal disorders take place during formation of the egg or the sperm and are not hereditary. The best known of these disorders is Down syndrome named after Langdon Down, the British physician who first identified it. About 1 of every 800 live births results in this syndrome, with the incidence increasing with the mother's age. Persons with Down syndrome have a distinct appearance with a small head, flat eyes, high cheekbones, and sometimes, a protruding tongue. Several of these features suggested an Oriental appearance and led to the condition being called Mongolism, a term that is now completely out of favor. Most persons with this syndrome range in IQ from 35–55, with some having IQs close to 70. Until the 1970s, clinicians were pessimistic about the potential of children with Down syndrome, but they are now viewed as capable of learning and accomplishing many things in their lives (Comer, 1995, p. 682).

Prenatal complications are another possible cause of retardation. Most brain growth takes place during fetal development, that is, before birth. Many difficulties may affect brain development during this phase, including decreased oxygen supply to the developing fetus and exposure to alcohol, drugs, and other toxins. In the case of fetal alcohol syndrome, for example, the infant weighs less than normal, develops slowly, and may show other deficits. The brain of the fetus or infant is also vulnerable to viral infections such as measles, rubella, mumps, HIV, and herpes, which may impair cognitive processes (Borich & Tombari, 1995).

Classifying Persons with Mental Retardation

Persons are diagnosed or classified on the basis of both intelligence tests and tests of *adaptive functioning*. The latter measure the extent to which a person has learned basic skills such as personal care, feeding, toileting, language, pedestrian skills, and skills having to do with getting along with other people. These adaptive skills are learned by most people without formal training (Borich & Tombari, 1995). Most states rely more on the IQ score in diagnosing mental retardation than on measures of adaptive behavior (Morgenstern & Klass, 1991).

There is wide variation in intellectual ability within the group of persons classified as retarded. They are subdivided into four groups: the mildly, moderately, severely, and profoundly retarded. As shown in Table 2–2, the large majority are classified as mildly retarded. These individuals can learn basic adaptive skills, such as dressing and feeding themselves, and can perform many kinds of work tasks. They can marry, live independently with some supervision, and hold jobs. For example, McDonald's has found that these workers can do many kinds of routine jobs.

As we go down the scale, individuals are less capable and require more help and supervision. There is also greater probability that the person will show some physical defect or deformity. Persons who are profoundly retarded may have limited mobility, and communication is generally limited to some simple gestures and vocal intonations. Some of these individuals are cared for in large institutional settings, but there is a trend toward placing them in smaller group homes with 15–20 residents. See Table 2–2 for further information about the expected performances of individuals at various levels of retardation.

The education of persons with retardation begins with a mapping out of target behaviors. Self-care, social behavior, and basic academic and vocational skills are usually the main areas of concentration. Within each area, specific skills are divided into simple components that the person is capable of learning. Learning then proceeds in a step-by-step fashion, gradually building the simple components into more skilled performance (Coleman et al., 1984). The advantage of this gradual approach is that the person experiences success frequently in the learning process.

It should be stressed that most persons with retardation can learn a variety of social and vocational skills and need not be institutionalized. Those with mild retardation are the most capable, and they are taught within the public school system. There are, in fact, about 750,000 such youngsters being educated in America's public schools (Drew, Logan, & Hardman, 1988). Others may be placed in special schools in the community. At school, they are taught elementary reading, writing, and arithmetic to the fullest possible extent. The less capable students may devote relatively more time to learning the basic skills of daily living such as washing, eating, brushing teeth, buttoning buttons, and so on. Some are eventually placed in sheltered workshops where they may do light assembly, packaging, and other jobs for modest pay. Often, payment is on a piecework basis. However, the jobs are real jobs, and the pay is real money. This means that the worker can experience the satisfaction that comes from making a contribution to society.

TABLE 2-2 Behavioral Expectancies of Individuals with Retardation by Level of Severity*

Level of Retardation	Percentage of the Retarded	Preschool Behavior (Under Age 6)	School Performance	Adult Functioning	Social Adjustment
Mild IQ Range 50–69	85%	Slightly slow in walking, talking, and caring for self, but not very different from average children; often not identified as retarded before entering school	Can learn academic skills at between the third- and sixth-grade level	May become self-supporting and has potential for sheltered or competitive employment; some supervision may be needed	Able to interact with others but with some poor social skills; makes friends; marriage a possibility
Moderate IQ Range 35–49	10%	Noticeably slow in learning self-help skills, but eventually learn to walk and talk on a single level	Can learn academic tasks up to second-grade level; survival skills can be learned	Capable of employment in highly supervised settings; very rarely suitable to independent living; live in supported settings	Can interact with others but may appear awkward and slow to understand; marriage rarely attempted
Severe IQ Range 20–34	4%	By age 6, may have learned to walk and feed self; speech limited; may not be toilet trained at this phase	May be able to learn basic self-care skills and some speech	Capable of simple tasks in home or sheltered workshop; some permanent care is needed	Social interactions generally very limited
Profound IQ Below 20	1%	May have some minimal ambulatory skills at age 6; communication usually by nonverbal techniques; may not be toilet trained	May be able to learn some basic movements and positions; some are bedbound, helpless	Not capable of employment; permanent care needed; may be institutionalized	Little or no social awareness

*Based on various sources including Patton, Payne, and Beirne-Smith (1990).

In the recent past, many children with retardation were considered uneducable, and little effort was put into teaching them academic skills. Educators are now coming around to the view that we should avoid a pattern of very low expectations for these students. Dover (1990) recommended that certain principles be followed with regard to instruction. The first of these is that programs focus on instructional goals as primary objectives, and that medical and psychological goals be provided only when there is a clear need for them. In other words, *learning comes first*. The failure to learn should lead to a search for better techniques of instruction. Another principle is that the goal of instruction should be independence. Dover also recommended that communication training receive heavy emphasis. Students must learn to communicate if they are to gain access to desired activities, make their needs known, or get the attention of teachers and other individuals. Perhaps the main idea is that exceptional learners should be classified primarily on their needs to learn certain skills. This means that children are not blind, deaf, mentally retarded, or learning disabled but instead are students who need instruction in mobility, pedestrian skills, signing, reading recognition, money management, and so on.

There has been significant improvement in the outlook for persons with retardation since 1970 when the President's Committee on Retardation concluded that the potential contribution of many such persons was being wasted because of a shortage of adequate schools and facilities. Since then, there has been a sharp reduction in the number of retarded people simply being warehoused in large custodial institutions. Increasingly, persons with retardation are included in regular schools and in community programs.

THE HOMELESS

For most people, home is associated with warmth, protection, and sharing life experiences with loved ones. It is a place of safety, a refuge from the pressures and demands of the outer world. The thought of being homeless, of having no place to call one's own, is almost inconceivable to most of us. Nevertheless, this is precisely what has happened to thousands of Americans. Men, women, and children all over the country are finding shelter in bus and train terminals, parks, alleyways, abandoned buildings, caves, packing cases, and other unlikely places. The more fortunate among them spend the night in a mission or Salvation Army shelter where a shower and hot meal are provided.

Homelessness in the United States is an embarrassment considering that it exists in the context of great wealth. Although some homeless have always been with us, their numbers increased dramatically in the mid-1980s. As rapidly as shelters opened, they were filled to capacity. In New York City, a "right to shelter" policy threatened to drain the budget (Bassuk, 1995, p. 318). Policymakers across the country wanted to know how many people needed shelter, but attempts to count the homeless yielded widely divergent results:

> Government estimates were lowest with a 1984 count of 250,000–350,000 homeless persons (U. S. Department of Housing and Urban Development, 1984).
>
> Groups advocating for the homeless came up with counts as high as 3 million (Bassuk, 1995).
>
> A survey of soup kitchens and shelter users in 1989 in 178 cities reported an estimate of 500,000–600,000 (Burt & Cohen, 1989).
>
> Subsequently, a shelter and street count by the U. S. Census Bureau (1991, April 12) reported that there were 228,372 homeless people, a number that was doubted by some experts since it seemed too low.

These estimates, discussed by Bassuk (1995), vary so enormously that they provide no basis to plan for the needs of this population. Why do the number differ so much? The counts varied depending on several factors. One factor is who does the counting. It appears that government agencies may produce low numbers to minimize the extent of the problem. Advocacy groups, on the other hand, may tend to exaggerate the numbers to dramatize the problem and, possibly, increase public support to help the homeless. We are not suggesting that anyone is actually making up numbers. The fact is that researchers may use different techniques for counting the homeless and may define homelessness more or less stringently. In any case, the homeless are somewhat elusive in the sense that they move from street to shelter to housing in a nomadic fashion. Some homelessness consists of brief episodes, but other cases constitute virtually permanent lifestyles. We should not forget the "couch people" who have moved in with friends and relatives and who are not included in the homeless tallies (Daley, 1987).

Who Are the Homeless?

Marin (1987) noted that the word *homeless* is applied to so many different kinds of people with so many different problems that it is almost meaningless. He listed some of the groups packed into the category of "the homeless" as follows:

- *The mentally ill,* including drug addicts, alcoholics, and deinstitutionalized psychiatric patients, probably the largest single subgroup of homeless
- *The physically disabled* whose benefits do not enable them to afford permanent shelter
- *The elderly* on fixed incomes insufficient to meet their needs
- *Runaway children,* some of whom have been abused

♦ *Immigrants,* both legal and illegal, who have not been able to find permanent shelter
♦ *Tramps and hobos,* who have chosen "the road" as a way of life for a variety of personal reasons

Another category of homeless has been identified as the *situationally homeless.* These are people "whose homelessness has resulted from a change in circumstances, such as unemployment, spousal abuse, eviction, or urban redevelopment" (Breakey, 1987, p. 42). Their problems are chiefly financial and stem from difficult circumstances rather than major disabilities such as alcoholism or mental illness. It seems likely that poor women and their children have a disproportionately large representation in this category (Hagen, 1990). Low income, unemployment and underemployment, along with family violence, especially wife battering, are some of the factors that put women out of their homes. Holden (1986) reported that families, usually young women with two or three children, are the fastest growing segment of the homeless population, making up about 20% of the total.

Some causative factors, cited by Hope and Young (1986), are unemployment, particularly among young people and minorities; deinstitutionalization of mental patients; and the grim shortage of affordable housing. This latter problem is possibly the most important in explaining why the poverty of the 1980s so often took the form of having no permanent residence. There has been a dramatic reduction in low-cost housing due in part to the process of gentrification. This refers to the redevelopment of rundown areas of our cities so as to attract middle- or upper-class residents. Low-cost housing is converted to high-priced condominiums, old hotels that once catered to transients are torn down or upgraded, and so on. The problem reflects a limitation of our capitalist system: It is not profitable to build new low-cost housing, so it doesn't get done. Without government subsidy, it is unlikely that the need for low-cost housing will be met.

Attitudes Toward the Homeless

Americans tend to divide society into winners and losers. The homeless are even bigger losers than those consigned to the welfare system. Often they are seen as lazy, weak, defective persons who are content to live off of handouts from hardworking, decent people. It is not surprising, then, that homeless people are sometimes treated with contempt. Some towns have passed ordinances making it illegal for the homeless to sleep at night in public places. In other communities, the police tell the homeless to move on, sometimes even providing one-way bus tickets to facilitate the move. "To put it as bluntly as I can," said Marin (1987, p. 47), "for many of us the homeless are *shit.* And our policies toward them, our spontaneous sense of disgust and horror, our wish to be rid of them in all of this has hidden in it . . . our feelings about excrement."

Although negative feelings toward the homeless may prevail, they are by no means universal. Some express a deep compassion for the plight of the homeless. Marin (1987) listened to the life stories of the homeless and found a pattern that usually began with ordinary life. Then a catastrophic event occurred, which in turn led to a series of smaller events until homelessness became inevitable. In this view, the homeless are not different from the rest of us. They have suffered a loss or injury and have had homelessness thrust upon them.

Helping the Homeless

The system of services for the homeless as it existed in the 1970s was totally insufficient to meet the growing need. For example, rescue missions were set up 50 or more years ago when most clients were male alcoholics. Rescue missions are shelters supported by religious groups that typically operate under a rigid set of rules. They vary greatly in size, ranging from 15-bed shelters to huge barracks-style arrangements that accommodate hundreds (Hope & Young, 1986). Except for some large Salvation Army shelters that have hired social workers, missions are generally staffed by religious converts who are intent on saving others from perdition and/or alcoholism.

The voluntary sector also provides a network of shelters run by churches, synagogues, and nonprofit community agencies. As the need for shelters increased, many congregations decided to open church doors to those who needed a place to sleep. From these sorts of informal beginnings, some churches went on to set up formal shelters that sometimes provide supportive counseling. Voluntary groups such as Traveler's Aid and the YWCA and YMCA have also provided shelters. Shelters run by churches and voluntary agencies always seem short of funds; some shelters close during the summer months, and others have had to close doors permanently.

During the early 1980s, it became increasingly obvious that private voluntary agencies could not by themselves do the job of helping the homeless. Nevertheless, municipal governments showed a marked reluctance to increase expenditures for this purpose. Vigorous activity on the part of advocates along with glaring publicity was required to prod cities into action. New York, Los Angeles, Philadelphia, Washington, DC, Chicago, and other large cities all acted to support additional shelters. Typically, the city selects unused public buildings and then contracts with a private group to actually run the shelter. In practice, city shelters tend to be larger, more violent, and more bureaucratic than private ones (Hope & Young, 1986). They also tend to cost more to operate than private shelters (Krauskopf, 1984).

Additional help for the homeless was provided by the federal government in 1983. After prolonged prodding by advocates, Congress appropriated $100 million for emergency services to be dispensed by the Federal Emergency Management Administration (FEMA). Lesser amounts were appropriated in subsequent years. Some of the money goes to soup kitchens and other forms of emergency help. FEMA also distributes grants to voluntary umbrella organizations such as the United Way and the National Conference of Catholic Charities. According to Hope and Young (1986), most of those who work with the homeless believe that federal funding, although welcome, has been grossly inadequate.

In summary, it seems fair to say that the services provided to the homeless were late in coming, still have the quality of hasty patchwork, and remain inadequate to meet the need. It can also be said that the underlying problems have not been addressed in a large-scale way. Hope and Young (1986) argued that the rights to life, liberty, and the pursuit of happiness are empty abstractions unless animated by rights to housing and basic sustenance. A true safety net, they maintain, should be a first step.

Currently, the general public does not appear to be greatly concerned about the plight of the homeless. The term *compassion fatigue* has sometimes been applied by the popular press to describe prevailing public attitudes. As Bassuk (1955, p. 319) noted, "Regardless of the numbers, the very existence of people on the streets in a society as affluent as ours is a travesty. As the homelessness epidemic has become a chronic disfigurement, the public has increasingly inured itself to the desperate plight of the growing numbers of individuals and families." The "insidious spread" of homelessness, Bassuk continued, "should cause at least enough alarm to make us question our priorities . . . "

PERSONS LIVING WITH HIV/AIDS

Although AIDS, an acronym for the Acquired Immune Deficiency Syndrome, does not presently claim nearly as many lives as do heart disease and cancer, there is no other disease that raises such intense fears and concerns among the general public. The threat of AIDS, a contagious disease, has altered patterns of sexual activity and is the center of intense controversy about what steps should be taken to prevent the spread of the disease.

What Is AIDS?

AIDS is a serious viral disease that damages the body's natural immune defenses. The disease begins when the human immune deficiency virus, HIV, enters the bloodstream, but this cannot be detected for 6 weeks or even longer in some cases. At this early stage, many infected people experience no ill effects, although some show mild symptoms such as fatigue, swollen glands, and possibly a rash. These initial symptoms disappear, but the virus quietly multiplies. During the middle stage of the disease, which may begin after 5 years, the immune system declines in strength, and treatment with AZT, DDI, and other antiviral drugs may be started. Years may elapse before the final or terminal phase is reached. This occurs when the immune system is weakened to the extent that it can no longer fight off invading bacteria, viruses, and parasites. Death may be caused by pneumonia, unusual cancers, or any of a variety of other "opportunistic" diseases. For years, people weren't considered to have AIDS until they showed overt signs of serious illness, but the federal government is revising its standards to include those whose blood tests show a serious level of deficiency but who are as yet symptom-free (Enkholm, 1991).

The AIDS Epidemic

Within a period of a few years, AIDS grew from a clinical oddity to a major epidemic. When the first cases of AIDS were reported in 1981, epidemiologists at the Centers for Disease Control (CDC) in Atlanta began tracking the disease. They determined that the first cases of AIDS probably occurred in 1977. By 1982, the syndrome had appeared in 15 states with the majority of victims being homosexual or bisexual men (Institute of Medicine, 1986). As of 1993, The World Health Organization (1993) estimated that over 13 million people worldwide had become infected with HIV. This included over 1 million in North America, 500,000 in western Europe, and another 1.5 million in Latin America and the Caribbean. Hardest hit was Africa, with over 8 million infections. The data suggested that an increasing number of infections were due to heterosexual intercourse (Merson, 1993).

In the United States, it is estimated that up to 897,000 persons were living with HIV infection as of 1993, including 150,000 women. About 227,000 persons had died of AIDS by this time. Prevalence rates were generally highest among minorities, with 3% of young black males with HIV and 1% of black women in their 30s (Rosenberg, 1995).

Who Are the Victims of AIDS?

The victims of AIDS fall into the following categories:

- Sexually active homosexual and bisexual men, 65%
- Present or past users of intravenous drugs, 17%
- Homosexual and bisexual men who are also intravenous drug users, 8%
- People with hemophilia or other coagulation disorders, 1%
- Heterosexual contacts of someone with AIDS or at risk for AIDS, 4%
- Infants born to infected mothers, 1%

The remaining cases do not fall into any of these groups, but researchers believe that transmission occurred in similar ways (U. S. Department of Health and Human Services, 1987).

Individuals who are HIV positive are more likely to be people of color, residents of inner cities, and economically disadvantaged than is the general population. They include women, mainly African American or Latino, who did not insist on condom use and were infected by a male lover. Also included are the 1500–2000 babies who are born with the virus each year (Enkholm, 1991).

How Is the Disease Transmitted?

It seems clear from the categories of victims that the major means of transmission is sexual contact, particularly anal intercourse and other sexual practices that may result in semen-to-blood or blood-to-blood contact. Anal intercourse is a high-risk activity because the lining of the rectum is thinner and more easily torn than the thicker protective lining of the vagina. Anal intercourse can therefore result more easily in direct semen-to-blood exchange. Although in a small percentage of cases the virus has been transmitted from an infected male to a female, it is not known if these cases involved oral or anal intercourse.

Needle sharing among intravenous drug users is another major means of transmission. This practice can result in small amounts of blood from an infected person being injected directly into the bloodstream of the next user. The risk of contracting AIDS through a blood transfusion has been significantly reduced since May 1985 by screening all blood donations for the AIDS virus.

Preventing the Spread of AIDS

Educational campaigns about AIDS by private and governmental agencies are aimed at both the general public and those in high-risk groups. The intent is to encourage people to discontinue practices that spread the disease. Specifically, sexually active people are being advised to refrain from sexual contact with those whose health status is unknown and to avoid practices that may result in blood-to-blood or semen-to-blood exchanges. Male homosexuals who have had contact with a number of partners are being advised to assume that they have been exposed to the virus and to refrain from sexual contact involving the exchange of bodily fluids. Drug users are being urged not to share needles and to enter treatment programs that will help them become drug-free (New York State Department of Health, 1986). Some state agencies are offering voluntary free testing for those who wish to determine if they have been exposed to the AIDS virus. Another preventive effort, which has aroused much controversy, is the campaign to encourage the use of condoms in sexual intercourse. Schools are making greater efforts to educate children about the dangers of sexually transmitted disease and, in some areas, are actually dispensing condoms to students. At the same time, the media are considering lifting the ban on the advertising of condoms.

We find ourselves in complete agreement with Merson (1993) who argued that prevention is the key to reducing the horrific effects of AIDS. At the same time, we have to face up to the fact that our prevention message is not getting through to young adults. Recent data have shown that among persons between 18 and 25, there was actually an increase in the rate of HIV infections between 1986 and 1992 (Rosenberg, 1995). During the same period, the rate for older white males leveled off. What is disturbing about the data is that the risks are well known to younger adults. Apparently, many are choosing to engage in unsafe sex even though the methods of preventing infection are understood and widely publicized. Clearly, we must redouble our efforts to persuade young adults and minorities to avoid unsafe sexual practices.

Care for AIDS Victims

A wide spectrum of human services has been developed for AIDS victims, including the following:

- ◆ Informational hotlines—for example, the Centers for Disease Control National Hotline (900-322-7514)—give out information on community AIDS groups around the country
- ◆ Educational materials provided by federal, state, and local governments
- ◆ Counseling for AIDS patients, families, and those at risk for AIDS
- ◆ Assistance in locating medical, dental, and other health services
- ◆ Transportation to medical care
- ◆ Assistance with insurance coverage, housing, and civil rights issues

Walker (1987) pointed out that every AIDS patient has an average of eight close relatives and intimates. This means that millions of lives have already been disrupted by AIDS in one way or another. There is clearly a great need to provide support not only to the AIDS patients but also to their close associates. Across the country, approximately 300 community-based organizations have started to provide support groups for patients' families. The Gay Men's Health Crisis in New York City has programs for both the parents and partners of those with the disease. Similar support groups exist in Minneapolis, Denver, San Francisco, and other large cities. Some groups are without formal leaders, whereas others are led by trained mental health professionals.

Families have a difficult time dealing with any seriously ill patient, but AIDS families are particularly hard hit. Walker (1987) observed that some families were shocked to learn that a member had been leading a secret life. The links to homosexuality and drug abuse caused some family members to feel stigmatized, secretive, and possibly, angry at the victim. Families must learn to live with grief, cope with feelings of shame, and face their anger at the patient. The act of talking is the beginning of the process of working through these intense feelings.

AIDS and the Health Care System.   The increasing number of AIDS victims is taxing the capacities of public hospitals and clinics, especially in larger cities. The high costs of taking care of AIDS sufferers are due, in part, to several factors.

- The illness tends to require the services of diverse medical specialists because so many bodily systems may be affected.
- The medications used are themselves costly but may cause side effects that, in turn, need to be treated with additional costly therapies.
- Home care for the dying becomes difficult or impossible because potential caregivers may also be debilitated, leading to sometimes lengthy hospitalization.
- AIDS victims are living longer, with the course of the disease running around 12 years from initial infection to terminal phase.
- The illness does not run a smooth course. Symptoms may come and go in an unpredictable fashion, and there may be stable periods. This means the victim may require multiple hospital admissions (Strauss, Fagerhaugh, Suczek, & Weiner, 1991).

In short, it appears that AIDS is developing many of the cost factors associated with other chronic diseases such as cancer and heart disease. The cumulative effect of these chronic diseases is to tax the health care system beyond its present capacity. This situation has put various subgroups of health care consumers in competition with one another for the limited funds available for research and treatment. AIDS victims are placed at a disadvantage in this competition because they are perceived by some as having made personal lifestyle choices that brought about their present predicament. The argument runs that the rest of us should not be required to pay for the consequences of their choices. Well aware of negative public attitudes, AIDS activists have created a powerful national lobby devoted to increasing government and private investment in AIDS research and treatment.

In an ideal world, all human lives would be treated as equally valuable and, therefore, be regarded as deserving the same quality of medical care. It is unlikely that this ideal will be realized any time soon in the United States. It runs counter to the values of many Americans who would provide better care to those who are perceived as most deserving—that is, those who make an economic contribution to the community. A more practical problem is that we may not have the resources to provide high-quality medical care for everyone. The sharing of available resources would mean a reduction of services for those now enjoying high-quality care. It seems doubtful that the affluent will be willing to do this for the sake of homeless people, addicts, or AIDS victims.

The authors' view is that we must take steps to slow the development of all chronic diseases, including AIDS, and do our utmost to prevent these diseases from occurring in the first place. This means the development of programs of prevention aimed at improving the environment and at altering our behavior to stop the spread of disease.

SUMMARY AND CONCLUSIONS

This description of some target populations gives an idea of the magnitude of the task facing human services today. Of course, one cannot add up the number of people included in each population because there is overlap among the groups. An individual may be poor, physically disabled, elderly, *and* an alcoholic. In fact, there is a strong tendency for poverty and advanced age to be disproportionately associated with both mental and physical disorders. A member of a low-income family is twice as likely to become disabled as a member of a middle-class family. It is also true that nearly half of the adult disabled population is at or near the poverty level. Even considering this overlap among groups, it has been estimated that one in every six Americans, or 36 million, is disabled in some way (Bowe, 1980). Even more alarming is the increase in the number and percentage of Americans who are chronically ill, over 65, or disabled.

It is not known how the United States will respond in the future to this greatly increased need for services. It is apparent that there has been a distinct shift in national priorities during the past decade. The earlier commitment to solve social problems, particularly those associated with poverty and racism, has given way to a focus on other priorities. The prevailing trend is to hold down or reduce spending for social programs. In one sense, the pattern is a familiar one. Historically, periods marked by concern for the less fortunate members of society have alternated with periods of relative neglect. No one knows how long the current trend will continue. Certainly, many programs have been cut, and the impact has been keenly felt by human services workers and the populations they serve.

One possible approach to reducing costs of human services involves the increased use of prevention programs. Millions of dollars are spent on facilities and services for criminals, mental patients, alcoholics, and drug addicts, yet relatively little money is invested in programs designed to prevent individuals from joining these target groups in the first place. Similarly, larger sums are spent on welfare benefits than on programs that might keep some people off the rolls. Obviously, a person who has been trained for a well-paying job is unlikely to need long-term welfare support. The initial cost of a successful prevention program would be more than made up in the long run. Unfortunately, politicians and others concerned with funding have proved very resistant to investing in prevention programs. These issues will be discussed in more detail in Chapter 8.

It is likely that new approaches to target populations will increase proportionately with the growth in population. However, some groups, particularly the elderly and disabled, will increase at a disproportionate rate. The net effect is that a greater percentage of the population will be in need of services, which will be provided by a relatively smaller number of human services workers. This is the dilemma that will face human services in the near future.

ADDITIONAL READING

Beaver, M. L. (1983). *Human service practice with the elderly.* Englewood Cliffs, NJ: Prentice Hall.

Bloom, B. L. (1984). *Community mental health: A general introduction* (2nd ed.). Pacific Grove, CA: Brooks/Cole.

Bowe, F. (1980). *Rehabilitating America.* New York: Harper & Row.

Burgdorf, R. L., Jr. (Ed.). (1980). *The legal rights of handicapped persons.* Baltimore, MD: Paul Brookes.

Comer, R. J. (1996). *Fundamentals of abnormal psychology.* New York: W. H. Freeman.

Costin, L. B., Bell, C. J., & Downs, S. W. (1991). *Child welfare: Policies and practices* (4th ed.). New York: Longman.

Cox, H. G. (1988). *Later life: The realities of aging.* Englewood Cliffs, NJ: Prentice Hall.

Davison, G. C., & Neale, J. M. (1996). *Abnormal psychology* (6th ed.). New York: Wiley.

Dell Orto, A. E., & Marinelli, R. P. (Eds.). (1995). *Encyclopedia of disability and reha-bilitation.* New York: Macmillan.

DiIulio, J. J. (1991). *No escape: The future of American corrections.* New York: Basic Books.

Gallagher, B. J. (1987). *The sociology of mental illness* (2nd ed.). Englewood Cliffs, NJ: Prentice Hall.

Helfer, R. E., & Kempe, R. S. (1987). *The battered child* (4th ed.). Chicago: University of Chicago Press.

Hopper, K., & Hamberg, J. (1984). *The making of America's homeless: From skid row to new poor—1945–1984.* New York: Community Service Society.

Inciardi, J. A. (1987). *Criminal justice* (2nd ed.). New York: Harcourt Brace Jovanovich.

Johnson, A. B. (1990). *Out of Bedlam: The truth about deinstitutionalization.* New York: Basic Books.

Julian, J., & Kornblum, W. (1986). *Social problems* (5th ed.). Englewood Cliffs, NJ: Prentice Hall.

Patton, J. R., Payne, J. S., & Beirne-Smith, M. (1990). *Mental retardation* (3rd ed.). Columbus, OH: Merrill.

Popple, P. R., & Leighninger, L. H. (1990). *Social work, social welfare, and American society.* Needham Heights, MA: Allyn & Bacon.

Robinson, N. M., & Robinson, H. B. (1976). *The mentally retarded child* (2nd ed.). New York: McGraw-Hill.

Torrey, E. F. (1988). *Nowhere to go: The tragic odyssey of the homeless mentally ill.* New York: Harper & Row.

Wilson, J. Q., & Petersilia, J. (Eds.), (1995). *Crime.* San Francisco: ICS Press.

REFERENCES

AARP (American Association of Retired Persons). (1986). *A profile of older Ameri-cans.* Washington, DC: Author.

AARP (American Association of Retired Persons). (1995). AARP Bulletin: Special Report. Washington, DC: Author.

Anglin, D. M. (1988). The efficacy of civil commitment in treating addiction. *Journal of Drug Issues, 18,* 527–547.

Asch, A. (1984a). The experience of disability: A challenge for psychology. *American Psychologist, 39,* 529–536.

Asch, A. (1984b). Personal reflections. *American Psychologist, 39,* 551–552.

Bassuk, E. L., & Gerson, S. (1978). Deinstitutionalization and mental health services. *Scientific American, 238,* 46–53.

Bassuk, E. L. (1995). Dilemmas in counting the homeless. *American Journal of Orthopsychiatry, 65,* 318–319.

Bazell, R. J. (1973). Drug abuse: Methadone becomes the solution and the problem. *Science, 179,* 772–775.

Beaver, M. L. (1983). *Human service practice with the elderly.* Englewood Cliffs, NJ: Prentice Hall.

Blumstein, A. (1995). Prisons. In J. Q. Wilson & J. Petersilia (Eds.), *Crime* (pp. 387–419). San Francisco: ICS Press.

Borich, G. D., & Tombari, M. L. (1995). *Educational psychology: A contemporary approach,* New York: Harper Collins.

Bowe, F. (1980). *Rehabilitating America.* New York: Harper & Row.

Braginsky, D. D., & Braginsky, B. M. (1975, August). Surplus people: Their lost faith in self and system. *Psychology Today,* pp. 68–72.

Breakey, W. R. (1987). Treating the homeless. *Alcohol Health and Research World, 11,* 42–46, 90.

Brenner, H. (1973). *Mental illness and the economy.* Cambridge, MA: Harvard University Press.

Brieland, D., Costin, L. B., & Atherton, C. R. (1980). *Contemporary social work* (2nd ed.). New York: McGraw-Hill.

Burgdorf, R. L., Jr. (Ed.). (1980). *The legal rights of handicapped persons.* Baltimore, MD: Paul Brookes.

Burt, M. R., & Cohen, B. E. (1989). *America's homeless: Numbers, characteristics, and the programs that serve them.* Washington, DC: Urban Institute Press.

Caputo, R. K. (1989). Limits of welfare reform. *Social Casework, 70,* 85–95.

Carlson, E. (1995, June). *Chater sees no crisis now, but warns of strain in next century. AARP Bulletin, Special Report.* Washington, DC: American Association of Retired Persons.

Carson, R. C., Butcher, J. N., & Coleman, J. C. (1988). *Abnormal psychology and modern life* (8th ed.). Glenview, IL: Scott, Foresman.

Clear, T. R., & Braga, A. A. (1995). *Community corrections.* In J. Q. Wilson & J. Petersilia (Eds.), *Crime* (pp. 421–444). San Francisco: ICS Press.

Coleman, J. C., Butcher, J. N., & Carson, R. C. (1984). *Abnormal psychology and modern life* (7th ed.). Glenview, IL: Scott, Foresman.

Comer, R. J. (1995). *Abnormal psychology* (2nd ed.). New York: W. H. Freeman.

Connell, C. (1995, July 28). Worried about Medicare. *The Standard Star, Gannett Suburban Newspapers,* p. 3B.

Costin, L. B., Bell, C. J., & Downs, S. W. (1991). *Child welfare: Policies and practices* (4th ed.). New York: Longman.

Crispell, D., & Frey, W. H. (1993, March). American maturity. *American Demographics,* pp. 31–42.

Daley, S. (1987, June 17). "Couch people": Hidden homeless grow. *The New York Times,* pp. B1, B4.

Davison, G. C., & Neale, J. M. (1996). *Abnormal psychology* (6th ed.). New York: Wiley.

DeJong, G., & Lifchez, R. (1983). Physical disability and public policy. *Scientific American, 48,* 240–249.

DiIulio, J. J. (1991). *No escape: The future of American corrections.* New York: Basic Books.

Dover, R. B. (1990). Defining mental retardation from an educational perspective. *Mental Retardation, 28,* 147–154.

Drew, C. J., Logan, D. R., & Hardman, M. L. (1988). *Mental retardation* (4th ed.). Columbus, OH: Merrill.

Egeland, B., Clochetti, D., & Taraldson, B. (1976). Child abuse: A family affair. *Proceedings of the N. P. Masse Research Seminar on Child Abuse,* 28–52.

Enkholm, E. (1991, November 17). Facts of life: More than inspiration is needed to fight AIDS. *The New York Times,* pp. E1, E3.

FBI crime index rose by 6% in 1986. (1987, July 26). *The New York Times,* p. 21.

Federal Bureau of Investigation. (1995). *Uniform crime reports.* Washington, DC: U. S. Government Printing Office.

Fenderson, D. A. (1984). Opportunities for psychologists in disability research. *American Psychologist, 39,* 524–528.

Forst, B. (1995). Prosecution and sentencing. In J. Q. Wilson & J. Petersilia (Eds.), *Crime* (pp. 363–386). San Francisco: ICS Press.

Freeman, R. B. (1995). The labor market. In J. Q. Wilson & J. Petersilia (Eds.), *Crime.* San Francisco: ICS Press.

Frum, D. (1995, August 14). Welcome, nouveaux riches. *The New York Times,* p. 15.

Fuchs, V. R. (1991). Are Americans underinvesting in their children? *Society, 28,* 14–22.

Gallagher, B. J. (1987). *The sociology of mental illness* (2nd ed.). Englewood Cliffs, NJ: Prentice Hall.

Gannett News Services. (1991, September 27). Census: 1 in 7 were poor in 1990. *The Standard Star,* p. 22A.

Garfinkel, I., & McLanahan, S. S. (1986). *Single mothers and their children.* Washington, DC: Urban Institute Press.

Gliedman, J., & Roth, W. (1980). *The unexpected minority: Handicapped children in America.* New York: Harcourt Brace Jovanovich.

Goffman, E. (1963). *Stigma: Notes on the management of spoiled identity.* Englewood Cliffs, NJ: Prentice Hall.

Goldstein, A. (1994). *Addiction: From biology to drug policy.* New York: W. H. Freeman.

Gramm, P. (1993, July 8). Mandatory jail sentences work. *The New York Times,* p. A19.

Greenwood, P. H. (1995). Juvenile crime and juvenile justice. In J. Q. Wilson & J. Petersilia (Eds.), *Crime* (pp. 445–488). San Franciso: ICS Press.

Grief, G. L. (1985). *Single fathers.* Lexington, MA: Lexington Books.

Group for the Advancement of Psychiatry, Committee on Aging (1971, November). *The aged and community mental health: A guide to program development* (Vol. 8, Series No. 81). New York: Author.

Hagen, J. L. (1990). Designing services for homeless women. *Journal of Health and Social Policy, 1,* 1–16.

Hay, J. W., & Ernst, R. L. (1987). The economic costs of Alzheimer's disease. *American Journal of Public Health, 77,* 1169–1175.

Hershey, R. D. (1988, July 9). Rate of joblessness at lowest point in last 14 years. *The New York Times,* p. 1.

Hershey, R. D. (1995, November 4). Job growth was sluggish last month. *The New York Times*, p. A37.

Holden, C. (1986). Homelessness: Experts differ on most causes. *Science, 232,* 569–570.

Holmes, S. A. (1994, October 28). Ratio of inmates reach one million in a 2-decade rise. *The New York Times*, pp. A1, A25.

Hooyman, N. R., & Kiyak, H. A. (1991). *Social gerontology: A multidisciplinary perspective.* Needham Heights, MA: Allyn & Bacon.

Hope, M., & Young, J. (1986). *The facts of homelessness.* Lexington, MA: Lexington Books.

Houghton, J. F. (1980). One personal experience: Before and after mental illness. In J. G. Rabkin, L. Gelb, & J. B. Lazar (Eds.), *Attitudes toward the mentally ill: Research perspectives* (pp. 3–10). Rockville, MD: National Institute of Mental Health.

Houghton, J. F. (1982). First person account: Maintaining mental health in a turbulent world. *Schizophrenia Bulletin, 8,* 547–552.

Inciardi, J. A. (1987). *Criminal justice* (2nd ed.). New York: Harcourt Brace Jovanovich.

Institute for Social Research. (1979, Winter). *Newsletter.* Ann Arbor: University of Michigan.

Institute of Medicine, National Academy of Sciences. (1986). *Mobilizing against AIDS: The unfinished story of a virus.* Cambridge, MA: Harvard University Press.

Jaegerman, M. (1993, February 4). Price tag: Psychotherapy. *The New York Times*, p. C2.

Johnson, A. B. (1990). *Out of bedlam: The truth about deinstitutionalization.* New York: Basic Books.

Joint Commission on Mental Health of Children. (1970). *Crisis in child mental health: Challenge for the 1970s.* New York: Harper & Row.

Julian, J., & Kornblum, W. (1986). *Social problems* (5th ed.). Englewood Cliffs, NJ: Prentice Hall.

Kahn, R. L., & Antonucci, T. C. (1982). Applying social psychology to the aging process: Four examples. In J. Santos & G. R. Vandenbos (Eds.), *Psychology and the older adult: Challenges for training in the 1980s.* Washington, DC: American Psychological Association.

Kaufman, J., & Zigler, E. (1987). Do abused children become abusive parents? *American Journal of Orthopsychiatry, 57,* 186–192.

Kramer, R. (1994, Autumn). In foster care, children come last. *City Journal*, pp. 63–70.

Krauskopf, J. (1984). *New York City plan for homeless adults.* New York: Human Resources Administration.

Kupfer, A. (1988). What to do about drugs. *Fortune, 117,* 39–41.

Lazare, D. (1990, January 23). The drug war is killing us. *The Village Voice*, pp. 22, 24–26, 28–29.

Lyons, R. D. (1984, October 30). How release of mental patients began. *The New York Times*, pp. C1, C4.

Marin, P. (1987, January). Helping and hating the homeless. *Harper's Magazine*, pp. 39–49.

Martinson, R. (1974). What works?—Questions and answers about prison reform. *The Public Interest, 35,* 22–54.

McFadden, R. D. (1987, December 1). Child abuse is higher in mental units, study says. *The New York Times,* pp. B1, B6.

Merson, M. H. (1993, May 28). Slowing the spread of HIV: Agenda for the 1990s. *Science, 260,* pp. 1266–1268.

Miller, G. (1987, June 16). The continuing crisis in foster care. *Congressional Record, 133,* E2410–E2411.

Morgenstern, M., & Klass E. (1991). Standard intelligence tests and related assessment techniques. In J. L. Matson & J. A. Mulnick (Eds.), *Handbook of mental retardation* (2nd ed., pp. 195–210). New York: Pergamon Press.

Musto, D. F. (1987). *The American disease* (expanded ed.). New York: Oxford University Press.

Narrow, W. E., Regier, D. A., Rae, D. S., Manderscheid, R. W., & Locke, B. Z. (1993). Use of services by persons with mental and addictive disorders: Findings from the N.I.M.H. epidemiologic catchment area program. *Archives of General Psychiatry, 50,* 95–107.

National Institute of Mental Health. (1974). *Teenage delinquency in small town America* (Research Report 5, DHEW Publication No. ADM 75–138). Rockville, MD: Alcohol, Drug Abuse, and Mental Health Administration.

New York State Department of Health. (1986, March 1). *Acquired immune deficiency syndrome: 100 questions and answers* (pamphlet). Albany, NY: Department of Health.

O'Connor v. *Donaldson,* 422 U. S. 563 (1975).

Patton, J. R., Payne, J. S., & Beirne-Smith, M. (1990). *Mental retardation* (3rd ed.). Columbus, OH: Merrill.

Pear, R. (1984, August 3). Rate of poverty found to persist in spite of gains. *The New York Times,* pp. A1, B8.

Pear, R. (1991, October 18). Social security benefits to go up 3.7%. *The New York Times,* p. B8.

Pear, R. (1995, March 14). Welfare and food stamp rolls end six years of increases. *The New York Times,* p. A18.

Pepper, B. (1987). A public policy for the long-term mentally ill: A positive alternative to reinstitutionalization. *American Journal of Orthopsychiatry, 57,* 452–457.

Petersilia, J. (1987). *Expanding options for criminal sentencing.* Santa Monica, CA: Rand Corporation.

Physician Task Force on Hunger in America. (1985). *Hunger in America: The growing epidemic.* Boston: Harvard University School of Public Health.

Plum, K. C. (1987). Moving forward with deinstitutionalization: Lessons of an ethical policy analysis. *American Journal of Orthopsychiatry, 57,* 508–514.

Popple, P. R., & Leighninger, L. H. (1990). *Social work, social welfare, and American society.* Needham Heights, MA: Allyn & Bacon.

President's Committee on Mental Retardation. (1970). *The decisive decade.* Washington, DC: U. S. Government Printing Office.

Rabinovitz, J. (1995, June 20). Court allows welfare cuts in Connecticut. *The New York Times,* pp. B1, B5.

Regier, D. A., Narrow, W. E., Rae, D. S., Manderscheid R. W., Locke, B. Z., & Goodwin, F. K. (1993). The de facto U. S. Mental and Addictive Service System: Epidemiologic catchment area prospective 1-year prevalence rates of disorders in services. *Archives of General Psychiatry, 50,* 85–94.

Richardson, S. A. (1976). Attitudes and behavior toward the physically handicapped. *Birth Defects: Original Article Series, 12,* 15–34.

Robinson, N. M., & Robinson, H. B. (1976). *The mentally retarded child* (2nd ed.). New York: McGraw-Hill.

Rorvik, D. M. (1979, April 7). Do drugs lead to violence? *Look,* pp. 58–61.

Rosenberg, P. S. (1995, November 24). Scope of the AIDS epidemic in the United States. *Science, 270,* 1372–1375.

Rovner, J. (1995, June). Social security lauded for its achievements—But what of the future? *AARP Bulletin, Special Report.* Washington, DC: American Association of Retired Persons.

Sack, K. (1991, May 15). New York is pressed to pare welfare as home-relief rolls grow. *The New York Times,* pp. 81, B2.

Schmolling, P. (1975). Civil rights for mental patients: The road to neglect? *Hospital and Community Psychiatry, 26,* 168–170.

Schmolling, P. (1993). Social policy issues in narcotics abuse. *Journal of Health and Social Policy, 5,* 49–65.

Schmolling, P. (1994, January 16). States are on right welfare track. *The Standard Star, Gannett Suburban Newspapers,* p. 3E.

Schottenfeld, R. S. (1989). Involuntary treatment of substance abuse disorders—Impediments to success. *Psychiatry, 52,* 164–176.

Schwarz, J. E., & Volgy, T. J. (1992). *The forgotten Americans.* New York: Norton.

Shapiro, J. P. (1995, August 14). Sins of the fathers. *U. S. News and World Report,* pp. 51–52.

Social Security Administration. (1991). *Social Security Bulletin, 54*(9). Washington, DC: U. S. Department of Health and Human Services.

Strauss, A. L. Fagerhaugh, S., Suczek, B., & Weiner, C. (1991). AIDS and health care deficiencies. *Society, 28,* 63–73.

The White House. (1989, September). *National drug control strategy.* Washington, DC: U. S. Government Printing Office.

Three of 100 males in correction system, U. S. says. (1987, January 2). *The New York Times,* p. A17.

Tobin, S. S., & Lieberman, M. A. (1976). *Last home for the aged.* San Francisco: Jossey-Bass.

Toner, R. (1995, July 16). Resolved: No more bleeding hearts. *The New York Times,* pp. 1, 16.

Toner, R., & Pear, R. (1995, July 23). Medicare, turning 30, won't be what it was. *The New York Times,* pp. 1, 24.

Tumulty, B. (1992, January 11). Jobless rate hits 5-year high. *The Standard Star,* p. 16A.

Turnbill, H. R. (1982, August). *Oversight on Education for All Handicapped Children Act, 1982.* Testimony before the Senate Subcommittee on the Handicapped, 97th Congress. Available from the Senate Committee on Labor and Human Resources, Washington, DC.

U. S. Bureau of the Census. (1991). *Marital status and living arrangements, 1991.* (Current Population Reports, P-20, No. 450). Washington, DC: U. S. Government Printing Office.

U. S. Bureau of the Census. (1991, April 12). Census Bureau releases 1990 decennial counts for persons enumerated in emergency shelters and observed on the streets (Press Release). Washington, DC: U. S. Department of Commerce News.

U. S. Department of Health and Human Services. (1987, Winter). *Facts about AIDS* (pamphlet). Washington, DC: Author.

U. S. Department of Health and Human Services, National Center on Child Abuse and Neglect. (1988). *Study findings: Study of national incidence and prevalence of child abuse and neglect.* Washington, DC: U. S. Government Printing Office.

U. S. Department of Housing and Urban Development. (1984). *A report to the secretary on the homeless and emergency shelters.* Washington, DC: Office of Policy Development and Research.

U. S. Department of Justice (1992). *Sourcebook of criminal justice statistics, 1991.* Washington, DC: Author.

U. S. Department of Labor, Manpower Administration. (1970). *Win for a change.* Washington, DC: U. S. Government Printing Office.

Ventura, S. J. (1994, October). Data on teenage pregnancies. *Statistical Bulletin, 75,* 10–17.

Verhovek, S. H. (1995, September 21). States are already providing glimpse at welfare's future. *The New York Times,* pp. A1, B10.

Walker, L. (1987, June 21). What comforts AIDS families. *The New York Times Magazine,* pp. 16–22, 63, 78.

Waller, P. (1991). The politics of child abuse. *Society, 28,* 6–13.

Weicker, L., Jr. (1984). Defining liberty for handicapped Americans. *American Psychologist, 39,* 518–523.

Weiler, P. G. (1987). The public health impact of Alzheimer's disease. *American Journal of Public Health, 77,* 1169–1175.

Weinstein, J. B. (1993, July 8). The war on drugs is self-defeating. *The New York Times,* p. A19.

Weiss, R. D., & Mirin, S. M. (1987). *Cocaine.* Washington, DC: American Psychiatric Press.

Wilson, J. Q. (1977). *Thinking about crime.* New York: Vintage.

Wilson, J. Q. (1990). Against the legalization of drugs. *Commentary, 89,* 21–28.

Wilson, J. Q. (1995). Crime and public policy. In J. Q. Wilson & J. Petersilia (Eds.), *Crime* (pp. 489–507). San Francisco: ICS Press.

Wines, M. (1995, September 24). The social engineers let welfare go unfixed. *The New York Times,* pp. E1, E14.

Wolfe, B. L. (1991). Treating children fairly. *Society, 28,* 23–28.

World Health Organization (WHO). (1993). *The HIV/AIDS pandemic: 1993 overview.* Geneva: Author.

Yoshikawa, H. (1994). Prevention as cumulative protection: Effects of early family support and education on chronic delinquency and its risks. *Psychological Bulletin, 115,* 28–54.

Human Services in Historical Perspective

INTRODUCTION

Who is responsible for helping the disadvantaged within a society? The family? Religious organizations? The government? Is helping to be viewed as a basic human right or as a societal gift? Throughout history, societies have responded to these questions in various ways. If a society does accept some responsibility for helping its disadvantaged, additional questions quickly emerge. Which groups of people and types of problems should be helped, to what extent, and how?

How a given society answers these questions is based on its dominant values, attitudes, and beliefs. If a society believes that its poor or elderly members should be helped, then it will develop some system or method to provide the needed care for these target populations. Another society may give priority to its physically or mentally disabled members and develop services focused on these groups but excluding others.

The present range and diversity of human services are quite large. Throughout history, many people and events have influenced the development and direction of the field. As societies have changed through the ages, values and beliefs have often been replaced or at least modified by new ones. The developing human services systems of today are to some extent an outgrowth of our previously held societal values and beliefs concerning helping. It is likely that the quality, methods, and availability of human services in the future will be greatly influenced by current attitudes toward helping. Through knowledge of the past, we can better understand the present and also be in a more favorable position to shape the future.

For clarity and to help you understand more fully the historical development of the interrelated aspects of the human services field, this chapter is divided into several sections. The first section provides a general overview of the historical roots of the human services field by tracing the development of early societal beliefs and helping practices. The next section traces changing societal attitudes and helping practices that have contributed to the development of human welfare services. The following section examines the historical development of mental-health services. The chapter concludes with a brief discussion of future trends in the human services field.

PREHISTORIC CIVILIZATIONS

The earliest records of helpful treatments can be traced back to the Stone Age of approximately half a million years ago. Through cave drawings and the remains of primitive skulls, scientists know about a medical treatment called **trephining**. In this procedure, a small section of the skull was bored out, probably by means of sharp stones or other such crude instruments. This hole cut from the skull was supposed to allow a route of escape for the evil spirits that were believed to inhabit the afflicted person's body, thereby curing the person. Scientists have surmised that this treatment was administered to people who evidenced certain forms of observable deviant behavior. It should always be remembered that what constitutes deviant behavior is a product of what the norm for behavior is at a given point in time.

In this early era, most human problems were attributed to devils, demons, or other evil spirits. Belief in the supernatural or **demonology** was the dominant belief system of the age, and various procedures or rites were used to exorcise evil spirits. The belief in the supernatural arose from early humans' attempt to explain the universe. All natural phenomena such as earthquakes or floods were attributed to the work of evil spirits. These ancient people also accepted the related belief, called **animism,** that spirits inhabit various inanimate objects such as rocks, trees, or rivers. The shaman, or medicine man who performed rites of exorcism, can now be viewed as the earliest human services worker. It was commonly believed that these individuals understood the secrets of the supernatural and possessed certain religious or mystical qualities that enabled them to help afflicted individuals.

Life during prehistoric times was at best a matter of pure survival against the hostile environment. Human problems centered around gathering food and having a relatively safe place to sleep. Poverty meant not being able to locate or secure food, and sometimes the weaker individuals were simply left to perish. In situations involving the physically disabled or infirm elderly, the tribe or extended family unit would usually share or provide for these individuals. However, how important afflicted people were to the tribe often determined the amount of assistance they received. In some instances, individuals separated from other tribes were taken in and befriended. Newcomers usually had to prove their worth in some manner in order to be allowed to stay with the tribe. The family was the primary source of help, but religion played an increasing role in the evolution of human services.

EARLY CIVILIZATIONS

Prior to 450 B.C., the world was believed to be governed by supernatural spirits. There were no major organized attempts to understand human problems and behavior from a scientific point of view. However, significant changes in beliefs were about to emerge that would alter the earlier supernatural explanations for human behavior.

During the Golden Age of Greece, a number of philosophers began to put forth new beliefs concerning human nature. One of these was the Greek physician Hippocrates (460–377 B.C.), who disagreed with the belief that supernatural spirits were the sole cause of human disease. He believed rather that most diseases were chiefly physiological or organic in origin. He shared the point of view earlier postulated by Pythagoras that the brain was the center of intelligence and that mental disorders were due specifically to the malfunctioning of the brain (Coleman, 1976).

Another contribution made by Hippocrates was his development of a system of psychiatric labels for patterns of deviant behavior. These labels included melancholia, mania, and epilepsy. To more clearly appreciate the radical change in belief advocated by Hippocrates, one must consider that the previous explanation for epilepsy was that it was a sacred or divinely ordained disease. Hippocrates claimed this disease was caused by a blockage of air in the veins due to secretions of the brain (Hoch & Knight, 1965). The treatments advocated by Hippocrates differed considerably from the earlier skull-cutting procedures. His treatments often involved vegetable diets, exercise, and pursuing a tranquil lifestyle.

Whether Hippocrates had the correct physiological explanation or treatment is not of critical historical importance here. The theory that diseases could be explained by natural—as opposed to supernatural—causes is of major importance. This change in belief systems regarding the origin of diseases influenced another significant change. Since deviant behavior or psychological problems could now be viewed as diseases of organic origin, they could now be considered part of the domain of medicine (Rimm & Somervill, 1977). As such, physicians, rather than priests, medicine men, or other religious healers, performed the necessary treatments. This separation of treatment responsibilities was one of the first steps toward developing the system of specialization that has continued to the present time in human services.

In the ancient Rome of 150 B.C., another physician, Asclepiades, advocated treatment procedures for mental disorders that stressed a medical and humane approach. His recommended treatments often involved massages and baths to soothe excited or nervous patients, with wine to calm the nerves. He actively denounced the cruel and severely harsh treatments that were still popular at this time, such as housing patients in totally dark cells, beating them with chains, bloodletting, castrating, and subjecting patients to prolonged periods of starvation.

Galen (130–200 A.D.), a Greek medical writer, was able to compile, systematize, and integrate a considerable amount of material from many complementary fields. His topics included medicine, anatomy, physiology, and logic. In addition, he made a major contribution to the understanding of abnormal behavior by developing a system of classifying the causes of mental disorders. He believed all disorders were either physical or mental. He felt these disorders could originate from such things as injuries to the head, fear, shock, or emotional disturbances.

The early civilizations presented some striking contradictions in helping attitudes and services. Although many advances were being made and many individuals were attempting to struggle against fear, ignorance, and superstition, the use of cruel treatment procedures was still prevalent. Even as many advocated more humane and philosophical beliefs concerning the nature of people, the practice of buying and selling slaves also existed. The poor and disabled often begged for alms along city streets. Although physicians were available for the sick, only those who could pay had access to them. The Romans and the Greeks viewed physical weakness or disability with little tolerance. Often the physically ill were taken out of towns to uninhabitated areas or deserted islands where they were left to struggle by themselves or die. Of course, this pertained predominantly to the poor or those without resources or family protection. As in most societies, the rich were treated one way and the poor another.

The period 200–475 A.D. marked a steady decline for civilization. As major plagues killed thousands upon thousands of people between the first and fourth centuries A.D., intense fear and anxiety spread throughout Europe and the Middle East. In this climate of fear, Christianity emerged and developed a large and zealous following. Medicine could not stop the plagues, so people turned to the comfort and solace offered by Christianity, which became the prime religion of the Western world. Religious figures replaced medical figures as the saviors from illness. The causes of disease were again explained in terms of loss of faith to demons. Evil spirits were viewed as the cause for most human misfortunes.

THE MIDDLE AGES

The Middle Ages date from the fifth century with the collapse of Rome at the hands of the barbarians advancing from the east. During this time, exorcism reemerged as the prevalent treatment for most disorders. The medical advances achieved by Greece and Rome were mostly forgotten (Fisher, Mehr, & Truckenbrod, 1974). Christianity became the dominant power throughout the Middle Ages.

As the Church became steadily more powerful and organized in the early part of the Middle Ages, it developed and provided a variety of human services. Monasteries often served as sanctuaries, refuges, and places of treatment for the mentally ill. The Church established institutions for the poor, provided residences for the handicapped, sponsored orphanages, and founded homes for the aged. Initially, these services were housed within church facilities, but later other nonreligious sites were founded.

In its earliest beginnings, the Church espoused the belief that the wealthy or those with adequate resources had a duty or responsibility to help the less fortunate. The less fortunate, in turn, began to expect assistance as an obligation or duty from the wealthy. Both the rich and the poor developed social roles and expectations for one another, and a clear distinction between the two classes was evident. It is important, however, to note that assistance given to the poor was set at the lowest subsistence or survival level. Much of contemporary human services philosophy can, in fact, be traced back to these early interpretations of religious values and teachings.

During this period, there was little interest in finding out why the disadvantaged were disadvantaged. The causes of poverty, for example, were of little interest to those providing human services. The rights and obligations for each class of society were clearly spelled out, and no further understanding was felt to be needed.

Initially, people believed that giving to the disadvantaged was important simply because others were deserving of and needed help. The Church gradually began to lose this emphasis on helping out of humanitarian concerns and replaced it with the notion that helping had to be done if one wanted to ensure a peaceful afterlife and achieve salvation. The Church preached that giving was a means of salvation, a means to an end. People would be rewarded in an afterlife for fulfilling their obligations in this life. Giving was seen as a necessary responsibility or duty of the wealthy that they often fulfilled reluctantly.

As the Church developed human services, the overall climate of the Middle Ages was marked by extreme cruelty and chaos. During the period 1200–1400, there was a strong increase in the belief in witchcraft, and in certain regions, mass outbreaks of flagellation (whipping) rituals occurred (Russell, 1972).

Although the Church tried to control all opposing beliefs and alternative religious movements, it was not completely successful. As people became disillusioned with the ability of the Church to protect them from misfortune, a variety of fanatical sects emerged throughout medieval Europe, and fear of witchcraft became a mass obsession. As Rimm and Somervill (1977) pointed out:

> Witches were viewed not only as degenerate beings in league with devils, but also as causes of sickness, disease, personal tragedies, and the stealing and killing of children. They were perceived as vicious instigators of terror, highly dangerous to a threatened and unstable society. (p. 16)

In the Middle Ages, the growth of financial sects represented a form of extremism, an impulsive act often characteristic of youth. In fact, the Europe of the Middle Ages was a youthful society. The death rate was extremely high, and people did not often survive past 40 years of age.

Beginning in the 13th century under Pope Innocent III, a religious tribunal was established. This tribunal, referred to as the *Inquisition*, was given the responsibility of seeking out and punishing any and all crimes associated with witchcraft or other forms of heresy. The methods employed by this ecclesiastical body to obtain confessions for accused crimes included intimidation, burnings, boiling suspects in oil or cutting their tongues out, and other inhumane forms of torture. The Inquisition, although it used cruel and inhumane measures, espoused the belief that the Church was providing service to society by getting rid of the causes of disease and famine. It also served as a means for the Church to exert its power and encourage loyalty by threatening those who did not conform with stated policies and beliefs.

Throughout the Middle Ages, a major power struggle existed between Church and State. Each faction wanted more power to govern without interference from the other. The Church developed a steady source of income by demanding that its parishioners donate approximately 10% of their incomes for church-related activities. The State viewed this steady source of income as a threat to its own base of power and sought many times to make it illegal to give money or services to those who could work.

Gradually, the disadvantaged came to be classified according to whether they physically could work or were unfit for work, such as the disabled, elderly, and children. Those individuals deemed legitimately unfit for work came to be known as the worthy poor, whereas the others were looked upon as being lazy and unworthy of assistance. Even though this steady clash for power existed, the Church was successful through most of the Middle Ages at preserving its domain, especially as far as providing human services to "worthy" individuals.

THE RENAISSANCE

As Europe emerged from the Middle Ages, it entered a period of rapid and turbulent change marked by the end of the feudal system, the birth of industrialization, and a decline in the power of the Church. As the government became more powerful and influential, individual states, cities, and towns developed more power. The middle class, composed mainly of tradespeople, grew, prospered, and became a more visible and distinct part of society.

By the 16th century, change had significantly altered the previously established religious, social, and economic order. The government, the Church and newly emerging business leaders shaped the nature and direction of societal change. Unfortunately, the rationale for change is often based upon the priorities and complex concerns of those in power and does not necessarily benefit all in society. These changing societal forces had a tremendous influence upon the direction and quality of human services. It is important to realize that what has become today a system providing an enormous range of services for the welfare of human beings from birth until death originally started out as simply providing food or shelter to people as a form of social welfare.

Having now provided a general overview of the early development of human services philosophy and practice, we will next examine the subsequent growth of human welfare services and then that of mental-health services.

HUMAN WELFARE SERVICES
SINCE THE RENAISSANCE

During the 16th century, the Protestant Reformation escalated the many struggles for power between Church and State. By the end of the 16th century, the State had finally established authority of the Church. As a result of diminished Church power, it became incumbent upon the State to take over many services formerly provided by the Church, which included providing for human services.

Under Henry VIII of England, the government formally took over the human services functions of the Church to provide for people who were not self-sufficient and established a system of income maintenance and public welfare. The official policy mandating this transition of power was outlined in the Statutes of 1536 and 1572. In 1601, the *Elizabethan Poor Law* established a system that provided shelter and care for the poor. This law also specified local responsibility for the poor and disadvantaged. It was first the responsibility of the family to provide for all human services. If the family could not provide such services, it then became the responsibility of the State to provide for disadvantaged individuals within their communities.

Although there were people with good motives and intentions, the Poor Laws were not initially created as a generous humanitarian gift from the State to aid its disadvantaged citizens; the Poor Laws were a means of social control following an era of mass frenzy, disease, famine, and economic instability that threatened to break apart the existing social structure.

As a result of these Poor Laws in England, a system for classifying the disadvantaged into three categories was established: (a) the poor who were capable of work; (b) the poor who were incapable of work due to age, physical disability, or motherhood responsibilities; and (c) orphaned or abandoned children who became wards of the State. The poor who could work were forced to work in state-operated workhouses. Massive overcrowding, filth, and inadequate food and sanitary conditions made these workhouses barely tolerable. If the individual was incapable of work and in need of food or shelter, he or she could be sent to an **almshouse** (poorhouse). The living conditions there were similar to those of the State workhouses. By comparison to the almshouse or workhouse, a more tolerable alternative was available for the more "fortunate" of the disadvantaged. In certain communities, it was possible for individuals or families to remain in their own dwelling and receive contributions of food and other items from their community. This circumstance was far less common than the other methods of providing services. Money was never given directly to the poor family, and any other essential services such as medical care were not generally available.

As this early, often crude, human services system evolved, procedures and rules were more clearly established and defined. Policies were established to decide who would be eligible for available services and who would have the authority to decide who got what and who went where. As the programs became more complicated, the government created a subsystem with sole responsibility for overseeing its public welfare system. Each community had its specified government welfare administrator, who made the local decisions regarding a person's eligibility for services. As the number of individuals who were in need of assistance increased, the local community bureaucracy became more impersonal. Indeed, this is still a problem with modern welfare systems. The form of welfare bureaucracy created in England during this period became the early forerunner of our modern welfare system in the United States.

The Industrial Revolution

By the 1800s, the Industrial Revolution was developing momentum. The Industrial Revolution began with the invention of a few basic machines and the development of new sources of power. The advent of industrialization created the mechanization of manufacturing and agriculture, changed the speed and methods of communication and transportation, and began the development of factory systems of labor. These events, in turn, caused dramatic changes in economic systems (Perry & Perry, 1988).

Large populations of unemployed individuals moved from rural areas to urban centers in search of work. Although new forms of labor were needed and work was available for some, the great majority of people still found themselves in poverty. As a result of the swell in the disadvantaged population within urban areas, many public institutions were created. The majority of the urban poor found themselves facing worse conditions than those they had left behind. Adequate living space was scarce, producing overcrowded and unhealthy conditions. Food was in short supply, and the urban environment provided little room to grow crops. Families often found themselves separated as members left in search of work.

Workers were generally seen by businessmen as commodities, to be used only when needed and disregarded when work was not immediately available. It was during this time that workers started to band together to share and provide what they could for one another. This banding together for the collective benefit of all resulted in the development of the early guilds and unions. In an effort to deal with the perceived threat to the social order brought on by these large numbers of disadvantaged people in urban areas, the government created more workhouses, debtors' prisons, houses for delinquents and orphans, and mental institutions.

The period of the Industrial Revolution brought about a new social philosophy that had a strong influence upon society's attitude toward the poor and disadvantaged. This new social philosophy, known as the **Protestant work ethic,** reinforced a set of values supporting the virtues of industrialization and condemned idleness as almost sinful.

Hard work, and thereby the accumulation of wealth, was interpreted as God's reward for leading a virtuous life. On the opposite end of this philosophy, poverty was often viewed as some form of punishment from God. This philosophy, as most notably preached by John Calvin, supported the notion that poverty-ridden individuals should remain in their disadvantaged conditions because God had divinely ordained this condition for them.

It was during the 1830s in England that the concept of **less eligibility** was established. This concept set forth the guideline that any assistance given to the disadvantaged must be lower than the lowest wage paid to any working person. Work was seen as an ultimate good and its absence, for any reason, was to be looked down upon. In theory, this concept sought to provide an incentive for all to work.

Another corresponding influence on society's attitude toward the disadvantaged was the concept of **laissez-faire economy,** introduced by the Englishman Adam Smith in 1776. His book *The Wealth of Nations* argued for an economy where government had virtually no influence and placed no restrictions upon the free marketplace. According to Smith, without government control, society would grow and prosper by itself based on people's individual merit and hard work. Supporters of this concept saw human services not as a right but as a misguided societal gift—a gift that they perceived would actually hinder overall economic production.

As previously described, many of these events and philosophies that were developing in England and Europe had a strong influence on societal attitudes toward helping in the United States. The economic value system emerging from England was again reinforced in the United States by the writing of another Englishman, Herbert Spencer. It was Spencer who interpreted Charles Darwin's writings on evolution in a provocative manner. His ideas, which came to be known as **social Darwinism,** applied theories of animal behavior to human behavior. Using Darwin's biological premise in regard to natural selection and coupling it with an economic argument, Spencer espoused the idea that those disadvantaged people who were unfit for society should not be helped; it was the natural order of things for them to help themselves or perish, as in nature. This, it was felt, would provide another incentive for people to work. Of course, this theory did not take into consideration those individuals who, for physical or other reasons, were unable to work. Additionally, this theory did not consider the many individuals who wanted work but for whom no work was available. In essence, social Darwinism only served to foster an attitude of indifference toward the poor.

Early Reform Movements in the United States

As the many institutions for the disadvantaged grew in size, workers were needed to supply the various types of helping services. One positive effect of the growth of these public institutions was that it helped formalize the system of "professional" helpers. Conditions within institutions were intolerable. The large number of people housed in small spaces created unbearable overcrowding. Lack of heat in winter, instances of brutality, inadequate food, and many other examples of inhumane treatment generated a good deal of concern by private citizens over these conditions and led to a series of attempts at social reform.

Many of the social reformers of the mid-19th century did not focus their efforts on a single injustice but instead called for a voice of reason and humane concern in every area of human welfare. In the late 1800s and early 1900s, the movement toward human welfare made great advances. In this period of heavy immigration to the United States, many thousands of newly arrived immigrants found themselves homeless and displaced in their new country. It was during this time that settlement houses were developed to provide immigrants with the essentials of life and to help them to get a foothold in American society.

The **settlement house movement** was a reflection of early human services philosophy. Settlement house workers embraced the view that it was the responsibility of society to help. They also advocated a major shift in helping attitudes and human services thinking to the belief that many of the problems confronting individuals are created by environmental circumstances rather than by personal inadequacy. This point of view has recently come to be known as the human services perspective. The founders of the movement expressed the idea that one must work toward improving the social conditions that exist within society. To accomplish this goal, a system providing for basic human services must be created to facilitate an adequate quality of life. It was further believed that a truly successful human services system should provide opportunities for all people to improve their lives and realize their potentials.

One notable early settlement house was Hull House, founded in Chicago by Jane Addams. It was here, many authorities believe, that contemporary social work was born. Using Hull House as the primary hub of her human services activity, Addams managed to create a small but comprehensive network of human services in her Chicago neighborhood that included basic adult education classes, kindergartens, and an employment bureau. In the following years, many other settlement houses were founded throughout the country. They served as a training ground for those providing social work services.

The early 1900s in the United States marked the resurgence of another significant human services movement. Often referred to as the progressive or social justice movement, its aim was to bring about social change through political action and legislative reform. This movement, which reflected liberal reform ideas, was embraced by many factions of society including the unions. Accepting the earlier idea that the social environment is a major factor in creating people's problems, the reformers advocated a series of economic reform including a minimum wage standard, a pension system for older workers, an 8-hour day and a 6-day workweek, as well as laws providing for unemployment insurance and the regulation of child labor. Many successful changes occurred despite the prevailing conservative outlook. The government began to assume greater responsibility for the provision of human services. During this period, a growing number of Americans became aware that a system of human services is integrally connected to the economic system and the role of the government. A comprehensive system providing for human services requires the support and interconnectedness of all institutions within society.

The Depression and World War II

The stock market crash of 1929 and the Great Depression dramatically changed the lives of many Americans. With huge numbers of unemployed workers and a depressed economy, the need for expansion of human services was evident. With millions of people unemployed, the relationship between environmental circumstances and human problems could not have been made any clearer.

As pointed out in Chapter 1, the federal government under the direction of President Franklin Delano Roosevelt established a series of government aid programs called the *New Deal*. These programs attempted to make work available where possible and to provide direct assistance to those people incapable of work. Examples of such programs were the Works Progress Administration, which provided jobs; the Civilian Conservation Corps, which provided training; and Aid to Dependent Children, which provided direct government aid.

In 1935, a major governmental response to the existing social conditions was the Social Security Act. This legislation established a form of social insurance and protection for individuals against an unpredictable economy. This measure not only helped to alleviate the current social conditions but was also calculated to aid and protect future generations. This human services legislation subsequently provided for a wide array of health and social welfare services.

It has happened throughout history that people's attitudes change but sometimes have a difficult time being completely erased. There are always those who cling to previous ideas and attitudes for both good and bad motives, as well as those who advocate change for similarly varied reasons. The 1940s in the United States witnessed a reemergence of the trend toward conservatism. Public criticism was again heard, denouncing the governmental system of providing for human services as helping to create a form of "welfare state." Conservatives felt that too much aid would rob people of the incentive to help themselves. However, as conservatives and liberals debated how much assistance is beneficial, returning World War II veterans created a further need for a variety of human services. As Chapter 1 has indicated, this clash between conservative and liberal thinking is still very evident today.

The 1960s

The 1960s were characterized by social unrest in the United States. The Vietnam War was being waged overseas and many Americans at home participated in marches and demonstrations to protest the ills they felt existed within the system. This was a turbulent, sometimes violent period marked by protests at many college campuses across the country. Widespread and organized efforts of this kind resulted in an eventual end to the war and advanced the civil rights movement and the war on poverty. These latter movements were successful in bringing national attention to the plight of minorities and the poor. New legislation was enacted that resulted in the establishment of many programs and services. Although the civil rights movement and the war on poverty did create increased economic and educational opportunities for the disadvantaged, they did not eliminate poverty and discrimination in the United States.

In the 1970s and 1980s, human welfare services in the United States have grown considerably. A massive number of programs exist that provide for human services throughout the life cycle. In the midst of such an array of services, the need for services of these types still remains great. Debates continue to rage over which programs are truly helpful and worthy of funding and which should be trimmed from our federal or state budgets. This controversy over social policy is discussed in more detail in Chapter 7.

Table 3–1 summarizes the development of human welfare services. We next examine the corresponding growth of mental-health services.

MENTAL-HEALTH SERVICES SINCE THE RENAISSANCE

The historical development of our system of mental-health services in certain instances paralleled the development of our system of human welfare services, as previously described. It is now apparent that having an adequate food supply, shelter, income, and other necessities of life has a direct bearing on one's mental health. Of course, our contemporary knowledge and understanding of how environmental factors influence human problems is much better than it was in the past. Previously, individuals deemed mentally ill faced a grim future without any substantial alternatives. In the sections that follow, we examine the people and events that have helped to shape our societal attitudes and treatment of the mentally ill.

Early Mental Asylums

Early institutions created to house the behaviorally deviant were commonly referred to as **asylums.** The word *asylum,* when used in this context, refers to a place of refuge that provides protection, shelter, and security. Although many mental patients did view the asylum as a place of refuge or safety, a good number probably did not. It was society that viewed the asylum as a form of protection and shelter from those people labeled as deviants.

TABLE 3–1 Development of Human Welfare Services

1300s–1500s (Europe/Middle Ages)	1500s–1700s (Europe/Reformation)	1800s–1890s (United States)	Early 1900s–1950s (United States)	1960–Present (United States)
Church and State engage in power struggle. Church becomes major provider of human welfare services. Monasteries serve as places of refuge for the disadvantaged, mentally retarded, homeless, mentally ill. Poor are classified as worthy versus unworthy. Helping is viewed as a means to salvation.	Government establishes basic system of helping under Henry VIII of England. System of income maintenance and public welfare is established. Elizabethan Poor Laws establish a system to provide shelter and care for poor. Care for disadvantaged is considered a local responsibility. Poor are viewed as morally inadequate and deficient. Almshouses/poorhouses and state-operated workhouses develop.	Industrialization grows. Protestant work ethic emerges. Individual states establish and sponsor helping programs. Industrialization creates large numbers of poor and unemployed. Workhouses, debtors' prisons, and houses for delinquents and orphans increase in number. Social reform movement spreads. Private charities provide sources of helping. Settlement house movement develops. Union workers' movement develops. Minimum wage laws are passed. Environmental factors are seen as contributing to disadvantaged.	Federal government begins to assume responsibility for the provision of human services. Great Depression creates huge numbers of unemployed and disadvantaged. Federal government under FDR establishes New Deal program and expands provision of human services; provides direct aid and programs such as the Works Progress Administration, Aid to Dependent Children, the Civilian Conservation Corps. Social security program is established.	Economic Opportunity Act is passed. Medicare and Medicaid are created. War on poverty begins. An array of training and retraining programs for the disadvantaged are provided. Community mental-health movement begins. Large institutional settings are reduced in favor of smaller community programs. Conservative trend to return the provision of human services back to individual states begins. Debate rages over reinstitutionalization.

The early public mental institutions in Europe and the United States were located within communities, and the community was primarily responsible for the governance and maintenance of the institution. As communities tend to be different from one another, so too did these institutions differ from one another. No universal guidelines for patient care or procedures were established among this broad network of community mental institutions, and mistreatment and abuse frequently occurred.

One noteworthy exception, among others, to the generalized inhumane treatment and lack of concern toward mentally ill was the mental hospital established in 1409 in Valencia, Spain. This hospital is probably the oldest mental hospital still functioning today (Andriola & Cata, 1969). As a rule, patients were readily discharged after they were seen as able to return to society. Patients were treated with relative dignity, and a system of voluntary admissions was established. The example set by this hospital is even more striking when one considers that the Inquisition and witch-hunting mania were also prevalent during this era.

One of the earliest public asylums and the one most typical of the overall character of these institutions was St. Mary's of Bethlehem (Bedlam), created in 1547. Although originally intended to be humanitarian in nature, this institution, as well as others to follow, was little more than a dungeon in which the behaviorally deviant were locked up and subjected to cruel, often ghoulish, treatment. Inadequate food, insufficient clothing, filth, infectious disease, and overcrowding were commonplace. The more difficult patients were subjected to treatments that consisted of days, weeks, or months spent in mechanical restraints or chained to the walls and denied food or water. The majority of patients were either mentally retarded, aged, physically ill, or accused or convicted of crimes. Little attention was given to individual cases, and the patients could just as easily have been sent to a prison or poorhouse as to a mental institution.

The Era of Humanitarian Reform

During the next 200 years, similar conditions existed in institutions for the insane in this country, such as Pennsylvania Hospital founded in 1752 and Williamsburg Hospital founded in 1773 (Bloom, 1977). During the late 1770s and early 1780s, a reform movement began that would alter significantly, although briefly, the existing conditions in mental institutions. This movement toward humane treatment of the insane has been referred to as the era of humanitarian reform and the moral treatment movement. This movement, which had its earliest beginnings in Europe, had great influence upon institutions in the United States in the late 18th and early 19th centuries.

Following the French Revolution in 1792, physician Phillipe Pinel became the director of La Bicétre, a mental institution in Paris. It was here that Pinel, inspired by the idea that the insane might be curable, unchained some prisoners, and provided adequate food, clothing, and other necessities of life to all. Although reform was clearly evident, Pinel and other early reformers still advocated the use of harsh measures as sometimes useful tools of treatment. However, the reforms of Pinel are considered by many to be the first major revolution in mental-health care (Wahler, Johnson, & Uhrich, 1972).

This reform movement, begun in France, spread to England. In 1813, the British physician Samuel Tuke, the director of the York Retreat, initiated a similar series of reforms. In the United States, other physicians also advocated similar improvements. It was during these early years of reform that physicians gained most in prestige and prominence in their evolving interest and later specialization in treating the behaviorally deviant.

Even though the early reforms advocated by Pinel, Tuke, and others had an impact upon the institutions of the day, by the middle 1800s in the United States public awareness and interest in the plight of the mentally ill had waned. Without such interest, the institutions once again fell back into a period characterized by neglect and widespread mistreatment. It was in the mid-19th century that Dorothea Dix became a prominent figure in the evolution of human services. Through her efforts, the earlier reform movement that began in Europe and lost temporary impetus in the United States was again revived and gained its greatest foothold in the United States. Dorothea Dix was instrumental in gathering enough public support to make greatly needed changes in the inhumane conditions in the asylums as well as in prisons and many poverty-related shelters.

Following a personal investigation of asylums and prisons throughout the country, Dix wrote many articles for newspapers outlining the plight of the disadvantaged. She contacted legislators and began a successful lobbying effort to inform and educate the public concerning these conditions within the institutions. As Bloom (1977) indicated:

> Before [Dix's] career came to an end, 32 state mental hospitals had been built in the United States, care of the mentally ill had been removed from the local community, and the professional orientation toward the insane had been changed from seeing them as no different from paupers or criminals to seeing them as sick people in need of hospital care. (p. 11)

The creation of a system of large state psychiatric hospitals to replace predominantly poorly run smaller community institutions was seen as an improvement in care for the mentally ill. However, this progress was followed by new problems. Believing the large psychiatric hospital to be the answer, the public seemed to lose concern for this population. In the following years, a gradual and steady rise in new admissions to these hospitals once again resulted in overcrowding, mismanagement, and mistreatment.

During the early 1900s, advocates of the social justice movement, who had been active earlier in other areas of human welfare, turned their attention to abuses within mental institutions. Having no desire to dismantle these institutions, they sought rather to change the system of patient treatment and procedures. New policies creating individual treatment plans were established. This appeared to be a more humane and responsible way to administer treatment. Each patient would be treated individually, taking into consideration his or her prior history. This policy seemed a step in the right direction, but it unfortunately created other abuses within the system. Too much arbitrary power and authority were given over to the professionals and bureaucrats overseeing these systems. Of course, there were patients who benefited from more individualized consideration, but generally, the large and unchecked state system often ignored individuals' rights and denied the possibility that the State could be wrong in certain instances.

Freud's Influence

By the 1920s and 1930s, Sigmund Freud's classic theories concerning human behavior were well established and widely accepted. Having had to endure considerable criticism in the earlier years of his developing work in response to his emphasis on human sexuality, his later refined theories had a major impact on most facets of society. Although Freud did not work directly in institutions, he had a strong influence on the prevailing treatment approach. His theories were so widely accepted by the public that the mental institutions of the 1930s adopted his approach to treatment and became psychoanalytically oriented. His contributions were so influential that many consider the second mental-health revolution to have begun with public acceptance of his work (Wahler et al., 1972).

As we will discuss in Chapter 4, many criticisms of certain aspects of Freud's theories still continue today. One such criticism by those who employ a human services perspective is that Freud's psychoanalytic theories focus too narrowly on the inner person, excluding the environmental factors that impact upon and influence human behavior.

Freud's impact, though considerable, did not lead to significant changes in the institutional system of care for the mentally ill. Steady deterioration in this system continued. Although there are exceptions, most hospital staffs were generally overworked, understaffed, and poorly trained. Patients were often neglected and many remained in hospitals for years.

The Trend Toward Deinstitutionalization
and Decentralization

Beginning in the early 1950s, certain changes began to develop in several hospitals as the result of growth in the field of **psychopharmacology.** It was now possible through the use of drugs to effectively reduce a patient's bizarre behavior, thereby affording other opportunities for treatment. Many patients previously viewed as untreatable were now able to return to the community while continuing with drug treatments at home (Pasamanick, Scarpitti, & Dinitz, 1967). Many controversies surfaced regarding the alleged widespread misuse or abuse of such drugs. Critics claimed that patients who were not in need of such drugs were given them routinely to keep them under control. Others pointed out that drugs may cause side effects that are as bad as the illness being treated.

Deinstitutionalization became a major policy in institutions during this time. There was a growing belief that people could be treated more successfully in familiar community settings. It appeared to some that deinstitutionalization was implemented more because of financial concerns than for treatment reasons. It was felt that it was just too expensive to keep people institutionalized on a round-the-clock basis, and treatment was initially thought to be less expensive in community settings.

Another change appearing at this time in the large state hospitals was **geographic decentralization.** This procedure, which initially began as a change focused on administrative admissions procedures, was eventually to have a significant effect upon the role of mental patients and their communities. Through this new administrative procedure, patients were placed in hospital wards based on their place of residence prior to admission. Patients were housed and treated with other patients from their own community rather than dispersed throughout the hospital system. Prior to this change, state hospitals generally remained isolated and removed from the communities they served. Through geographic decentralization, communities became more aware of the patients residing therein. Many problems have resurfaced regarding this issue, as many communities have openly voiced fear and dissatisfaction with having mental-health facilities or programs located within their borders.

The Community Mental-Health Movement

The 1960s was an important era for the field of mental health. Many professionals have in fact referred to this decade as the third mental-health revolution (Hobbs, 1964; Wahler et al., 1972). The changes occurring in this period marked another significant shift in human services philosophy as characterized primarily by the community mental-health movement.

To more fully appreciate the sweeping changes advocated by the community mental-health movement of the 1960s, one must look at the various issues that preceded this movement. The community mental-health approach came into being as a result of a growing disenchantment with the traditional large state psychiatric hospital system of the 1950s. Many reformers pointed to what they perceived as the failings of the existing system. Here are some of their criticisms of the traditional system.

1. The traditional system focused exclusively on the treatment and rehabilitation of existing mental illness rather than on the prevention of mental illness.
2. Many of the state psychiatric hospitals were too far away from the communities in which their patients resided.
3. Services were fragmented, with poor coordination between hospital and community agencies.

4. The traditional system emphasized long-term individual therapy to the exclusion of innovative clinical strategies, such as outreach programs, crisis hotlines, and family therapies, that might have been helpful to a greater number of individuals.
5. Nontraditional sources of personnel such as generalist human services workers were not being used despite a growing worker shortage.

The Joint Commission on Mental Illness and Health (1961, p. 2) evidenced the thrust of the community mental-health movements as it recommended that the objective of modern treatment should be the following:

1. To save patients from the debilitating effects of institutionalization as much as possible.
2. If patients require hospitalization, to return them to home and community life as soon as possible.
3. Thereafter to maintain them in the community as long as possible.

In 1963, the Community Mental Health Act was signed into law. This legislation reflected a growing philosophy that mental-health services should be located in the community with the government allocating funds for the creation of these comprehensive community mental-health centers. In Chapter 2, we examined the specific services offered by these centers. Deinstitutionalization was encouraged, resulting in a major shift of mental patients from the large mental hospitals to these community mental-health centers.

The community mental health movement has its advocates and its opponents. There are those who assert that, although the number of patients in the large institutions has decreased and the average length of stay has been reduced considerably, the tendency to readmit patients over and over again to the institutions has correspondingly grown (Wahler, 1971). Other watchful observers of the movement have pointed to instances in which patients have been placed in community settings without adequate supervision. Opponents of the movement indicate that the initial community centers often resembled the traditional hospital organization. The difficulty of developing new mental-health services grew out of a situation in which the workers were already socialized and evolved from the old hospital system (Perlmutter & Silverman, 1972).

Advocates of the movement point to the healing power of the community and the need to normalize the method of treatment as much as possible. If the goal of treatment is eventually to return the patient to a functioning life in the community, the community must be an integral part of the treatment.

The Advent of Generalist Human Services Workers

Another important development in the decade of the 1960s was the formal recognition of the role of generalist human services workers as reflected in the new careers movement. The title **generalist human services worker,** most recognized and utilized today, was originally titled **paraprofessional worker** in the 1960s. In addition, several other titles were also popular during this period of time, including lay therapist and new professional. The 1964 Economic Opportunity Act and the Schneuer Subprofessional Career Act of 1966 provided the impetus and the government funds to recruit and train entry-level workers for a range of positions within the human services field. These related pieces of legislation, coupled with other antipoverty amendments, created approximately 150,000 jobs for generalist human services workers (Reissman, 1967).

The rapid growth of the paraprofessional movement arose from a perceived worker shortage as the new community health centers sought initially to use personnel in more innovative ways. Albee (1960) pointed out the critical shortage of trained mental-health professionals. He predicted an even greater shortage in the future and advocated the creation of a new kind of mental-health generalist worker who could be educationally prepared in a shorter period of time. Through the creation of 2- and 4-year training programs based in colleges, it was believed that aspiring workers could receive enough broad-based education and general human services skills to function on a generalist level alongside the more highly trained professionals. Many of the basic tasks previously performed by psychologists, psychiatrists, or social workers—such as intake interviewing and setting fee schedules—could be delegated to the generalist human services worker, thus freeing the professional to focus selectively on more advanced clinical aspects of treatment and diagnosis that often required more extensive graduate preparation. Chapter 6 provides a closer examination of the diverse functions and roles of generalist human services workers. Table 3-2 on page 159 contains a listing of changes in the mental health movement through history.

Although no single description would adequately encompass the diversity of roles of generalist human services workers, there is agreement on some important common characteristics of the generalist, including the following:

1. The generalist works directly with clients or families (in consultation with other professionals) to provide a variety of services.
2. The generalist is able to work in a variety of settings that provide human services.
3. The generalist is able to work with all of the various professions in the field, rather than affiliating with any one of the professions.
4. The generalist is familiar with a variety of therapeutic services and techniques, rather than specializing in one.

Some of the more common work activities of generalist human services workers include but certainly are not limited to:

- Helping clients in their own environments with various services.
- Helping people get to existing services (as in simplifying bureaucratic regulations and acting as client advocate).

- ◆ Acting as assistants to various specialists (e.g., psychiatrists, psychologists, nurses).
- ◆ Carrying out activities for agencies and programs such as budgeting, purchasing, and personnel matters.
- ◆ Gathering information and organizing and analyzing data.
- ◆ Providing direct care for clients who need ongoing services.
- ◆ Working with various community groups to create needed programs and develop resources.

Since the 1960s, new and expanded roles have been created for generalist human services workers. Gartner (1971), Wahler et al. (1972), and Alley, Blanton, and Feldman (1979), among others, have traced the evolving functions and roles of these workers. The role of the generalist human services worker, once narrowly defined as merely custodial in nature, had grown by the 1970s to include a wide range of therapeutic activities. As Minuchin (1969) noted, the paraprofessional movement initiated a reexamination of professional roles and tasks, which resulted in a renewed interest in environmental factors as opposed to the intrapsychic view of maladaptive behavior. As a result, the human services field of the 1970s through today emphasizes the use of generalist human services workers in roles reflecting the importance of a patient's social and environmental needs.

THE 1990s AND BEYOND

The many tasks and problems facing our human services system today are similar to those faced in previous times. Poverty, unemployment, and mental illness still exist. What is different, however, is that new methods and approaches are needed to deal with the problems that are now a part of our highly complex contemporary society. The civilization of today is unlike any other in history. The rate of change is so rapid and the changes themselves so complex that it is almost impossible for anyone to keep pace with the developments occurring in the field. Societal change, although beneficial in certain respects, has also created significant stress, anxiety, and insecurity for many. As the trend toward specialization increases, more and more people find that their previously acquired skills rapidly become obsolete. Although scientific achievements have increased the life span, the threat of global nuclear war, the AIDS epidemic, and the massive drug problem have given rise to widespread concerns about what type of future awaits us.

In an effort to keep pace with the society of today, the human services system has also become highly complex, specialized, and at times fragmented. As the need for human services appears evident, the conservative trend of the 1990s is toward reduced federal spending for such services. This trend has severely impacted many nonprofit agencies that previously depended on such support. Agencies must develop new sources of funding such as the development of grants from foundations and other private funding sources. In addition, an increasing number of agencies are reaching out to attract and utilize volunteers to help maintain various programs and services affected by reduced funding. As Chapter 7 examines further, the shortage of funds is becoming an increasingly large issue in the 1990s and will continue to be so well into the future. And as our earlier discussion in Chapter 1 indicated, the movement toward privatization of agencies is yet another trend of the 1990s.

Over the past 25 years, with the change from hospital care to community care, there has been a dramatic increase in the use of paraprofessionals or generalist workers in the human services field. At present, they are the single largest group delivering direct care to the mentally ill. One of the more recent trends, which is likely to continue for quite some time, is the establishment of bachelor's degree and master's degree programs in human services. Many programs formerly titled Mental Health Technology or Mental Health Assistant have been changing to adopt the more generic title of Human Services. Within the human services field itself, there is a movement toward the development of generic guidelines that would create a national certification process. This certification would seek to obtain a standard for required basic competencies within the field.

Current population trends indicate an increase in the rate of immigration into the United States. Demographic data suggest that we can expect over a million new arrivals each year in the 1990s (Hernandez, 1989). Our human services system will be hard pressed to meet the needs of this culturally diverse population of people, many of whom possess little or no formal education and see no immediate job opportunities. The great diversity in cultural backgrounds has already initiated many changes in the provision of services and has caused a reexamination of the role of western and nonwestern treatment strategies. Multicultural counseling programs and ethnic sensitivity training are already a part of our current training system, and they are likely to continue on a larger, more formalized scale throughout the 1990s and beyond. Chapter 5 examines the various issues of multicultural awareness in further detail.

Another important population trend in the United States is what many gerontologists refer to as "the graying of America." This refers to the growing number of people in our society aged 65 and older. More than 15% of the population is now over 65, and future trends indicate that by the year 2040 more than 25% of our entire population will be 65 years old or older (Harris, 1990). To understand this trend more clearly, consider that there are currently more people living in the United States over the age of 65 than the total population of the country of Canada. Future trends indicate a growing need to provide specialized services pertaining to the physical and emotional needs of later life.

Clendenin and Kohlberg (1987) suggest that future employment trends are likely to be very problematic and disturbing. The work force may not have the necessary education and training to fulfill job requirements in

TABLE 3–2   Highlights and Legislation in the Mental-Health Movement

800–1300s	Church becomes major provider of services to the mentally ill.
1409	Oldest mental hospital still functioning today is established in Valencia, Spain.
1752	Pennsylvania Hospital for the Mentally Ill is founded.
1792	Phillipe Pinel, director of a French mental institution, believes the insane might be curable and initiates reforms.
1800s	Dorothea Dix and other social reformers help to establish the state psychiatric hospital system in the United States. National Society for Mental Illness (Hygiene) is established to study the care of the insane.
1920–1930s	Freud's theories concerning human behavior gain widespread acceptance.
1937	First International Committee for Mental Hygiene is formed. Hill-Burton Act provides funds for building psychiatric hospital units.
1946	National Mental Health Act establishes federal funds to develop training programs for mental-health professionals.
1948	World Federation for Mental Health is formed.
1950s	Major advances are made in the field of psychopharmacology.
1955	Congress creates Joint Commission on Mental Illness and Health. This committee evaluates the needs of the mentally ill and seeks to make resources available.
1961	World Psychiatric Association is formed.
1963	Mental Retardation Facilities and Community Mental Health Centers Construction Act is passed. Trend begins toward community care for the mentally ill and decentralization of the mental-health system.
1964	Economic Opportunity Act is passed. Passage of Schneuer Subprofessional Career Act gives impetus and funds to recruit generalists for training in human services and mental-health field.
1967	Federal government provides money for the staffing of mental-health centers.
1968	Community Mental Health Centers Act provides for comprehensive services for the mentally ill.
1970	Comprehensive Alcohol Abuse and Alcohol Prevention, Treatment, and Rehabilitation Act is passed.
1974	Juvenile Justice and Delinquency Prevention Act is passed.
1979	Mental Health Systems Act establishes bill of rights for the mentally ill and the right to refuse medication.

(continued)

TABLE 3–2   Highlights and Legislation in the Mental-Health Movement
(continued)

1984	Office of Prevention is established within the National Institute of Mental Health.
1986	Protection and Advocacy for Mentally Ill Individuals Act is passed.
1990	Americans with Disabilities Act is signed into law. It prohibits discrimination against people with disabilities.

high-tech society. Workers will need more than a high school diploma to meet the criteria for obtaining new jobs, and in many instances, a college education will be mandatory. The alarming high school dropout rate, especially in urban areas, and the high rates of illiteracy contribute greatly to an underprepared labor force. This issue is certainly multifaceted and complex, but clearly one part of the solution in the future will be to retrain workers as their skills become obsolete. We also need to train unskilled workers to take on more demanding jobs. Additional societal trends indicate a changing structure of the once typical American family unit. More and more families are now headed by a single parent or parents of the same gender. As the concept of family undergoes change, its impact upon society is not quite clear. Chapter 1 examined this change more extensively.

ADDITIONAL READING

Atchley, R. C. (1991). *Social forces of aging* (6th ed.). Belmont, CA: Wadsworth.

Campbell, R. J. (1989). *Psychiatric dictionary* (6th ed.). New York: Oxford University Press.

Dana, R. H. (1981). *Human services for cultural minorities*. Baltimore, MD: University Park Press.

Ennis, B., & Seigel, L. (1973). *The rights of mental patients*. New York: Avon.

Green, J. W. (1982). *Cultural awareness in the human services*. Englewood Cliffs, NJ: Prentice Hall.

Hampton, J. K. (1991). *The biology of aging*. New York: William C. Brown.

Harris, H. S., & Maloney, D. C. (Eds.). (1996). *Human Services: Contemporary issues and trends*. Boston: Allyn & Bacon.

Hofstadter, R. (1944). *Social Darwinism in American thought*. Boston: Beacon Press.

Iglehart, A. P., & Becerra, R. M. (1995). *Social Services and the ethnic community*. Boston; Allyn & Bacon.

Jones, L. Y. (1980). *Great expectations: America and the baby boom generation*. New York: Coward, McCann & Geohegan.

Katz, M. B. (1986). *In the shadow of the poor house: A social history of welfare in America*. New York: Basic Books.

Lustbader, W. (1990). Mental health services in a community health center. *Generations, 14*(1), 22–24.

Morales, A., & Scheafor, B. W. (1980). *Social work, a profession of many faces.* Boston: Allyn & Bacon.

Nash, K. L., Jr., Lifton, N., & Smith, S. E. (1978). *The paraprofessional: Selected readings.* New Haven, CT: Advocate Press.

Popple, P. R., & Leighninger, L. (1993). *Social work, social welfare and American society* (2nd ed.). Boston: Allyn & Bacon.

Reich, C. A. (1970). *The greening of America.* New York: Random House.

Schorr, A. L. (1986). *Common decency: Domestic policies after Reagan.* New Haven, CT: Yale University Press.

Schulman, E. D. (1991). *Intervention in human services: A guide to skills and knowledge* (4th ed.). New York: Macmillan.

Trattner, W. (1974). *From poor law to welfare state.* New York: Free Press.

Ward, M. J. (1946). *The snakepit.* New York: Random House.

Weinberger, P. E. (1969). *Perspectives on social welfare.* New York: Macmillan.

Woody, R. H. (1984). *The law and the practice of human services.* San Francisco: Jossey-Bass.

REFERENCES

Albee, G. W. (1960). The manpower crisis in mental health. *American Journal of Public Health, 50,* 1895–1900.

Alley, S. Blanton, Jr., & Feldman, R. (Eds.). (1979). *Paraprofessionals in mental health: Theory and practice.* New York: Human Sciences Press.

Andriola, J., & Cata, G. (1969). The oldest mental health hospital in the world. *Hospital and Community Psychiatry, 20,* 42–43.

Bloom, B. L. (1977). *Community mental health: A general introduction.* Pacific Grove: CA: Brooks/Cole.

Clendenin, J. L., & Kohlberg, W. H. (1987, September 20). The road ahead. *The New York Times Magazine.*

Coleman, J. (1976). *Abnormal psychology and modern life.* Glenview, IL: Scott, Foresman.

Fisher, W., Mehr, J., & Truckenbrod, P. (1974). *Human services: The third revolution in mental health.* New York: Alfred.

Gartner, A. (1971). *Paraprofessionals and their performance.* New York: Praeger.

Harris, D. K. (1990). *Sociology of aging* (2nd ed.). New York: Harper & Row.

Hernandez, H. (1989). *Multicultural education: A teacher's guide to content and process.* Columbus, OH: Merrill.

Hobbs, N. (1964). Mental health's third revolution. *American Journal of Orthopsychiatry, 34,* 822–833.

Hoch, P. H., & Knight, R. P. (Eds.). (1965). *Epilepsy: Psychiatric aspects of convulsive disorders.* New York: Hafner.

Joint Commission on Mental Health Illness and Health. (1961). *Action for mental health.* New York: Basic Books.

Minuchin, S. (1969). The paraprofessional and the use of confrontation in the mental health field. *American Journal of Orthopsychiatry, 34,* 722–729.

Pasamanick, B., Scarpitti, F. R., & Dinitz, S. (1967). *Schizophrenics in the community.* New York: Appleton-Century-Crofts.

Perlmutter, F., & Silverman, H. A. (1972). C.M.H.C.: A structural anachronism. *Social Work, 17,* 78–84.

Perry, J. A., & Perry, E. K. (1988). *The social web* (5th ed.). New York: Harper & Row.

Reissman, F. (1967). Strategies and suggestions for training paraprofessionals. *Community Mental Health Journal, 3,* 103–110.

Rimm, D. C., & Somervill, J. W. (1977). *Abnormal psychology.* New York: Academic Press.

Russell, J. B. (1972). *Witchcraft in the Middle Ages.* Ithaca, NY: Cornell University Press.

Wahler, H. J. (1971). What is life all about or who all needs paraprofessionals? *The Clinical Psychologist, 24*(3), 11–14.

Wahler, H. J., Johnson, R. & Uhrich, K. (1972). *The Expediter Project: Final report to National Institute of Mental Health.* State of Washington: Department of Social and Health Services.

Theoretical Perspectives

INTRODUCTION

A theory is a statement that attempts to explain connections among events. It is not in itself a fact, but a concept that brings facts together into a sensible overall picture. There is nothing mysterious about the process of making, testing, and using theories. Even quite young children construct useful theories about events in their daily lives. These take the form of ideas such as, *If I say I'm sorry, Mommy won't hit me* or *If I do good at school, my parents will give me a present.* These ideas are based on observations of previous events. On a simple level, they enable the child to understand, predict, and sometimes control the environment.

The process of theory making goes on throughout life. The fact is that the individual is constantly being bombarded with incoming stimuli. Without mental structures to classify and organize these events, the individual would be overwhelmed and unable to function in an organized way. In this sense, theory making is absolutely essential to successful living.

Just as personal theories enable the individual to function effectively, scientific theories enable the human services worker to function effectively. In this chapter, we look at a number of major theories that help workers understand the causes of disorders and plan effective action to either prevent or treat these disorders. We begin by discussing the nature of scientific theory. We then examine two general theoretical frameworks for helping: the medical model and the human services model. This is followed by a detailed look at three more specific theoretical viewpoints that can be applied within the broader frameworks. These are the psychoanalytic, the humanistic, and the behavioristic systems of therapy. The chapter includes a brief look at some nontraditional paths to fulfillment and closes with an account of systems theory, which some believe holds great promise as a theoretical viewpoint for the future.

SCIENTIFIC THEORY

There is no hard-and-fast distinction between personal and scientific theories. All theories are intended to help us make sense of the world around us. The distinguishing features of scientific theories are that they are consciously formed, tested, and shared with other researchers. One purpose of scientific theories is to serve as a guide to future research. Ideally, theories should be continually tested and modified to fit newly discovered facts.

Of course, scientists often fall short of this ideal. Many theories once accepted by reputable authorities are now completely discredited. Sometimes incorrect theories are based on faulty, or limited, observations. For example, a number of early investigators attributed criminal behavior to inherited tendencies (Lombroso-Ferrero, 1911). In this view, the criminal was a "born type" who could be distinguished from "normals" by certain physical traits, such as a low forehead, an unusually shaped head, eyebrows growing together above the bridge of the nose, and protruding ears. Modern investigators found that this theory did not account for criminals who lacked these physical characteristics and that it ignored data that linked criminal behavior to poverty and certain social conditions.

Theories can be no better than the facts on which they are based. Some investigators are not above faking data to "prove" a point. It was recently reported, for example, that a distinguished British psychologist had falsified—actually made up—data that supported his contention that intelligence is inherited. We can only hope that this kind of gross faking is rare. On the other hand, it is by no means unusual for a scientist to be biased in favor of cherished beliefs. In fact, everyone shows this sort of bias at times. People are more likely to accept evidence that support their beliefs than evidence that goes against these beliefs. Because theories often serve as guides to action, the blind acceptance of an incorrect theory may have harmful consequences. The only remedy against the hazards of bias is to be receptive to *all* of the relevant facts in a situation.

THEORIES ABOUT HUMAN DISORDERS

Now that we have presented a general idea of what theories are and what purposes they serve, our focus shifts to the main concern of this chapter— theories about human disorders. Very simply, these are theories that try to explain why and how certain disorders come about. Based on this understanding, each theory proposes certain treatments designed to alleviate the disorder in question. Theories, then, are not merely matters for dry academic discussion; they also have a powerful impact on what the helper does for or to the client.

Traditionally, human disorders are divided into two main types: physical and mental or psychological. The latter will be emphasized because these are of main concern to the human services worker. All of the major theories to be reviewed offer reasonable explanations of how and why psychological disorders occur. However, the explanations are quite different from one another. Why are there so many different explanations? There are several possible answers to this question. One is that human behavior is so complex that no single theory can explain every disorder. Another answer is that each theory tends to focus on certain kinds of abnormal behavior. A third point, related to the other two, is that different theories tend to focus on different levels of observation. Before proceeding to the specific theories, it is necessary to clarify what is meant by *levels of observation.*

Three Levels of Observation

Each theory tends to focus on one of three general levels of observation: the biological, the psychological, or the social level. In other words, researchers tend to specialize in the study of events at one particular level.

From the *biological* point of view, an organism is viewed as a physical or biochemical system. Disease, physical damage to the body, or inadequate development of internal organs may all hamper an individual's ability to get along in the outside world. For example, some forms of mental retardation are due to abnormal development of the brain and nervous system. It is also known that one form of senility is due to a breakdown in the blood vessels of the brain. Physical abnormalities are the main province of medical science. The medical approach to treatment (to be described) employs medication, surgery, and other physical methods to cure, or least ameliorate, disorders.

From the *psychological* point of view, the individual attempts to gain gratification of needs and goals by interacting with the outer environment. In order to adapt successfully, the person must behave in ways that suit the immediate situation. The person's skills, motives, needs, emotions, and ways of handling stress all play a role in this adaptive struggle. Obviously, some individuals are more successful than others in attaining satisfactions. Some of the psychological problems familiar to the human services worker are clients' low self-esteem, lack of skills, and self-defeating ways of trying to achieve stated goals in life.

The *social* level refers to the powerful influences of family, schools, neighborhood, and society. To the human services worker, one of the most important social variables is socioeconomic status. This includes specific factors such as income, level of education, and the prestige value of one's occupation. High-level executives, administrators, and professionals rate higher on this scale than do blue-collar workers and welfare recipients. The majority of those who receive help from human services are concentrated in the lower income levels.

There is controversy, and some confusion, about applying these three levels of observation to specific disorders. There are biological, psychological, and social theories about alcoholism, schizophrenia, criminality, and many other disorders. Various investigators proclaim that one level is more important than the other two in causing these disorders. There is, for example, intense debate about the relative importance of inherited physical traits in predisposing an individual toward one disorder or another. The fact is that all three levels may be involved in the development of a certain disorder.

Multiple Causes

In both medical and social sciences, it is now generally accepted that many disorders have more than one cause. For example, on the biological level, the immediate cause of tuberculosis is infection by a certain bacterium.

Since this is a common bacterium, the following question arises: Why do some people come down with the disorder, whereas others do not? The answer is that the victim is often in a physically run-down state in which the body's normal defenses against infection have been depleted. Further investigation usually shows that a number of psychological and social factors play a role in getting the victim into this state. For example, the lifestyle of the patient often seems to have a frantic, overactive quality. Social factors are implicated by the fact that the incidence of tuberculosis is far higher in poor than in affluent communities. Obviously, then, biological, psychological, *and* social factors may all be involved in causing a particular disorder.

Political Implications of Theory

The controversies among theories are not merely matters of factual evidence but also involve underlying political and economic factors. For example, it makes a difference if the behavior problems associated with poverty are attributed to (a) psychological defects such as laziness or lack of intelligence or (b) the impact of society, which has stacked the cards against the poor. In the first case, the individual is held fully responsible for his or her poor circumstances. In the second, the person is seen as the victim of social and economic factors beyond his or her control. Obviously, a more sympathetic response goes along with this second point of view.

MODELS OF DYSFUNCTION

This brief introduction to theory paves the way for discussion of two general models of dysfunction: the **medical model** and the **human services model.** The term *model* in this context refers to a general theoretical point of view about the causes of disorders. Perhaps the earliest model was the religious or magical perspective, which emphasized evil spirits as the cause of illness. The medical model, with its scientific emphasis, gradually replaced the spiritual notion of causation. The medical model emphasizes biological factors, such as bacterial, viral, or genetic agents, in causing diseases. More recently, the human services mode, with its focus on social factors, has challenged the medical model. We will first take a detailed look at the medical model.

THE MEDICAL MODEL

As applied to psychological disorders, this model stresses the causative role of factors *within* the individual. Adherents of the medical model do not claim that all so-called mental disorders are due to biological or organic factors. In fact, they make a distinction between *organic* and *functional* disorders.

The organic disorders are caused by physical abnormalities of the brain, nervous system, and other internal systems. Epilepsy, senility, some kinds of retardation, and certain psychotic states are examples of disorders in which some physical abnormality has been found to play a role. Organic disorders may be caused by inherited defects, chemical imbalances, viral infections, malnutrition, and various drugs and poisons. Disorders associated with physical damage are likely to be longstanding, whereas those associated with drugs may represent temporary disorders of brain function.

The functional disorders, in contrast, are due to psychological factors operating within the individual. These might include poorly controlled drives and impulses, unrealistic ideas, and unresolved conflicts. Addictions, antisocial tendencies, neuroses, and some psychotic reactions are classified as functional disorders. This means that the major causes are presumed to relate to the personality of the individual rather than to any physical defects. There are some disorders, such as the schizophrenias, that cannot be classified with great confidence because of doubt about the causes.

Medical Procedure

Regardless of whether a disorder is organic or functional, the procedures of medical practice can be applied to it. This means that a certain psychological disorder can be approached as though it were a physical disorder like measles or tuberculosis. The first step in medical and psychiatric practice is to arrive at a **diagnosis,** which means to classify and label the disorder according to the presenting symptoms. Next comes the formulation of a treatment plan, which may include medication, shock therapy, psychotherapy, and/or confinement to a mental hospital. The treatment is related to the **prognosis,** which is an educated guess about what degree of recovery can be expected for the patient.

For example, a young man became despondent over losing his fiancée to someone else. He made the rather dramatic suicidal gesture of threatening to jump from the roof of an apartment building but let himself be talked down by the police. He was taken to a community mental-health center and admitted to a ward for observation and treatment. He was diagnosed as suffering from a depressive reaction. The treatment plan included brief counseling sessions to help ventilate his feelings of hurt, loss, and anger. In addition, he was put on a mood-elevating drug. In view of his history of good functioning, the prognostic outlook was favorable. This is the medical model in action: A psychological or emotional reaction is handled with the basic procedures of medicine.

Treatment Approaches of the Medical Model

Because the medical model is accepted by many professionals employed in mental hospitals, prisons, schools, mental retardation centers, and other settings, the human services worker needs to understand something about the treatments derived from this model.

By far the most common treatment approach is drug therapy, sometimes called chemotherapy. Recent decades have seen the development of a wide variety of powerful drugs that are capable of modifying mood and emotional states. The major tranquilizers, for example, are a class of drugs first introduced to this country in the 1950s. They quickly became a major treatment modality in psychiatric clinics and hospitals when it was found that they suppress or ameliorate some of the disturbed behavior of psychotic patients. They are likely to be used when a patient shows extreme tension, aggressiveness, delusions, hallucinations, or insomnia. Without producing a cure, they often make the patient more manageable by staff. Thorazine, Mellaril, and Stelazine are the trade names of three of the most frequently used drugs of this type.

Another popular treatment approach involves the use of minor tranquilizers to reduce tension and anxiety. In the 1960s, Roche Laboratories introduced two drugs that were members of the chemical family called benzodiazepines: Librium and Valium. These drugs soon captured a large share of the market for psychotropic medications, prompting other drug companies to produce and market similar drugs (Lickey & Gordon, 1991). In 1975, about 85 million prescriptions for benzodiazepines were written in this country. This was followed by a wave of concern in the medical community about the possible overprescription of these medications. As professionals became worried about the risks of abuse, including addiction and dependence, the rate of prescription began to decline. It was found that withdrawal from the drugs may bring serious complications, including an anxiety state more severe than the original anxiety disorder (Miller & Mahler, 1991). However, during the 1980s, there was a gradual return to high consumption of these drugs, until the current level of 60 million annual prescriptions was reached. Most of the prescribing is done by general practitioners rather than by psychiatrists. The drugs provide a handy means of pacifying patients who complain of tension, anxiety, mild depression, and insomnia.

Another relatively recent drug therapy is the use of **lithium carbonate** for persons suffering from manic-depressive disorders. It is particularly useful in controlling the excessive elation, irritability, and talkativeness of the manic phase. Another group of mood-altering drugs is the antidepressants, which have been effective in combating certain types of severe depressive states.

Table 4–1 lists the generic and brand names of some of the frequently prescribed **psychoactive** medications. New drugs are constantly being

TABLE 4–1 Major Types of Psychoactive Medications

Type of Drug	Generic Names	Brand Names	Major Uses	Possible Side Effects
Major Tranquilizers	Chlorpromazine Phenothiazines Haloperidol	Thorazine Stelazine Mellaril Prolixin Compazine Haldol	Sometimes called antipsychotics, these medications help control severe anxiety, agitation, delusions, hallucinations, hostility, and hyperactivity associated with schizophrenia and other psychotic states.	Confusion, restlessness, insomnia, euphoria, exacerbation of psychotic symptoms, muscle weakness, and fatigue. Prolonged use may result in tardive dyskinesia, a neurological disorder featuring involuntary muscular movements.
Minor Tranquilizers	Benzodiazepines Meprobamates	Valium Librium Serax Centrax Restoril Xanax Miltown Equanil	These antianxiety medications are widely prescribed by primary care physicians when anxiety, irritability, and agitation—symptoms often related to situational stress—become severe enough to interfere with daily functioning.	Drowsiness, dizziness, headache. Since these drugs depress the central nervous system, reflexes are slowed. Caution must be taken when driving and operating machinery. Dangerous when used in combination with alcohol and other CNS depressants. Some patients may become addicted to these drugs.
Antidepressants	Tricyclics MAO inhibitors Combination agents	Elavil Sinequan Tofranil Aventyl Nardil Parnate Limitrol Triavil	These medications generally lift mood and are used to combat severe depressions. They have been found to be particularly effective in endogenous depression—having no apparent situational cause. The MAO inhibitors are often used in patients who do not respond favorably to treatment with tricyclics.	Anxiety, restlessness, exacerbation of psychosis, dry mouth, blurred vision, skin rash, fatigue, sensitivity to sun.
Second-Generation Antidepressants	Fluoxetine Setraline Paroxetine	Prozac Zoloft Paxil	Although the major use is still to elevate mood, these medications are increasingly being used to treat eating disorders, including obesity, and obsessive-compulsive disorders.	May cause nausea and headaches but are reported to have fewer undesired effects than the earlier antidepressants.

Type	Generic	Brand Names	Use	Side Effects
Antimanic	Lithium carbonate	Eskalith Lithane Lithonate	Primarily used to treat manic episodes and bipolar affective disorders. It is also being used in some cases of schizophrenia.	Levels of lithium in the blood must be monitored and carefully regulated, as it can act as a toxic agent impairing various bodily processes. Overdosage may produce serious complications and may be lethal.
Sedative-hypnotic	Barbiturates	Triazolam Halcion Phenobarbital Seconal Amytal Numbutal Penthothal	Used to produce a calming effect and to induce sleep. Can be used to treat convulsive disorders.	Extreme dullness and drowsiness. May be deadly when taken with alcohol or other CNS depressants. May be habit forming.
Anticonvulsant	Phenytoin sodium Primodone	Dilantin Mysoline	Used to help control epileptic seizure disorders.	Insomnia, nervousness, motor twitchings, headache, nausea, vomiting, and many other symptoms.
Stimulant	Amphetamines	Benzedrine Dexedrine Methedrine Ritalin	Have been used in treating overweight and narcolepsy (uncontrolled fits of sleep), and have a paradoxical effect on hyperkenetic or hyperactive children, calming them down.	Insomnia, restlessness, talkativeness, loss of appetite, paranoid ideation, and possible aggression and anxiety.
Antialcoholic	Disulfiram	Antabuse	Used as an aversive therapy in treatment of alcoholism. When alcohol is taken while a person is using Antabuse, a potent negative reaction occurs including nausea, vomiting, racing heart, and flushing.	Use is contraindicated in people with certain physical disorders; may be carcinogenic with prolonged use, and may cause nervous system toxicity.

marketed, and it is likely that the table will need updating by the time you see it. All human services workers in medical settings are advised to prepare their own table of medications commonly used in their service. An essential reference book is the *Physicians' Desk Reference* (PDR), a comprehensive text on all kinds of drugs that is updated annually. We suggest that students learn how to use it.

The Prozac Revolution.   During the past several years, a second generation of antidepressants has gained enormous popularity. Chemically different from the **MAO inhibitors** and **tricyclics,** these medications alter the sensitivity of two neurotransmitters, norepinephrine and serotonin. Here is how they work.

Signals are carried from sending neurons to receiving neurons by means of neurotransmitters, which are actually chemicals released from nerve endings of the sending neurons. A pumplike mechanism in the nerve endings acts to recapture the neurotransmitter. The purpose of the pump is to prevent the neurotransmitter from remaining in the synapse too long. One theory holds that among depressed people this reuptake mechanism is *too* effective, resulting in an insufficient amount of certain transmitters and reduced signaling. The **second-generation antidepressants** indicated in Table 4–1 act specifically to increase the amount of available serotonin at the synapse, thereby increasing transmission of signals. The medication acts promptly, and it isn't clear why it usually takes about 2 weeks for the depressed patient to experience improved mood. In any case, the three leading second-generation antidepressants—Prozac, Zoloft, and Paxil—accounted for more than 60% of antidepressant drug sales during recent years (Cowley, 1994). The most popular, Prozac, has been prescribed for over 11 million people throughout the world and racked up over $1 billion in sales during a recent 6-year period. These medications are now also being prescribed for eating disorders, as well as for persons who feel somewhat miserable but have no clear-cut disorder.

The popularity of these medications has prompted concern among professionals and the public at large. Many people believe the drugs are being glamourized and overused and that possible dangers have been ignored. Prozac, introduced in 1987, was soon under attack by professionals who reported cases in which patients began experiencing violent or suicidal tendencies after taking the drug (Comer, 1995, p. 334). The negative publicity surrounding Prozac reduced its popularity during the early 1990s, but Dr. Peter Kramer's (1993) book, *Listening to Prozac,* served to increase interest once again. Although some patients were admittedly not affected by the drug, others were able to experience a new outlook on the world and a new, more positive way of interacting with others.

We have focused on these medications because of the important questions they raise:

Will the use of these and other psychoactive medications reduce the
need for counselors and psychotherapists?

Will extended use of these drugs "rob people of the adaptive use of de-
spair" and interfere with their "realistic connection" to external
events (Comer, 1995, p. 335)?

Should these medications be prescribed for persons who have no definite psychological disorder but who just want to feel better?

Will extended use of these drugs take away the pain and vulnerability
that people need to grow and to be creative?

We have no pat answers to these difficult questions but offer them for class
discussion.

Drugs are only one type of medical model treatment. A number of convulsive therapies have been developed for use with psychiatric patients. The
most common of these in current use is the famous, or infamous, **electroconvulsive therapy** (ECT). Used extensively in private psychiatric hospitals,
it involves administering an electric shock at the patient's temples for a
brief (0.1–0.5 second) duration. Treatments are given several times a week
and may continue for 5 or 6 weeks. ECT is used mainly to treat patients
who are depressed, especially when there is no obvious external stress such
as loss of job or divorce. Probably no other form of therapy evokes such
negative feelings as this one. Despite modern trappings, it appears to many
to be some kind of medieval torture. During the 1950s, there were many
reports of abuse and sloppy administration of the procedure. It was used
with a wide variety of disorders, and results were often unfavorable. Recent
refinements of the technique have reduced side effects and increased its
effectiveness.

Another medical-type treatment called **psychosurgery** has also been
sharply criticized by human service workers. The most frequently used procedure of this type is the **lobotomy**, which involves cutting nerve fibers con-
necting the frontal lobes to other parts of the brain. Literally thousands of
these operations were performed on mental patients during the years before the introduction of major tranquilizers. It was used mainly with patients who were so aggressive that they presented severe management
problems. Unfortunately, the procedure often produces serious irreversible
side effects such as lethargy, childish behavior, and mental dullness.

Valenstein (1986) has provided a fascinating history of psychosurgery.
He tells the story of how it came about that "tens of thousands of mutilat-
ing brain operations were performed on mentally ill men and women in
countries around the world" (p. 3). By the 1960s, it was apparent that these
lobotomies were causing severe damage to the victims. These operations,
now thought bizarre and obsolete, were part of the mainstream medicine
of their time. They were due in part to the readiness of many psychiatrists
to believe in simple, biological approaches to the treatment of the mentally
ill. Valenstein also shows that the physicians who developed and promoted
this procedure were driven by intense ambition to deceive themselves and

others about the value of their "cure." These events clearly show the need for clinical testing of new, potentially harmful procedures before they are allowed to be used on a large scale.

Other therapies related to medical approaches, such as rehabilitation and occupational therapy, are described in Chapter 6.

Criticisms of the Medical Model

A number of authors have cried out against the injustices that arise from the medical/psychiatric approach to mental illness. Szasz (1973), for example, charged that his psychiatric colleagues were guilty of persecuting mental patients under the guise of treating them. In particular, he questioned the validity of labeling certain individuals as mentally ill when, in fact, they were merely suffering from problems in living. Mental illness, he went on, is a myth, not a genuine disease at all. The underlying purpose of labeling (diagnosing) certain people as mentally ill is to provide society with a convenient means of getting rid of undesirable deviates. These are typically people who have committed no real crime but are bothersome, annoying, or frightening to other people.

Along the same lines, Kovel (1980) charged that psychiatry's focus on the psychological aspects of the patient "is a handy way of mystifying social reality" (p. 73). The same author argued that psychiatrists exert social control over social misfits by telling them they have a case of this or that and then imposing a treatment plan. What is left out of the process is acknowledgment of the damaging role of poverty, poor housing, lack of opportunity, unemployment, and other social ills.

A Psychologist Questions the Medical Model.   Psychologist Laurence Simon (1994) voiced some deep concerns about the medical model in a newsletter sent to his colleagues. He said that he was weary of calling the victims of abuse, who came to him for help, "sick" or "mentally ill." The act of diagnosing a person, Simon argued, creates barriers to understanding that person and conflicts with the therapist's desire to see the client in humanistic terms. Labeling someone as mentally ill tends to invalidate that person's perceptions and feelings. Simon invited his colleagues to meet with him to discuss these issues. In response, he received many calls from therapists who were pleased that someone had given voice to their own doubts, confusion, and anger. Some psychologists believed that they were not really employing a medical procedure when they worked with "patients" in psychotherapy, but they had no alternatives to this terminology. In the end, no one agreed to get involved in meeting to deal with these concerns. They were frankly afraid of challenging the **status quo.** Therapists who refused to assign a diagnosis on insurance forms felt they risked losing clients and, thereby, risked reducing their income. Others felt that they could not freely express their doubts about the medical model to their supervisors in the settings in which they worked.

Simon (1994) proposed an alternative to the medical model based on a psychoeducational approach. His psycho"therapy" is a noncoercive process in which the client is helped to evaluate past experiences, perceive the present more accurately, and then determine future goals based on this understanding. Clients are helped to distinguish realities from fantasies and to find meaning in their lives, but they are not diagnosed or judged. Client and therapist are essentially equals, sharing some psychological processes but each viewing the world based on his or her unique life experiences. In this psychoeducational form of therapy, clients learn to apply "scientific" rules of evidence to their own values, beliefs, and attitudes. They also study the impact of society, job, school, and family on their lives and are provided with the tools needed to evaluate their personal history. If all goes well, the process frees clients to think, feel, and act in a genuine way and allows them to choose their own lifestyle.

THE HUMAN SERVICES MODEL

The **human services model** received its major impetus during the 1960s. It was closely associated with social movements devoted to bettering the lives of oppressed minority groups. Human services workers thought of themselves as warriors and sometimes even as revolutionaries. Impatient with the medical model and its emphasis on the inner person, these workers wanted to bring about great social changes by improving the environment. In particular, they focused on the harsh external conditions that oppressed the lives of the poor. These workers were not interested in formulating complex theories. Their attitude was pragmatic—that is, based on a spirit of practical problem solving (Fisher, Mehr, & Truckenbrod, 1974). The idea was if something worked, use it.

The basic assumption of this model is that maladaptive behaviors are often the result of a failure to satisfy basic human needs. The first step in intervention is not diagnosis but an assessment of the victim's life situation with a view to discovering what needs are not being met. The person may be in need of decent housing, medical attention, a job, or a more adequate diet. Others may be lacking these essentials and may also be extremely lonely and in need of social interaction. It is not surprising that emotional problems are intensified by such factors as unemployment, loneliness, and low social status. Society, not the individual, is seen as the culprit. Therefore, society must be prodded to provide the needed goods and services.

Hansell's Theory

One of the most elaborate theories used by human services workers is Hansell's motivation theory (Hansell, Wodarczyk, & Handlon-Lathrop, 1970). He and his colleagues theorized that people have to achieve seven basic attachments in order to meet their needs. If a person does not achieve each attachment, he or she goes into crisis or state of stress. Here is a list of the seven basic attachments, along with signs of failure of each one.

1. Food, water, and oxygen, along with informational supplies. Signs of failure: boredom, apathy, and physical disorder.
2. Intimacy, sex, closeness, and opportunity to exchange deep feelings. Signs of failure: loneliness, isolation, and lack of sexual satisfaction.
3. Belonging to a peer group such as social, church, or school group. Signs of failure: not feeling part of anything.
4. A clear, definite self-identity. Signs of failure: feeling doubtful and indecisive.
5. A social role that carries with it a sense of being a competent member of society. Signs of failure: depression and a sense of failure.
6. The need to be linked to a cash economy via a job, a spouse with income, social security benefits, or other ways. Signs of failure: lack of purchasing power, possibly an inability to purchase essentials.
7. A comprehensive system of meaning with clear priorities in life. Signs of failure: sense of drifting through life, detachment, and alienation.

Human Services Interventions

Hansell's scheme readily lends itself to the task of helping the client in practical ways. The worker needs to find ways to satisfy some of the client's unmet needs. The client's complaints are related to the signs of failure just described. Sometimes, the nature of the unmet need is blatantly obvious, but at other times, it may be quite subtle. The client is not always able to cooperate with the helper. For example, the client may deny having a certain need or may feel demeaned by accepting the kind of help available. The aim of human services counseling is usually to link the client with sources of satisfaction. This might involve helping the client secure welfare benefits, find a job, join a club or social group, return to school, or locate a temporary shelter. The focus is on solving problems here and now. Past problems and bad experiences may be discussed, but they are not the main focus of counseling.

The human services worker is usually a generalist trained to work in a variety of agencies to provide across-the-board services to clients and their families (Southern Regional Education Board, 1978). By definition, a generalist is familiar with a variety of therapeutic approaches rather than specializing in one or two areas. The main goal of intervention is usually to identify the needs and problems of the client and then to provide resources to meet the needs and solve the problem. Of course, the worker is not usually able to meet needs in a direct, personal sort of way but is familiar with service providers in the community. These include doctors, ministers, lawyers, police, parole officers, mental-health professionals, and just about anyone else who may be able to help the client. If needed services are not available, the worker may be able to influence the community to set up new programs. More of this is discussed in Chapter 8.

A wide variety of roles may be played by the human services worker, each calling for special skills. The worker may be an advocate, a mobilizer, a teacher, or an administrator. The skills required by these activities are discussed in further detail in Chapter 5. The immediate point is that the underlying purpose is usually the same: identifying and meeting the needs of clients.

Human services workers have sometimes criticized mental-health professionals (psychiatrists, clinical psychologists, and social workers) for overlooking obvious practical solutions to human problems. One reason for this oversight is that these professionals are often trained in intricate psychological theories and treatment methods. They often see problems as reflecting deep emotional conflicts rather than poverty and other external factors. Psychoanalytic theories in particular confer status and prestige on therapists. One author suggested that the mundane problems of poverty hold little fascination for the middle-class professional, who would prefer to psychologize about the poor and prescribe the latest fashion in psychotherapy (Pelton, 1978).

ISSUES UNDERLYING CONFLICT BETWEEN MODELS

The conflict between adherents of the medical and human services models goes far beyond disputes over theory. A host of issues related to power, money, and licensing have not been fully resolved. For example, human services workers maintain that the criteria for delivering service should center around competence to do the job. They point out that **indigenous workers** who live in the community served are often more effective in helping residents than highly educated professionals. They also point out that generalist human services workers are often able to perform counseling and therapy just as effectively as traditional professionals. Without denying the usefulness of indigenous workers and paraprofessionals, traditional mental-health professionals are likely to emphasize the importance of advanced academic training, degrees, and licenses in determining job duties, salaries, and responsibilities. They see themselves as supervisors of workers with less academic training. Each side accuses the other of basing claims on narrow self-interest rather than considering the needs of the clients.

Although this topic is discussed further in subsequent chapters, we can state here that human services workers are steadily increasing in numbers and assuming more and more responsibility for delivery of services. With this growth has come an increased desire for professional training and status. What is emerging is a new breed of professional, trained not in medical model disciplines but in human services.

THE HOLISTIC TREND IN MEDICAL THEORY

As we have seen, the traditional medical model views disease as a departure from a biological norm and, accordingly, stresses biological or physical approaches to treatment. Increasingly, this model is being criticized for its limited scope and for overlooking the social settings in which disease occurs. The *holistic* approach, which considers all aspects of a person's life, is gaining favor among both physicians and human service workers as an alternative model. It is based on the idea that environmental, social, and psychological factors may all contribute to illness or to health. It follows that health promotion need not be limited to biological or physical interventions. Practitioners of holistic healing attempt to find a balance between a person's mind, body, and spirit in a given environment. In specific cases, the holistic ideal may translate into any of the following kinds of treatment: changes in diet, meditation, relaxation, biofeedback, and stress reduction (Popple & Leighninger, 1990). Because it emphasizes lifestyle factors, the holistic approach lends itself to prevention of illness. Holistic programs, aimed at promoting healthier lifestyles, have been established in industrial, hospital, and school settings.

Psychoneuroimmunology (PNI).   This is a new field of study that has already provided evidence that supports the basic ideas of the holistic model. PNI attempts to find connections between psychological states, the nervous system, and the immune system. To use somewhat outdated terminology, it is the study of interactions between the mind and the body. As Lerner (1994, p. 137) explained, "emotional states . . . and behavior patterns may profoundly affect not only our symptoms but the progress of our disease itself." Experimental studies have shown that acute stressors (e.g., electric shock, bright lights, extreme temperatures, or overcrowding) often cause suppression of the immune system in animals. The immune system is our first line of defense against disease: It consists of complex mechanisms that detect and destroy foreign invaders such as bacteria and viruses. It also defends against cancer cells that originate within the body. Early findings, reviewed by Lerner (1994), indicated that humans under stress also undergo a weakening of the immune system, putting them at increased risk of infectious disease and tumor growth. These findings help explain the repeatedly found connection between disease and stressful life events that we discussed in Chapter 1. Lerner (1994) expressed astonishment at the lack of attention paid to emotional factors by some conventional doctors in the treatment of cancer and other serious disorders.

Alternative Medicine.   Lynn Payer (1988), a leading medical journalist, compared medical practices in the United States with those of several modern European nations. She found that American medicine is more aggressive than that of England, France, and Germany. American doctors perform more invasive diagnostic examinations and more surgery than others. For example, an American woman has two or three times the chance of having a hysterectomy as her counterpart in Europe. When drugs are used, they are likely to be prescribed at higher doses, and more powerful drugs are preferred. In contrast, physicians in Europe are more likely to use "soft" medicine based on the healing power of nature, including the use of spas, herbs and plants, and special diets. There is also a greater emphasis on spiritual healing than is found in conventional treatment in this country.

Some Americans are questioning the value of the harsh, invasive methods so often employed by their physicians. Deep anesthesia, surgery, radiation, and chemotherapy often produce serious undesirable effects along with their benefits. Up to one-third of American patients have been seeking alternative methods. Some seek alternatives when they have not been helped by traditional medicine, but an increasing number are simply bypassing the regular doctor. Still other patients seek alternative treatments for certain conditions and regular treatment for other conditions (Ricks, 1995). There is a large menu of unconventional methods from which to choose. For example, asthma, chronic pain, drug addiction, and other disorders may be treated by means of **acupuncture,** a traditional Chinese method in which needles are inserted into the skin at certain critical points. Chinese doctors believe that a system of meridians, or energy pipelines, runs through the body. The points at which the needles are placed are like valves where the energy levels can be adjusted. Although some may question whether these meridians really exist, there is little doubt that acupuncture has proved its value in controlling pain and nausea. Other uses are now being seriously researched (Lerner, 1994). Also growing in popularity is Chinese herbal medicine, which has a very long history of use in the Far East.

A number of doctors are now providing nutritionally oriented alternatives to more conventional drug-oriented approaches. Medical schools have long been criticized for failing to educate doctors in nutrition, but they are beginning to make up for this deficiency. It is well known that poor nutrition, particularly the high-fat/high-sugar diet of Americans, contributes to heart disease, high blood pressure, diabetes, and other ills. Thus, it makes sense to seek improved health through better nutrition. Perhaps the most dramatic example of this approach was provided by Dr. Dean Ornish (1990) who showed that a combination of strict, low-fat diet, meditation, and stress reduction could actually reverse heart disease in many patients. A wide variety of other disorders are also being treated by means of herbs, diet, and special nutrients. It is believed that certain foods, such as garlic, can boost the immune system or otherwise help the body fight disease.

Visualization or imagery therapy has received a good deal of attention in the popular media in recent years. For example, one story described how a cancer victim, who happened to be a nurse, vanquished 27 tumors with the help of imaginary knights on white horses (Ricks, 1995). She pictured giant white horses with mounted knights stabbing at cancer cells. Although given only months to live, 27 of the 28 tumors disappeared during the formal visualization therapy. The tumor that remains is now benign. In this form of therapy, patients are first taught to relax and then to develop their own images for fighting the disease. Apparently, this technique makes use of the power of suggestion. There is much evidence from religious healing, experimental studies, and other sources that our expectations can sometimes be used to alleviate anxiety and promote healing (Frank & Frank, 1991). The so-called *placebo effect* refers to the strong influence that inactive "medications," such as sugar pills, may have on a patient's condition. Again, it is the patient's expectations that may influence the effect of a given pill.

There are so many other alternative approaches, such as homeopathic medicine, Hindu methods of healing, and aroma therapy, that we could not possibly detail them all here. Critics have conceded that some of the alternative methods have been proven to be effective, but others may have dubious value in regard to a particular disorder. It is up to the consumer to carefully evaluate the evidence pertaining to a particular therapy before getting involved with it.

The holistic trend in medicine may provide the means of reconciling the medical model with the human services model. This is because the holistic approach recognizes the importance of environmental factors in human disorders. On a practical level, the acceptance of alternative methods of healing will mean a greater role for nonmedical therapists in the treatment of physical illnesses.

SCHOOLS OF THERAPY

This section highlights three perspectives most commonly used in group and individual approaches to psychological problems. These are the psychoanalytic, the humanistic, and the behavioristic schools or systems of therapy.

A "school" in this context is a group of workers who study certain disorders and use similar methods of study. Although the members of a school may disagree about various points, they share certain basic ideas about the causes of psychological disorders. These basic beliefs, in turn, dictate their approach to helping.

New schools typically arise when a group of young researchers begins to question established beliefs. The early psychoanalysts, for example, challenged the prevailing psychiatric opinion of the 1800s that mental disorders were always due to physical defects of the brain or nervous system. The pioneers of analysis studied disorders known as **neuroses** that seemed to be due to emotional rather than physical factors. The psychoanalytic movement, which grew out of this early work, eventually became the dominant approach to mental health during the middle decades of this century. More recently, the psychoanalytic school itself has been challenged by adherents of opposing schools. These later developments cannot be fully appreciated without understanding the basic ideas of psychoanalysis.

THE PSYCHOANALYTIC VIEWPOINT

The development of **psychoanalysis** is very much associated with Sigmund Freud and his followers. Actually, many of Freud's insights, such as the idea of the unconscious mind, had already been discovered by others (Murray, 1988). There is no doubt, however, that Freud was responsible for shaping psychoanalysis into a coherent system of thought. Under Freud's direction, psychoanalysis became one of the influential movements of modern times.

Major Freudian Concepts

The major idea that evolved from psychoanalysis was that neurotic symptoms are the result of conflicts within the patient. Neurotic symptoms include **phobias,** which involve an intense fear of a specific stimulus such as enclosed places; **obsessions,** which involve the repeated intrusions of certain unwanted thoughts into consciousness; and **compulsions,** which require the patient to repeatedly perform some ritualistic act such as hand washing. These and similar complaints are the result of a conflict between a person's sexual and aggressive urges on one hand and society's demands for control of these impulses on the other (Maddi, 1972). The neurotic

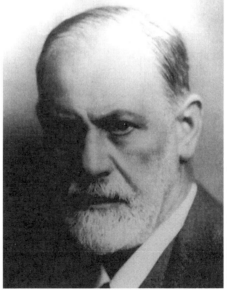

© ARCHIV/Photo Researchers, Inc.

Sigmund Freud

symptoms represent attempts to resolve the conflict. For example, a patient may suffer from a compulsion to wash hands many times a day. This may be an attempt to reduce guilt about urges to masturbate or perform some other "unclean" act. The person is not consciously aware of the underlying desire. According to Freudian theory, the desire must be made conscious and the conflict resolved before the symptoms will go away.

In Freudian terms, the personality is made up of three subsystems: the id, the ego, and the superego. The **id** is the seat of primitive instincts such as sexual and aggressive drives. This part of the personality wants what it wants now. It is the first system to appear in the development of the child. The **ego** is gradually developed to help the child attain gratification in a realistic and socially acceptable manner. The ego employs reason and logic and is concerned with helping the person survive in the world. The **super-ego,** similar to the conscience, is an outgrowth of the taboos and moral values of the society as interpreted by the parents. It aims to inhibit desires that are regarded as wicked or immoral. These three forces are in constant interaction, one factor that makes the theory very complex.

When the ego, the "executive" of personality, is confronted with id impulses that are threatening to get out of control, anxiety and guilt feelings are aroused. In some instances, the anxiety is reduced by coping with the impulses in a satisfactory way. A young person may, for example, decide to gratify sexual urges in the context of marriage. When a realistic resolution of conflict is not available, the ego employs a **defense mechanism** to reduce tension. For example, the entire conflict may be repressed—that is, blocked from awareness. Or the desire may be expressed in some disguised or symbolic way. For example, aggressive urges may be discharged in sports and games, or erotic feelings may be expressed in artistic pursuits.

Therapeutic Concepts

Early in his career, Freud began to work with Josef Breuer, a Viennese physician who pioneered in treating neurotics. Breuer treated a number of patients whose symptoms were "hysterical" in nature—that is, due to emotional rather than physical factors. Some of these patients suffered memory losses or paralysis of certain organs but had no physical defect that could account for the symptoms. Breuer treated them with hypnosis, the method used by earlier therapists. Under hypnosis, patients were often able to recall painful experiences, called traumas, associated with the onset of the symptoms. Breuer found that if the patient could relive the painful emotions associated with the trauma, the symptoms often disappeared. This was the beginning of the "talking cure," a method based on uncovered feelings and experiences buried in the unconscious.

Free Association.   Freud carried on the talking cure with new patients. He gradually developed the technique of **free association,** in which the patient lies on a couch and is encouraged to say anything that comes to mind, no matter how embarrassing it may seem. The basic aim was to bring into conscious awareness any memories or thoughts that had been repressed—that is, pushed into the unconscious because of their threatening nature. While free associating, clients sometimes "blocked," or became unable to bring emotionally charged thoughts into conscious awareness. Freud regarded this as a sign of resistance, which can be defined as any tactic or behavior that works against the production of unconscious material. All clients resist therapy at one time or another. Freud recognized that resistances must be approached with caution because they protect the patient from unbearable anxiety. Overcoming resistances became a regular part of analytic therapy.

Transference.   Freud found that during therapy his clients sometimes experienced feelings, attitudes, and defenses toward him that were derived from previous significant relationships. These feelings and attitudes seemed to have been transferred from the past to the present. The client reacted to Freud as though he were mother, father, or some important figure. Occasionally, patients seemed to fall in love with him and wanted very much to please him. Or sometimes the client would be very hurt if strong feelings were not reciprocated.

According to Freud's theory, **transference** reactions imply that the client is generalizing from past experience. If the mother were warm and overprotective, the client assumes that the analyst will also behave in this way. Over the years, analysis of transference became a central feature of psychoanalysis because it provided a vehicle for resolving old conflicts. Analysis of transference made it possible for analysts to work toward a radical change in the personality of the client.

The goals of psychoanalytic therapy have change greatly over the years. The aim of the early work was simply to relieve neurotic symptoms, whereas later analysts aimed to bring about significant personality change. In this sense, psychoanalysis is the most ambitious system of therapy and one reason that therapy may take many years.

Psychoanalytically Oriented Psychotherapy

The form of treatment developed by Freud came to be known as classical or orthodox psychoanalysis. It required three, four, or even five sessions a week and could go on for many years. Free association, dream analysis, and analysis of transference were the major technical methods. As the analytic movement grew and its practitioners emigrated to America and to other parts of Europe, the treatment was adapted to different cultures. Psychoanalysis became very popular in this country during the 1930s and 1940s, but it was streamlined to suit American needs and tastes. The number of sessions was reduced to one or two a week, an armchair was usually substituted for the couch, and there was relatively greater emphasis on solving present-day problems as opposed to delving into the past. Many psychiatric clinics and mental hospitals employed this modified analytic approach in treatment and training.

Early Revisionists: Adler and Jung

Owing in part to his forceful personality, Freud gained many followers during the early decades of this century. However, some of them found themselves unable to accept critical aspects of his theory. For example, two of his early followers, Alfred Adler and Carl Jung, disputed Freud's claim that repressed sexual drives were the primary cause of neurotic symptoms. To Freud's dismay, they both advanced major revisions of his theory and went on to organize psychoanalytic schools of their own. Both argued that Freud had not fully realized the importance of social and cultural factors in shaping personality. Beyond this area of agreement, Adler and Jung went on to construct widely divergent theories.

Adler's Individual Psychology.   Adler firmly believed that human beings are social beings first and foremost, and that personality is formed by patterns of relationships with others. Adler's best known concepts are those of **inferiority** and **compensation.** He taught that everyone suffers inferiority feelings to some degree because each of us was, in fact, inferior to adults during childhood. In addition, some individuals feel inferior to peers and siblings because of real or imaginary deficiencies. Some children are smaller, weaker, or uglier than others, whereas some compare themselves unfavorably in regard to intelligence or material possessions. The greater the intensity of inferiority feelings, the greater the need to compensate by striving to be superior. The person may seek power, strive for perfection, or develop some special skill or talent to the utmost. The ways in which a person strives for mastery become part of his or her style of life.

Adler developed an approach to treatment that was more direct than the classic approach. He sat opposite the patient and focused the discussion on the patient's attitude toward other people and society. He believed that most people who needed treatment were excessively selfish in their outlook on life. Neurotics, criminals, pampered children, and various social misfits had one feature in common: They thought only or primarily about themselves. The path to psychological health was to develop a strong "social interest." This meant being helpful to others, seeing them as worthy, and controlling one's urge to compete irrationally against others for power. In general, Adler's approach is very congenial to those with a human services orientation. He was very much interested in improving the lives of ordinary people and is credited with being one of the first to set up child guidance centers for the benefit of working-class families.

Jung's Analytical Psychology.   Jung is regarded as the most complex and difficult of the analysts, with some of his concepts verging on mysticism. More than any other analyst, he stressed the importance of the religious and spiritual side of human nature. He delved into occult writings and sought insights into the nature of humans by studying the dreams and myths of primitive peoples. *Man and His Symbols,* edited by Jung (1964), is a good introduction to this mysterious world.

Jung agreed with Freud that behavior is often influenced by ideas buried in the unconscious mind. He went on from there to suggest that the unconscious mind is made up of two layers. The first is the **personal unconscious,** which contains personal experiences that have been repressed or forgotten. The second layer is the **collective unconscious,** which contains experiences inherited from our ancestors. All of us share this collective unconscious, which includes images and ideas never experienced on a personal level. These ancient experiences are embodied in **archetypes,** which are significant racial memories passed from one generation to the next. Some of the archetypes include the Great Mother, the Hero, the Wise Old Man, and God—images that recur in every human society. These archetypes are based on common human experiences such as birth, love, conflict, and death. They can be recovered through dreams and fantasies, and they can be tapped to enhance creative abilities and to provide insights about our personal development.

Jung's approach to treatment stressed the client's need for personal growth. He observed that many of his patients, particularly those in their middle years, complained of a sense of stagnation in their lives. They had completed certain of life's tasks, such as raising their children, and now found themselves without any clear sense of direction. Jung used dream analysis and fantasy to help clients get in touch with their true selves. The images that appeared in fantasy productions were sometimes derived from personal experience and sometimes from the deeper layer of the collective unconscious. Each could provide clues about what was needed to get the personality moving toward growth and fulfillment. Jung's ideas about growth of personality influenced the humanistic theorists, to be discussed later.

Later Revisionists: The Neo-Freudians

The next generation of psychoanalytic thinkers included Karen Horney, Erich Fromm, Erik Erikson, and Harry Stack Sullivan. Though they remained in the psychoanalytic tradition, each departed considerably from the Freudian model. The theories of these neo-Freudians are too complex to be presented in detail. However, some of their major ideas can be briefly reviewed.

The neo-Freudians highlighted social factors in the development of personality. Horney, for example, believed that the child's dominant motive is not gratification of instincts but a striving for security and acceptance by others. When important persons in the family are perceived as hostile and ungiving, the child experiences painful feelings of anxiety. Horney discerned three major trends or tactics that children use to reduce this anxiety and increase security. Some children find themselves in a situation in which moving toward others makes them feel safe; these children may become submissive and self-effacing in their dealings with others. The second pattern shown by some youngsters is a moving away from others; these children seem to act on the premise that if they don't get too close to others, they won't get hurt. The third pattern is moving against others, which may take the form of rebellious and antisocial behavior. The other neo-Freudians developed somewhat different ideas but agreed with Horney's emphasis on social interaction.

The new revisionists all doubted Freud's assumption that adult personality was shaped by early childhood experiences. For example, Sullivan, who founded the interpersonal theory of psychiatry, believed that experiences during the juvenile and adolescent phases could have a profound impact on personality. He felt it was crucial for a youngster to have close friends and confidants during these difficult periods of life. Without close friends, the isolated child runs the risk of sexual difficulties and even serious psychiatric illness in early adulthood. Sullivan attributed his own serious psychological problems to loneliness and isolation during his juvenile years (Perry, 1982). He identified strongly with the young schizophrenic patients he treated at psychiatric hospitals. His treatment approach emphasized the creation of a therapeutic ward environment, and he was one of the first to train ward attendants and nursing personnel in the daily treatment of these patients. His approach is therefore of considerable interest to human services workers who are treating patients in mental hospitals.

Along with the other neo-Freudians, Erikson (1963) stressed the social aspects of human development. He taught that in each stage of life, the person tries to establish an equilibrium between the self and the social world. At each phase of development, the person is faced with a task or a crisis to be resolved. For example, the infant's basic task is to develop a sense of trust in self, others, and the world. Obviously, the infant is totally dependent on others for survival. In an atmosphere of insecurity, the child may develop a sense of mistrust that can retard progress and color later relationships with others. At each later phase, the person is faced with another crisis. Obviously, it would be helpful for the human services worker to have an understanding of the developmental tasks faced by clients at various stages. It is sometimes important to examine the choices a client made at previous stages of life and to consider how these affect current functioning.

Criticisms of Psychoanalysis

No other psychological theory has been subjected to such intense criticism as has psychoanalysis. Some of the early attacks were harsh and highly emotional in tone and may have been triggered by Freud's exposure of sexual problems in Victorian Europe. The day is past when professionals are shocked by frank discussions of sexual matters. However, certain other criticism are not based on outraged sensibilities but on serious doubts about the scientific credibility of psychoanalysis.

Many critics have noted that analysts often base conclusions on what patients remember about their past experience. As Freud himself discovered, there is no way to be sure if the anecdotal reports represent real events, fantasies, or some combination of fact and fancy. There is rarely any independent verification of the events reported by patients. Thus, there is some basis for the criticism that psychoanalysts have built a huge theoretical structure on a weak foundation.

Another serious criticism is that analytic theory lacks predictive value and relies on after-the-fact explanations (Hall & Lindzey, 1978). For example, it is not very helpful to be informed that a client attempted suicide due to a strong death wish because the "explanation" is circular. In other words, the strong death wish is inferred from the behavior itself. Other behaviors are explained in terms of complex interactions between id, ego, and superego. If a patient gives in to sexual impulse, this might be interpreted as a victory for the id over the superego. If the impulse is repressed, the superego has won. The problem is that psychoanalysis does not provide clear rules for predicting *in advance* if one or another part of the personality is going to dominate future behavior.

Another type of criticism centers around the general failure of analysts to report on the effects of their therapy. Considering the popularity of analytic thinking during the 1920s to the mid-1950s, there were very few reports of the outcome of the treatment. Those reports that did surface usually did not include a control group—that is, a comparison group of patients who received no treatments or some other treatment. Prochaska (1984) reviewed some of the relevant studies and concluded that there is still insufficient evidence to judge the effectiveness of analytic therapy. Certainly, there is little to support the claim that psychoanalytic therapy is superior to briefer forms of therapy. The failure of analysts to provide objective evidence about the effects of their therapy was one of the factors that led to its partial eclipse after the 1950s.

Perhaps the most scathing denouncements of Freudian theory have come from those with a human services orientation. Certain implications of Freudian theory can be seen as harmful to the interests of disadvantaged individuals. For example, Freud's idea that the child develops an irrational, unconscious mind early in life seems to imply that behavior is largely determined by these unconscious forces. Maladaptive or antisocial behavior is seen as the outcome of internal forces beyond rational control, which downplays the role of here-and-now environmental events. As Fisher et al. (1974) pointed out, mental-health workers with an analytic point of view focus their efforts on "curing" patients, a process that involves a long search into the past history of the patient. It is also accepted that diagnosis and treatment are lengthy and complicated, requiring considerable expertise and training. The therapy itself tends to require considerable verbal and intellectual skills on the part of the patient. Those who do not possess such skills or a capacity for reflection are looked upon as uninteresting and possibly untreatable cases. These and other aspects of the analytic approach were simply unacceptable to the social activists of the 1960s. They wanted to help people now, and they wanted to do it primarily by changing the environment rather than by changing the person.

Some Useful Applications of Psychoanalytic Concepts.   Now that the turbulent '60s and '70s are behind us, human services workers can examine psychoanalysis in a more dispassionate light. There seems no doubt that psychoanalysis is here to stay. Although no longer predominant, it is one of several therapeutic approaches actively competing for students, adherents, and clients. Certain analytic ideas have withstood the test of time and may be useful to human services workers.

The concept of defense mechanisms is probably the most wisely used concept in psychotherapy. It is often useful to consider how a client reacts to anxiety and guilt feelings and perhaps to discuss some alternative ways of dealing with these painful emotions. It is also helpful to the client to review those unpleasant past experiences that may be interfering with present functioning. Without becoming bogged down in the past, it may be important for both worker and client to understand how the client got into his or her current predicament. This review of the past may reveal some self-defeating behaviors that the client needs to modify in the future.

Regardless of theoretical bias, counselors and therapists acknowledge that certain Freudian themes come up again and again in therapy. These include the client's desire to be preferred by the parent of the opposite sex, sibling rivalry, guilt feelings about sex, and fear of closeness or intimacy with another. The therapist can benefit from psychoanalytic insights about these issues without accepting them as doctrine. Regardless of its faults, psychoanalytic theory is probably the most comprehensive theory available for the study of complex human relationships.

THE HUMANISTIC PERSPECTIVE

The **humanistic perspective** is not a school with a definite organization and clearly established leaders. It represents a kind of informal association of people who share certain basic philosophical notions. Some of these ideas were derived from existential philosophy, which focuses on the meanings a person gives to his or her experience in the world. The existential approach to therapy is sometimes regarded as a separate school in its own right. However, the humanistic and existential approaches are so closely related that, for present purposes, we will consider them together.

Philosophical Underpinnings

The humanistic orientation emphasizes the unique qualities of humans, especially their capacity for choice and their potential for personal growth. A major assumption is that the individual is free to choose alternatives in life.

Humanists deny the psychoanalytic belief that human behavior is dominated by animalistic drives. There is always a capacity for free will and choice even if the person *feels* trapped by circumstances or compulsive drives. A related assumption is that the person strives toward the highest possible fulfillment of human potentialities. There is potential for growth, or some kind of forward movement, in every human being. In this sense, humanists share a generally optimistic view of human nature.

The existential/humanist position is to some extent a reaction against the methods of modern science. Existentialists, in particular, argue that science tends to dehumanize people by regarding them as mechanical devices. In this view, science tends to pull people apart in a misguided attempt to see how they work. The person is divided into sensations, feelings, drives, perceptions, thoughts, physical systems, and so on. In this process of analysis, the unique quality of the individual is lost.

Furthermore, humanists maintain that this unique person cannot be understood by a distant objective observer. Real understanding requires getting into the frame of reference of the other person—that is, understanding how the other experiences and perceives the world. Some sort of dialogue between two persons is necessary for the understanding to come about. It is also assumed that both individuals engaged in a dialogue are likely to influence and change each other. The human being is never seen as a finished product but as always changing.

The following sections go into more detail about some of the concepts and treatment applications devised by humanistic theorists. Some of the major figures associated with the humanistic approach are Abraham Maslow, the psychologist cited in Chapter 1; Carl Rogers (1951, 1961), who founded client-centered therapy; Eric Berne (1964) and Thomas Harris (1967), who developed transactional analysis; and Fritz Perls (1969), the major pioneer of Gestalt therapy. Victor Frankl (1963) and Rollo May (1969) are prominent existential psychologists. We cannot go into detail about the ideas of each of these authors, but we can examine some of the basic concepts related to helping that most of them would endorse.

The Humanistic Approach to Helping

Humanists take a **holistic** view toward understanding their clients. This means that they want to understand the person as a whole, as opposed to breaking the personality into its components. The focus is on this person's private view of the world rather than on objective reality. What a person believes to be true influences behavior whether it is really so or not. If you are convinced that a person dislikes you, this belief governs how you relate to that person even though the other person may not really dislike you.

The humanistic therapist helps the client to clarify feelings, to think more deeply about problems, and to explore all important aspects of the current life situation. The helper provides an atmosphere in which this kind of exploration can safely take place. Unlike other significant people in

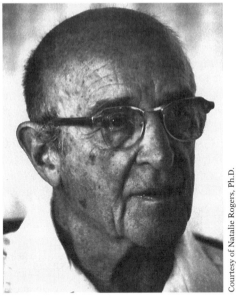

Courtesy of Natalie Rogers, Ph.D.

Carl Rogers

the client's life, the therapist has no desire to push the client in one direction or another. In other words, the helper does not want to mold or shape
the client into some preconceived image. Clients are therefore free to
search for their own special meanings and directions in life.

Implied in what has been said is that humanists are not sympathetic
toward the therapist who plays the role of doctor/expert. The humanistic
counselor does not study, direct, or analyze the client. Nor does the human-
ist assume a superior position from which to look down on the client.
Counseling is a dialogue between two individuals, each with his or her
unique experiences and perceptions. The helper does not have instant remedies or solutions to life's problems but helps clients struggle toward their
own answers.

Self-Actualization.   The humanistic approach to helping is based on the
concept that **self-actualization** is a primary motivating force in human behavior. Rogers (1959) defined this motivational force as "the inherent tendency of the organism to develop all its capacities in ways which serve to
maintain or enhance the organism" (p. 196). Crystals, plants, and animals
grow without any conscious fuss; the same kind of natural ordering process
is available to guide the development of the person (Whyte, 1960). Very
often, however, the forces of self-actualization bump up against conditions
that others impose (Meador & Rogers, 1984). In other words, the child may
be loved and approved only when behaving in certain specified ways—for
example, when good, cheerful, productive, successful, or competitive.
These conditions begin to warp the natural process of self-actualization.

Often, the child totally accepts these conditions because he or she has no basis on which to question them. In therapy, the person has the opportunity to resume growth in the atmosphere of acceptance provided by the therapist.

Maslow's (1954) concept of self-actualization is contained in this sentence: "What a man *can* be, he *must* be" (p. 46). This means that individuals must do what they are best equipped to do. One can maximize one's potential as a secretary, administrator, artist, politician, or mechanic. Skills, interests, background, and inherited tendencies all need to be considered in determining areas of maximal fulfillment. Serious difficulties may arise if the drive for self-actualization is thwarted. For example, if a person who wants to help disadvantaged people must work as an accountant or if someone with artistic ability is employed as a salesclerk, the need to fulfill potentials is not being satisfied. The individual may feel out of place and may be haunted by a sense of self-betrayal.

Responsibility.   Many people who seek counseling have been thwarted in their push for self-actualization by a tendency to live for others. All too often, they have been influenced by parents, teachers, or peers to pursue goals that are uncongenial to their true natures. Often, the growing child seeks approval from elders by living up to their demands and expectations. Some adults who seek help remain stuck in patterns of childish dependence. They have not fully accepted responsibility for finding their own path in life. Perls (1969) suggested that a prime goal of therapy is "to make the patient *not* depend upon others, but to make the patient discover from the very first that he can do many things, much more than he thinks he can do" (p. 29). He added that frustration is essential for growth because it helps individuals muster their own resources to discover that they can do well on their own. The therapist has to be alert to the manipulations of clients who may try to get the therapist to tell them what to do. The general thrust of humanistic therapy is to get the client to assume responsibility for thoughts, feelings, and direction in life. Only then is the person really free to pursue self-actualization.

The Self-Concept.   The **self-concept** is the core or center of the personality around which experiences are organized and interpreted. The "I" or the "self" includes how we see ourselves, how we think others perceive us, and how we would like to be. The self-concept begins to develop early in life. The child begins to evaluate certain experiences as good or bad and, quite naturally, takes on the values of parents, teacher, and peers. However, values imposed from the outside may require the child to ignore inner feelings. For example, if the child learns that anger or sexual urges are bad or not valued, the child may block these urges from awareness.

Rogers (1951) suggested that maladjustment occurs when the person denies awareness to significant experiences that do not fit the self-concept. When one's behavior and experiences do not mesh with the way one sees oneself, there is a lack of "congruence," which may lead to tension and anxiety. One goal of therapy, then, is to help the client experience and accept these denied experiences. The client may, for example, come to accept hostile feelings as okay in some situations. The hope is that this acceptance will reduce the tension and conflict.

Criticisms of the Humanistic Approach

Some critics believe that humanists exaggerate the benefits of the therapist's accepting attitude. It may take more than an attitude of positive regard to transform the client into a self-actualizing person. When Carl Rogers attempted to treat schizophrenics with this approach, the results were not especially impressive (Rogers, 1967). It may be unrealistic to expect one caring relationship to overcome years of negative life experiences.

Nor is it always helpful to emphasize that people have choices. Many poor, discouraged people do not see themselves as having many choices, and they really do not have the range of options available to affluent persons. They may need some practical kinds of help and some new opportunities before they can experience their potential for growth.

The humanistic approach does not seem to apply to patients who are not intellectually capable of making their own decisions. Young children and many persons with retardation or mental illness are not really able to make decisions about direction in life. The major decisions must be made by those responsible for their care. Although every client can be treated in a respectful way, it often doesn't make sense to treat the client as an equal. The behaviorist approach (to be discussed) seems to lend itself more effectively to treatment of people with limited potential.

Positive Aspects of the Humanistic Approach

The most useful aspect of the humanistic perspective it that is provides the human services worker with a sophisticated understanding of the helping relationship. Humanistic therapists have gone far beyond armchair speculation on this issue. Credit must be given to Rogers, his associates, and other humanists for providing solid research evidence about qualities in a relationship that facilitate positive change. Since this evidence is discussed in Chapter 5, there is no need to review it here. Suffice it to say that humanists have contributed significantly to improving the tools and skills of the counselor.

THE BEHAVIORISTIC MODEL

Unlike psychoanalysis, **behaviorism** did not begin as a method of treating psychological problems but has its roots in experimental studies of animal and human behavior. Dating back to the 1800s, it began as a reaction against psychological studies in which human subjects were asked to report on their sensations and perceptions. The early behaviorists felt that psychology wasn't getting anywhere by gathering vague reports of conscious experience. They argued that there was no way to verify a person's private experiences. They proposed, instead, that psychology be put on a firm scientific footing by studying overt behavior under such conditions that two or more observers could agree that a particular action or response had taken place. Psychology, they said, should focus on the effect of the environment on the behaving organism and should provide precise measurements of both the stimulating conditions and the resulting behavior. Private events such as dreams, fantasies, and thoughts would be ignored until techniques were invented to measure them in some verifiable fashion.

The early behaviorists believed that important laws governing behavior could be revealed by studying the behavior of animals—cats, dogs, rats, pigeons—in carefully controlled experimental situations. The emphasis was on conditioning, which involved situations that brought about a change in the behavior of the organism. Two general kinds of conditioning were identified and were designated as *classical* and *operant* conditioning. It is important for the counselor/therapist to understand both types because therapeutic approaches have been derived from each.

Classical Conditioning

Classical conditioning involves the study of reflexes—that is, responses elicited by certain stimuli in an automatic fashion. Such responses do not have to be learned or acquired by the individual. For example, an animal or person will respond with an eye blink if a puff of air is applied to the eye. Another automatic response in some creatures is to salivate when eating or chewing. Ivan Pavlov's (1927) studies of this salivary reflex in dogs are among the best-known experiments in the field of psychology. The basic experimental approach was as follows. Before conditioning, surgery was performed on the dog's cheek so that the saliva could be collected and measured precisely. During training, a bell, buzzer, or some other neutral stimulus was sounded just before food was given to the dog. As it ate, saliva would naturally begin to flow. The neutral stimulus and the food were presented over and over on subsequent feedings. Eventually, the dog salivated to the neutral stimulus even when no food was presented. Pavlov had succeeded in conditioning the response to a stimulus that would not elicit it before training. He observed that this conditioned response would eventually fade away—become extinguished—if the food were no longer presented.

Classical conditioning would be of limited interest if it applied only to dogs or salivary responses. Its importance stems from the fact that conditioning occurs in many real-life situations. In particular, the laws of classical conditioning seem to underlie the fear response. Many of us have been conditioned by life events to fear certain objects and situations such as

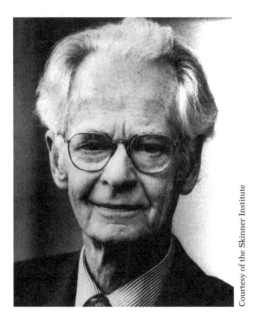

Courtesy of the Skinner Institute

B. F. Skinner

dogs, water, examinations, snakes, or enclosed spaces. Fears can also become associated with social situations involving persons of the opposite
sex, authority figures, crowds, and so on. Once a fear has become associated with a particular situation, it may not help very much to be told that
the fear is irrational or exaggerated. Behaviorists have developed some useful techniques, to be discussed, for helping people to overcome their fears.

Operant Conditioning

The other major type of conditioning, called either **operant** or instrumental, usually involves responses that are under voluntary control. This is in
contrast to the involuntary reflex involved in the classical method. In the
operant approach, the animal or person is moving freely in the environment. American psychologist E. L. Thorndike (1913) studied ways in which
the behavior of animals could be influenced by certain environmental in-
puts. He found that if a response is followed by a pleasant or satisfying
consequence, the response is likely to be repeated or strengthened. Similarly, if a response is followed by an unpleasant or punishing event, it is less
likely to occur. These simple principles were called the **law of effect.**

At present, B. F. Skinner is probably the best-known investigator of operant behavior. The basic principles can be demonstrated in the lab by
means of the Skinner box. This is nothing more than a chamber with a
lever and a food tray. A hungry rat placed in the box first explores its surroundings. Eventually, it pushes down the lever, which causes a pellet of
food to drop into the cup. The rat soon begins to press the lever more and
more frequently because this response is reinforced—that is, followed by a

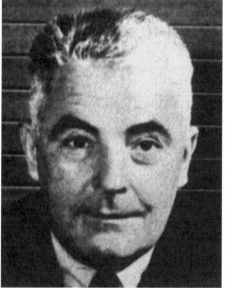

Archives of the History of American Psychology

John B. Watson

desirable or gratifying outcome. In everyday life, our behavior is constantly influenced by patterns of rewards and punishments. Children are trained by parents and teachers by means of good things to eat, grades, and expressions of approval. "Bad" or socially unacceptable behaviors may be followed by either punishment or the removal of desired rewards. The general pattern continues into adult life when others shape our behavior by rewarding certain performances with paychecks, promotions, or verbal praise, while discouraging other actions with various punishments and deprivations. The principles of operant conditioning have been applied to a number of therapeutic goals. Some will be reviewed in a subsequent section, but first we look at some early attempts to apply behaviorist principles to therapy.

John B. Watson and Little Albert

John B. Watson was an American psychologist who coined the term *behaviorism* and did much to make the new approach known to the general public. In his book *Psychology from the Standpoint of a Behaviorist*, which appeared in 1919, and in numerous magazines articles, he argued that the social environment was a powerful factor in conditioning personality and behavior. He boasted that given control over a child's early environment he could produce a lawyer, doctor, Indian chief, criminal, or just about any kind of adult.

The immediate importance of Watson is that he advanced the idea that behaviorism could be applied to the understanding and treatment of psychological disorders. His experiment with Little Albert, an 11-month-old boy, attracted a good deal of attention (Watson & Rayner, 1920). The purpose of the experiment was to show that an irrational fear, or phobia, could be acquired through conditioning. The experimental procedure was designed to condition a fear of a white rat in Little Albert, who previously was fond of rats and other animals. The experimenter, standing behind the boy, struck a steel bar with a hammer when Albert reached out to touch the white rat. The loud noise frightened the child and made him cry. After this procedure was repeated a few times, Albert became very fearful at the sight of the animal even without the loud noise. This newly acquired fear of white rats generalized to rabbits and other furry animals as well as to white furry objects such as a lady's muff.

Later, one of Watson's associates devised a method of treating such fears. Mary Cover Jones (1924) first conditioned a fear of a white rabbit in a child named Peter. She then presented the white rabbit at a distance when Peter was enjoying something to eat. Gradually, she brought the animal closer and closer, taking care not to evoke the fear response. The boy's fear was gradually eliminated, presumably because the once-feared stimulus was progressively associated with pleasant feelings.

The Behavioristic View of Abnormal Behavior

The experiments just described, and similar ones, demonstrated that phobias, irrational fears, and other types of abnormal behavior might be the result of learning and conditioning. The implications of these discoveries had a profound impact on the way in which behaviorists view abnormal behavior and "mental illness." They concluded that there is no basic difference between abnormal and normal behaviors because all behaviors are acquired by the same processes of learning and conditioning. The terms *abnormal* and *maladaptive* are simply labels applied to behaviors that are ineffective, self-defeating, or unacceptable to society. For example, one person may have learned through painful experience that stealing is followed by unpleasant consequences. Another person may have learned that stealing pays because the rewards are immediate and the punishment uncertain, absent, or tolerable. It merely clouds the issues to label some behaviors as antisocial or maladaptive. It is even worse to label certain persons as mentally ill or sick because it implies that they suffer from some mysterious defect of mind or spirit. Rather than labeling people, it might be more constructive to help them unlearn undesirable patterns of response and substitute new, more adaptive patterns.

The Growth of Behavior Therapy

In addition to Watson and his associates, a number of other workers began to apply behaviorist ideas to treatment. By and large, however, behavior therapies remained in the shadow of analytic approaches until about the mid-1950s. Since that time, the behaviorist approach has shown extraordinary growth and may soon become the dominant psychological approach to therapy.

Behavioral techniques have been employed in almost every kind of human services facility, including mental hospitals, community mental-health centers, correctional facilities, family service agencies, schools, and community settings (Sundel & Sundel, 1982). Behavioral therapies have been developed to treat a variety of problems including obesity, smoking, substance abuse, speech difficulties, bed-wetting, tics and similar nervous habits, sexual dysfunctions, and a variety of psychosomatic problems such as ulcer and high blood pressure. Before describing some of these techniques, we need to discuss the assessment procedure that precedes treatment.

Behavior Assessment. Behavioral treatment begins with a careful assessment of the problematic behavior rather than with the formal diagnosis required by the medical model. The origin of the behavior is considered along with the factors that currently maintain the behavior. This leads to the establishment of *behavioral objectives*—in other words, to specifying the behaviors to be changed and the new behaviors to be acquired. Behaviorists ridicule the pursuit of vague goals in therapy. For example, if a client complains of a lack of self-confidence, the behaviorist attempts to pin down exactly how the client behaves in specific social situations. The therapist might ask how the client would behave if he or she were a self-confident person. These behaviors then become the target behaviors, and a program is set up to help the client acquire them. One advantage of this approach to therapy is that the therapist and client have a clear idea of what they are trying to do.

The following sections describe some of the treatment methods devised by behavior therapists.

Systematic Desensitization. Systematic desensitization is probably the most widely used therapy based on classical conditioning. As currently practiced, it is an elaboration of the previously discussed method of treating fears and phobias developed by Watson and his associates. Of modern investigators, Joseph Wolpe (1958, 1969) did the most to refine the technique and to establish its therapeutic usefulness.

Treatment begins with an assessment of the stimuli or situations that evoke the fear response in the client. Water, open spaces, dogs, spiders, snakes, high places, or enclosed areas are some of the specific things or situations that may cause intense fear. The method can also be applied to social fears such as being rejected or criticized by certain people.

During initial sessions, the client is taught some variant of the progressive relaxation technique originally developed by Jacobson (1938). This technique helps the client learn to relax by alternately tensing and relaxing the major muscle groups of the body. The next phase of treatment involves making up an anxiety hierarchy—a series of scenes related to one of the client's fears. The scenes are graded in terms of how much fear they evoke.

For example, a student who is fearful of examinations might use a hierarchy in which the first scene involves being told by the professor that an exam is scheduled in 2 weeks. Further scenes bring this dreaded event closer and closer, until the final scene in which the student imagines receiving the exam itself. In treatment, each scene is imagined and paired with the relaxation procedures. When the client can imagine the least threatening scene without tension, the next scene is presented. Eventually, the client is able to imagine every scene in a relaxed manner.

The results of systematic desensitization have generally been quite positive, showing that the treatment generalizes to real-life situations. In some applications, the therapy takes place in real-life situations rather than in the therapist's office. For example, clients who are afraid to fly in an airplane may be taken through a real-life hierarchy of situations that ends with their actually getting into a plane and flying. Regardless of where treatment takes place, the basic aim of this approach is to substitute a desirable response (relaxation) for an undesirable response (tension/anxiety) in a gradual, step-by-step process.

Aversive Therapies.   Aversive therapies attempt to reduce an undesirable behavior by means of punishment. The undesirable behavior is followed by electric shock or another unpleasant stimulus. Aversive methods have been used to control head banging, self-mutilation, and other self-destructive behaviors. Applications have also been developed to treat sexual perversions such as child molestation, incest, and exhibitionism.

The basic approach is to associate the undesirable behavior with pain or extreme discomfort. For example, a 12-year-old retarded girl living in an institution was in the habit of hitting her ear with her arm and shoulder. Her ears were badly battered and needed frequent medical attention. She was referred to a behavior intervention ward, where any attempt to bang her ears was followed by a 1-second shock to the upper portion of her arms. She was connected to shock apparatus by means of wires that allowed immediate delivery of the shock. This procedure was effective in reducing the behavior. With further training, she was able to do without the machine, and she was eventually reassigned to another ward (Schaefer & Martin, 1975).

Aversive methods do not always work as well as in the preceding example. Sometimes their effect is temporary, and the treatment has to be repeated. In other instances, they may generate rage or excessive fear in the patient. Whenever possible, most therapists prefer to use positive reinforcers to influence behavior.

Token Economies.   Perhaps the most ambitious use of positive reinforcement of voluntary behaviors is the **token economy** used in some mental hospitals and other institutions. The aims is to encourage desirable behaviors by following them with some gratifying reward. Undesirable behaviors are usually discouraged by depriving the patient of a reward. As usual in behavior therapy, the first step is the establishment of target behaviors. These might include self-care, grooming, and housekeeping behaviors, as well as socializing with others and satisfactory performance on various jobs around the institution. A certain number of tokens can be earned for each behavior. Typically, the task and rewards are shown on a chart prominently displayed on the ward or section. The tokens can be redeemed at a commissary for cigarettes, candy, magazines, personal articles, and so on. In some settings, the patient can exchange tokens for a rental TV or even the freedom to leave the ward. Ayllon and Azrin (1965) described a token economy at a state mental hospital that was highly effective in modifying social and work behaviors in the patients. There is evidence that longer-term benefits also occur. Another reason for the increasing popularity of the approach is that the principles underlying the treatment are easy to understand. Workers and therapists can learn to apply the methods after a brief training program.

Recent Trends in Behavior Therapy

The methods described so far are based on traditional theories of learning and conditioning. Several new approaches have been put forth in recent decades. These include techniques based on social learning theory, cognitive behavior therapy, and biofeedback. The following sections provide brief summaries of these approaches.

Social Learning Theory and Modeling.   Social learning theorists point out that people can learn new responses simply by watching others perform them. For example, everyone has acquired some language and social skills by imitating others. A kid brother might learn something about how to approach girls by watching his older brother in action. Probably all of us have acquired certain actions or mannerisms by watching performers in movies or TV programs. This process of learning by imitation is called modeling by behaviorists.

Modeling has been used in a variety of clinical situations and has been found to be especially effective with children. One important benefit of certain modeling procedures is the reduction of fear in the observer. An example is the use of models to alleviate children's fear of surgery. Seeing a person do well in a difficult situation is encouraging to another who is faced with the same situation.

Assertion Training.   Social learning is also involved in the currently popular **assertion training.** This is designed to help people who have difficulty standing up for their rights in social situations. Some cannot say no in a firm, polite fashion and may end up being manipulated, pushed around, or abused by other people. Assertion training is not only for meek or shy people but may also benefit those who become so aggressive in social situations that they invite counterattack. Both the shy and overly aggressive

types need to learn to assert their rights and interests in a socially acceptable way.

The main technique of assertion training is behavioral rehearsal. The
client, usually in the context of a group, rehearses responses to social situations such as declining a date, saying no to the salesperson, or correcting a
waiter. In the safety of the therapy situation, the client has the opportunity
to rehearse various responses and receive feedback from the therapist and
group members.

The Cognitive Trend in Behavior Therapy.   In recent decades, some
behaviorists have departed from the tradition of sticking with the overtly
observable aspects of a learning situation. These cognitive behaviorists argue that much human behavior is influenced by thinking, particularly by
expectations of future reinforcements. Humans think about past experiences, reach conclusions, and plan future behavior in terms of complex
goals (Munsinger, 1983). The environment influences thinking, which in
turn influences what the person does in specific situations.

The cognitive/behavior approach to treatment owes a great deal to Albert Ellis's (1973) rational emotive therapy. He maintained that our
thoughts and beliefs have a powerful effect on how we behave and feel in
certain situations. If one's thoughts about a particular event are irrational,
it is likely that one is going to react in a foolish or maladaptive way. For
example, if a student believes it is *crucial* to be extremely competent in every one of life's tasks, then failure on an examination may be experienced
as some sort of catastrophe. The therapist helps the client by proposing a
more rational belief to substitute for the irrational one. The therapist may,
for example, suggest that it is desirable to do well on tests, but one failure is
not the end of the world. This might be followed by an exploration of the
reasons (e.g., poor study habits) for the poor performance, with suggestions for improvement.

Biofeedback.   Biofeedback is another relatively recent application of behavior theories. Based on a mix of operant and classical conditioning, biofeedback makes it possible for people to gain increased control over certain
physiological responses not previously under voluntary control. Research
has shown that humans and animals can learn to control some of their
internal functions, such as heart rate and blood pressure, if given feedback
about these responses. The feedback is provided by a machine that measures a certain physiological response in a precise way and converts the
information into a signal that the person can see or hear. The feedback
may, for example, take the form of a clicking noise, a tone, or a visual display such as an indicator dial.

Here is an example of how biofeedback might be applied in a clinical
setting. A client complains of severe tension headaches that are due to excessive contraction of muscles in the forehead. The therapist attaches to
the client's forehead electrodes that register the amount of activity or ten-

sion of these muscles. These signals are amplified by the biofeedback device and transformed into a tone of varying pitch. The pitch goes higher as the muscle tension increases and lower as tension is lessened. The client's task is to lower the pitch and keep it low. As muscle tension is reduced, the tension headache goes away. In subsequent training sessions, the client learns to reduce muscle tension without the biofeedback machine. Just how this learning takes place is still a subject for debate. The immediate point is that the technique often works.

Biofeedback has been used with some success to treat certain cardiac disorders, asthma, insomnia, migraines, speech problems, sexual dysfunction, and chronic anxiety. It is too early for any serious assessment of the effectiveness of biofeedback treatment. New techniques and improvements of older ones are constantly being reported. It can be said that the results so far have been promising and warrant further study. One significant advantage of biofeedback is that it does not carry the risk of side effects.

Criticisms of Behavioristic Approaches

Behavior therapy has been sharply criticized by civil rights advocates who point out that prisoners and mental patients have sometimes been subjected to behavior modification programs against their will. In some instances, inmates in institutions have been pressured to "volunteer" for such programs and have been given the distinct impression that noncompliance would be viewed as a failure to cooperate. This kind of threat must be taken very seriously when authorities have the final say about matters of parole or discharge. Even when participation is truly voluntary, the goals of treatment—the desired behavioral changes—are selected by staff, often with little or no input from the "subjects." Humanists doubt that a person can grow toward maturity and self-responsibility by being treated like a robot. Behaviorists view the matter of choice and free will in quite a different way than humanists. B. F. Skinner's (1971) *Beyond Freedom and Dignity* elaborates this view that freedom is an illusion.

Positive Aspects of Behavioristic Approaches

Despite these and other criticisms, behavior therapy is growing rapidly in popularity, is the object of intensive research efforts, and has produced useful treatments for a variety of human illnesses and problems. Certain behavioristic ideas can be usefully applied by human services workers dealing with different kinds of problems. One useful idea is simply the notion of establishing clear-cut behavioral objectives for the helping process. What is the goal of a session with a client? What objectives is a community organization trying to attain? What would have to happen to solve the problem or meet the need? If an unproductive situation seems resistant to change, it may be worthwhile to discover the reinforcing agents that maintain the situation. Once clear-cut objectives are established and a strategy for meeting these goals is decided on, it is relatively easy to measure progress toward the goal. Whenever possible, it is helpful to gather solid facts and data that indicate this progress.

WHICH THEORY IS BEST?

Instead of asking which theory is best, it might be better to ask which theory and treatment are the most useful in regard to a particular human problem. Theories are conceptual tools designed to help us understand complex situations. The tool is selected to suit the task to be done. Most helpers agree that certain theories seem to fit a particular client better than others. Probably the majority of skilled helpers are eclectic in approach. This means that they make use of several theories or parts of theories in their work rather than remain firmly devoted to one approach. From the eclectic point of view, it is acceptable to use the concept or treatment that seems appropriate to a particular situation. There is no requirement to be consistent in approach from case to case.

You may now feel somewhat bewildered by the variety of theoretical approaches that can be used in the helping process. Table 4–2 provides a condensed overview of the theories discussed in this chapter. It compares the five major theoretical perspectives along certain dimensions. In other words, it highlights, perhaps exaggerates, the differences between theories. It should help clarify the main points of comparison between these approaches.

ALTERNATIVE PATHS TO PERSONAL FULFILLMENT

This chapter has focused on what might be called the traditional approaches to psychological helping. These are the relatively well-established approaches that enjoy backing from governmental agencies, universities, and other organizations. You may be aware that there are also a number of unusual or alternative routes to psychological well-being. During recent decades, for example, there has been an explosion of interest in Eastern religions such as Buddhism and Hinduism. Spiritual leaders of these faiths, called gurus, have enjoyed considerable popularity, especially in large cities such as New York and San Francisco. Weiten (1986) suggests that this development is due to a need of Americans to turn inward in a quest for peace and serenity. We Americans live in an action-oriented society in which we tend to race about, fulfilling materialistic goals. The Eastern religions place relatively greater value on contemplation, intuition, and spirituality than on action and materialism. They offer the possibility of making contact with the inner self and perhaps experiencing oneself as part of a spiritual universe.

TABLE 4–2   A Comparison of Major Theoretical Approaches

	Medical Model	Human Services Model	Psychoanalytic Model	Humanistic Model	Behavioristic Model
Complexity of Theory	Complex	Simple	Very complex	Moderately complex	Relatively simple
Past/Present Emphasis	History used to arrive at diagnosis	"Here and now" solutions sought	Strong historical emphasis	"Here and now" emphasized	Present relearning
Assumed Causes of Disorder	Physical, bodily malfunctions	Unmet human needs	Internal conflict/ instinct vs. morals	Experiences that blocked self-actualization	Determined by previous conditioning
Therapeutic Approach	Medication, surgery, and physical treatments	Connect person with source of need satisfaction	Make conflict conscious	Create climate for growth, self-exploration	Change specific behaviors, habits, and thoughts
Length of Treatment	Varies depending on diagnosis	Short-term preferred	Very long-term (years)	Short to intermediate (months)	Usually short-term

Transcendental meditation is one application of meditative technique that has become popular in this country. The technique has been divorced from its Hindu religious base, simplified, and aggressively marketed to Americans. The meditator sits with eyes closed and focuses attention on a mantra, a specially assigned Sanskrit word. The exercise, which involves repetition of the mantra, is practiced twice daily for 20 minutes. There is evidence that meditation helps a person enter a relaxed state with calming of emotional responses (Wallace & Benson, 1972). Others maintain that these benefits can be achieved by simply resting or relaxing (Holmes, 1984).

A great many other approaches to self-realization have been proposed in recent years. Erhard Seminars Training (est), Scientology, and Silva Mind Control are three examples that have received nationwide attention. All have aroused intense controversy. Some graduates of these programs proclaim that their lives have been positively transformed. Others are less extravagant in their claims and say only that they received valuable insights and gained certain skills from participation. Critics, including Weiten (1986), believe that they are money-making operations based largely on "meaningless psychobabble" (p. 16) rather than on scientific evidence. We leave it to you to delve further into these controversies if you are interested.

SYSTEMS THEORY: THE MODEL OF THE FUTURE?

A major development in recent decades has been the widespread application of **systems theory** to scientific problems. A system, living or nonliving, can be defined as a group of related parts having some function or purpose in common. Miller (1978), in applying systems theory to living organisms, proposed that living systems are part of a sequence of larger systems (e.g., family, community, and nation) and are also composed of a series of smaller subsystems such as organs, tissues, and cells. Each system has a measure of independence from the larger system of which it is part, but it is also dependent on the larger system in some ways. For example, an individual has some independence from family but also remains part of the family in important ways. Each system has a boundary, transfers energy and information across the boundary, and is controlled by some decider system such as parents in a family (Baruth & Huber, 1984). Feedback mechanisms adjust the behavior of the system in somewhat the same way as a thermostat regulates the temperature in a heating system. By these mechanisms, individuals interact with one another so that each influences the other.

Perhaps the major application of systems theory to psychological treatment has been in the field of family therapy. It became apparent to the family therapists of the 1950s and 1960s that traditional theoretical approaches were of limited use in understanding family interactions. It was sometimes observed, for example, that when one member of the family showed improvement, another got worse. The traditional therapies, which had been developed largely in one-to-one treatment, did not provide clear explanations for these kinds of complex interactions. Systems theory was applied to the study of the family and soon became the dominant approach in this field. Systems therapists began to question the prevailing view that the member of the family with the presenting complaint or symptom was the sick one. They also doubted that this symptomatic member, usually a child or adolescent, should be the major focus of treatment. They came around to the view that the identified patient reflects disturbances in the entire family system. Rather than focus on a disturbed family member, these therapists treated the entire family and sometimes even brought in members of the extended family. It was found that present-day conflicts in the family sometimes reflected unresolved issues of previous generations.

One important application of systems theory to the understanding of family dynamics is the notion of circular causality in the family system. This means that interactions between members take place in a circular manner: The behavior of one influences a second, which in turn may influence a third, which may then return to affect the first (Baruth & Huber, 1984).

The usefulness of systems theory is by no means confined to family therapy. Glasser (1981) is one of several authors who have applied systems to individual therapy, and there have been numerous applications of this approach to specific clinical problems (e.g., Schmolling, 1983). Human services workers should also be aware that systems theory can illuminate their understanding of large organizations. After all, many human services workers spend much of their professional time as part of a service delivery system. An instructive and amusing introduction to understanding organizations from a systems point of view was provided by John Gall (1977).

Systems theorists are inclined to believe that their model will eventually come to dominate the behavioral sciences. This remains to be seen. There is no doubt that the influence of this approach is spreading rapidly.

DOES PSYCHOTHERAPY WORK?

This question is so broad that it is difficult to answer with precision. As we have seen, psychotherapy is not a single process applied to a specific disorder. It is up to future research to tell us which treatment strategy is best for what kind of problem. Nevertheless, Corey (1996) provided a useful summary of some of the major research findings of recent decades:

1. Many outpatients improve without formal psychotherapy, suggesting that they benefit from contacts with friends, family, and other primary social supports.
2. Psychotherapy is usually more effective than no therapy at all.

3. There is little evidence to support the superiority of one theoretical approach over another.
4. Certain factors common to various therapy systems account for much of the improvement found in clients. These include support factors, such as therapist warmth, and action factors, such as expectation of improvement.

This last finding clearly suggests that the content of the theories may be less important than these common factors.

Frank (1987, p. 293) argued that the effectiveness of all psychotherapies depends at least in part on their ability to combat the client's demoralization and discouragement. The therapist's ability to help depends on convincing the patient that the therapist understands him or her. Merely making sense of the patient's symptoms raises the patient's morale by combating feelings of confusion. Frank cast doubt on the assumption that the therapeutic power of a theory depends on how closely it approximates objective truth. The power of the explanation may rest on its capacity to make sense to the patient.

A related factor centers on the client's belief or faith in the efficacy of the therapy. This anticipation of good results is based on suggestion and is a potent general factor in all kinds of treatment. Of course, this effect is facilitated if the therapist has great confidence in his or her approach and conveys this feeling to the client.

Another set of factors, which are related to the skills, attitudes, and characteristics of the counselor, may also be as important as theory in determining effectiveness. The next chapter discusses these helper attributes in detail.

ADDITIONAL READING

Brammer, L., Shostrom, E., & Abrego, P. J. (1989). *Therapeutic psychology: Fundamentals of counseling and psychotherapy* (5th ed.). Englewood Cliffs, NJ: Prentice Hall.

Corey, G. (1996). *Theory and practice of counseling and psychotherapy* (5th ed.). Pacific Grove, CA: Brooks/Cole.

Frank, J. D., & Frank, J. (1991). *Persuasion and healing* (3rd ed.). Baltimore, MD: Johns Hopkins University Press.

Goldenberg, I., & Goldenberg, H. (1996). *Family therapy: An overview* (4th ed.). Pacific Grove, CA: Brooks/Cole.

Horney, K. (1950). *Neurosis and human growth.* New York: Norton.

Ivey, A. E., Ivey, M. B., & Simek-Downing, L. (1987). *Counseling and psychotherapy: Integrating skills, theory, and practice* (2nd ed.). Englewood Cliffs, NJ: Prentice Hall.

Jung, C. (Ed.). (1964). *Man and his symbols.* Garden City, NY: Doubleday.

Ornstein, R. E. (1976, October). Eastern psychologies: The container vs. the contents. *Psychology Today*, pp. 36–43.

Rogers, C. R. (1977). *Carl Rogers on personal power.* New York: Delacorte Press.

Rosen, R. D. (1977). *Psychobabble.* New York: Atheneum.

Schmolling, P. (1984). Schizophrenia and the deletion of certainty: An existential case study. *Psychological Reports, 54,* 139–148.

Skinner, B. F. (1971). *Beyond freedom and dignity.* New York: Knopf.

Sullivan, H. S. (1953). *Interpersonal theory psychiatry.* New York: Norton.

Yalom, I. D. (1980). *Existential psychotherapy.* New York: Basic Books.

REFERENCES

Ayllon, T., & Azrin, N. H. (1965). The measurement and reinforcement of behavior of psychotics. *Journal of the Experimental Analysis of Behavior, 8,* 357–383.

Baruth, L. G., & Huber, C. H. (1984). *An introduction to marital theory and therapy.* Pacific Grove, CA: Brooks/Cole.

Berne, E. (1964). *Games people play.* New York: Grove Press.

Comer, R. J. (1995). *Abnormal psychology* (2nd ed.). New York: W. H. Freeman.

Corey, G. (1996), *Theory and practice of counseling and psychotherapy* (5th ed.). Pacific Grove, CA: Brooks/Cole.

Cowley, G. (1994, February 7). The culture of Prozac. *Newsweek,* pp. 41–42.

Ellis, A. (1973). *Humanistic psychotherapy: The rational-emotive approach.* New York: Julian Press.

Erikson, E. H. (1963). *Childhood and society* (2nd ed.). New York: Norton.

Fisher, W., Mehr, J., & Truckenbrod, P. (1974). *Human services: The third revolution in mental health.* New York: Alfred.

Frank, J. (1987). Psychotherapy, rhetoric, and hermeneutics: Implications for practice and research. *Psychotherapy, 24,* 293–302.

Frank, J. D., & Frank, J. (1991). *Persuasion and healing* (3rd ed.). Baltimore, MD: Johns Hopkins University Press.

Frankl, V. (1963). *Man's search for meaning.* New York: Washington Square Press.

Gall, J. (1977). *Systemantics: How systems work and especially how they fail.* New York: Quadrangle New York Times Books.

Glasser, W. (1981). *Stations of the mind: New directions in reality therapy.* New York: Harper & Row.

Hall, C. S., & Lindzey, G. (1978). *Theories of personality* (3rd ed.). New York: Wiley.

Hansell, N., Wodarczyk, M., & Handlon-Lathrop, B. (1970). Decision counseling method: Expanding coping at crisis in transit. *Archives of General Psychiatry, 21,* 462–467.

Harris, T. (1967). *I'm O.K.—You're O.K.* New York: Avon.

Holmes, D. S. (1984). Meditation and somatic arousal reduction: A review of the experimental evidence. *American Psychologist, 39,* 1–10.

Jacobson, E. (1938). *Progressive relaxation.* Chicago: University of Chicago Press.

Jones, M. C. (1924). A laboratory study of fear: The case of Peter. *Journal of Genetic Psychology, 31,* 308–315.

Jung, C. (Ed.). (1964). *Man and his symbols.* Garden City, NY: Doubleday.

Kovel, J. (1980). The American mental health industry. In D. Ingleby (Ed.). *Critical psychiatry.* New York: Pantheon.

Kramer, P. (1993). *Listening to Prozac—A psychiatrist explores mood-altering drugs and the meaning of the self.* New York: Viking.

Lerner, M. (1994). *Choices in healing: Integrating the best of conventional and complementary approaches to cancer.* Cambridge, MA: MIT Press.

Lickey, M. E., & Gordon, B. (1991). *Medicine and mental illness: The use of drugs in psychiatry.* New York: W. H. Freeman.

Lombroso-Ferrero, G. (1911). *Criminal man.* New York: Putnam.

Maddi, S. (1972). *Personality theories: A comparative analysis.* Belmont, CA: Wadsworth.

Maslow, A. H. (1954). *Motivation and personality.* New York: Harper & Row.

May, R. (Ed.). (1969). *Existential psychology* (2nd ed.). New York: Random House.

Meador, B. D., & Rogers, C. R. (1984). *Person-centered therapy.* In R. J. Corsini (Ed.), *Current psychotherapies* (3rd ed., pp. 142–195). Itasca, IL: F. E. Peacock.

Miller, J. G. (1978). *Living systems.* New York: McGraw-Hill.

Miller, N. S., & Mahler, J. C. (1991). Addiction to and dependence on benzodiazepines. *Journal of Substance Abuse Treatment, 8,* 61–67.

Munsinger, H. (1983). *Principles of abnormal psychology.* New York: Macmillan.

Murray, D. J. (1988). *A history of western psychology* (2nd ed.). Englewood Cliffs, NJ: Prentice Hall.

Ornish, D. (1990). *Reversing heart disease.* New York: Random House.

Pavlov, I. P. (1927). *Conditional reflexes* (G. V. Anrep, Trans.). London: Oxford University Press.

Payer, L. (1988). *Medicine & culture: Varieties of treatment in the United States, England, West Germany, and France.* New York: Henry Holt.

Pelton, L. H. (1978). Child abuse and neglect: The myth of classlessness. *American Journal of Orthopsychiatry, 48,* 608–617.

Perls, F. (1969). *Gestalt therapy verbatim.* Moab, UT: Real People Press.

Perry, H. S. (1982). *Psychiatrist of America: The life of Harry Stack Sullivan.* Cambridge, MA: Belknap Press.

Physicians' Desk Reference (1996). 50th ed. Montvale, NJ: Medical Economics Company. Author.

Popple, P. R., & Leighninger, L. H. (1990). *Social work, social welfare, and American society.* Needham Heights, MA: Allyn & Bacon.

Prochaska, J. O. (1984). *Systems of psychotherapy: A transtheoretical analysis* (2nd ed.). Belmont, CA: Wadsworth.

Ricks, D. (1995, January 31). Alternative medicine attracts people of all ages. *The Standard Star, Gannett Suburban Newspapers,* p. 6C.

Rogers, C. R. (1951). *Client-centered therapy.* Boston: Houghton Mifflin.

Rogers, C. R. (1959). A theory of therapy, personality, and interpersonal relationships, as developed in the client-centered framework. In M. S. Koch (ed.), *Psychology: A study of a science* (Vol. 3). New York: McGraw-Hill.

Rogers, C. R. (1961). *On becoming a person.* Boston: Houghton Mifflin.

Rogers, C. R. (Ed.). (1967). *The therapeutic relationship and its impact: A study of psychotherapy with schizophrenics.* Madison: University of Wisconsin Press.

Schaefer, H. H., & Martin, P. L. (1975). *Behavioral therapy* (2nd ed.). New York: McGraw-Hill.

Schmolling, P. (1983). A systems model of schizophrenic dysfunction. *Behavioral Science, 28,* 253–267.

Simon, L. (1994). *Psycho"therapy": Theory, practice, modern and postmodern influences.* Westport, CT: Praeger.

Skinner, B. F. (1971). *Beyond freedom and dignity.* New York: Knopf.

Southern Regional Education Board (SREB). (1978). *Staff roles for mental health personnel: A history and rationale for paraprofessionals.* Atlanta: Author.

Sundel, M., & Sundel, S. S. (1982). *Behavior modification in the human services* (2nd ed.). Englewood Cliffs, NJ: Prentice Hall.

Szasz, T. (1973). *The myth of mental illness* (rev. ed.). New York: Harper & Row.

Thorndike, E. L. (1913). *Psychology of learning: Vol. 2. Educational psychology.* New York: Teachers College Press.

Valenstein, E. S. (1986). *Great and desperate cures: The rise and decline of psychosurgery and other radical treatments for mental illness.* New York: Basic Books.

Wallace, R. K., & Benson, H. (1972). The physiology of meditation. *Scientific American, 226,* 84–90.

Watson, J. B., & Rayner, R. (1920). Conditioned emotional reactions. *Journal of Experimental Psychology, 3,* 1–14.

Weiten, W. (1986). *Psychology applied to modern life: Adjustment in the 80s* (2nd ed.). Pacific Grove, CA: Brooks/Cole.

Whyte, L. (1960). *The unconscious before Freud.* London: Tavistock Publications.

Wolpe, J. (1958). *Psychotherapy by reciprocal inhibition.* Stanford, CA: Stanford University Press.

Wolpe, J. (1969). *The practice of behavior therapy.* New York: Pergamon Press.

The Human Services Worker

INTRODUCTION

In Chapter 4, we discussed the major theories of the human services/mental-health field. This chapter begins with the premise that theoretical knowledge alone is not sufficient for effective helping. Some workers know their theory but are ineffective in applying it. Other helpers seem to work well with clients but have very little theoretical background. In short, there is no definite relationship between the effectiveness of helpers and their knowledge of theory. Besides, it often happens that workers using the same theoretical approach vary greatly in effectiveness. What makes one helper more effective than another?

We explore this question in terms of the characteristics that have been shown to contribute to successful helping. These characteristics, attitudes, and skills have been identified mainly by humanistic psychologists, who have done a great deal of research on the nature of the helping relationship. Empathy, genuineness, and self-awareness are some of the helper characteristics that contribute to a good relationship with a client. In addition, this chapter reviews some of the basic skills, such as the ability to listen and communicate effectively, that are vital to the helper's success. The chapter closes with a discussion of the special skills required in group and community settings. Throughout this chapter, *worker, helper, counselor,* and *therapist* are used interchangeably, much as in the real world where human services workers who perform similar work are referred to by different terms depending on their location and setting.

DIFFERENT STYLES OF HELPING RELATIONSHIPS

As you will recall, the psychoanalytic, behavioristic, and humanistic therapies each have different goals, and each place emphasis on different aspects of the helping relationship. The therapist's use of the concept of *self* will vary greatly, based on the choice of theoretical model and therapy utilized. To understand this more fully, we will now examine the relationship between therapist and client in each of these perspectives.

The Relationship in Psychoanalytic Therapy

Psychoanalytic therapy seeks to bring unconscious material into the conscious and to strengthen the ego so that behavior is more reality based and driven less by primitive instinctual desires. The emphasis is on exploring the client's early past experiences in the hope of achieving a deeper level of self-understanding and insight (Kohut, 1984). The therapist who practices classical psychoanalysis seeks to maintain a sense of neutrality and objectivity with the client. There is very little self-disclosure by the therapist. The anonymous stance assumed by the therapist, sometimes called the blank-screen approach, is considered essential to the psychoanalytic method. The purpose is to develop a transference relationship, in which the client will project onto the therapist unresolved feelings that originated in the client's past significant relationships. It is believed that if the therapist remains neutral, the feelings that the client develops toward the therapist must be derived from the client's past relationships (Corey, 1991). For example, the client may begin to see the therapist as a stern, cold, controlling authority figure. In doing so, the client may be transferring to the therapist unresolved feelings derived from previous experience with his or her father.

In psychoanalysis, the client usually does most of the talking. The therapist's primary role is to listen, understand, and eventually interpret the meanings of the client's experience. A major purpose of this process is to uncover unconscious motives and to help clients achieve insight into their problems. The attainment of insight through the analysis of the transference is assumed to be necessary for the client to change in meaningful ways.

The Relationship in Behavior Therapy

Behavior therapy is a direct, active, and specific problem-solving approach to treatment. The focus is on the clients' current problems and life situation as opposed to their past history. Clients learn new coping skills and are urged to take specific action to reach desired goals, rather than to passively reflect upon prior experiences. Behavioral practitioners do not view the development of a special client/therapist relationships as being central or all important to this treatment approach. Instead, they contend that factors such as warmth, empathy, authenticity, permissiveness, and acceptance are considered necessary—but not sufficient—for behavior change to occur (Corey, 1991). The relationship is viewed primarily as a setting for the use of various behavioral strategies and techniques. The client becomes actively involved in the selection of his or her own goals, and the therapist applies specific techniques to help the client achieve those goals.

The helping relationship in this form of treatment has been characterized by critics as being somewhat rigid, overly directive, impersonal, and manipulative. However, many behavioral practitioners believe that establishing a good interpersonal relationship is highly desirable. Spiegler (1983) emphasizes that a good therapeutic relationship increases the chances that the client will be cooperative and receptive to therapy. Cormier and Cormier (1985) also stress that the behavioral approach should be based on a highly collaborative relationship between client and therapist. In fact, they view the process of selecting and achieving goals as a mutual, social-influence process in which relationship variables are involved.

The Relationship in Humanistic Therapy

The humanistic approach places a great deal of emphasis on the client/therapist relationship as a catalyst for personality change. The focus is on the clients' current life situation rather than on helping clients come to terms with their personal past (May & Yalom, 1989). Humanistic therapists practice a client-centered approach, in which the therapist does not actively establish goals or provide specific advice or direction to the client. The basic premise is that clients are capable of self-directed growth and have a great potential for resolving their own problems if provided with a helping relationship that facilitates such growth. The underlying belief of this approach is best summarized by Rogers (1961) when he states, "If I can provide a certain type of relationship, the other person will discover within himself the capacity to use that relationship for growth and change, and personal development will occur" (p. 33). The utilization of any directive techniques designed to get the client to "do something" are, at best, considered secondary to the development of this unique client/therapist relationship. This approach places great emphasis on the "personhood" of the therapist. Not only does the therapist need effective helping skills, but he or she must also have the ability to create a growth-producing environment and must possess the personal characteristics and attributes amenable to these conditions.

CHARACTERISTICS OF EFFECTIVE HELPERS

Although research has not yet indicated a "correct" method of helping, it has identified certain characteristics of helpers that are associated with successful helping. For example, the findings of Avila, Combs, and Purkey (1978), Brammer (1981), Truax and Carkhuff (1967), and Rogers (1961) indicate that effective workers possess certain personal characteristics that contribute to success. The discussion that follows examines these characteristics that contribute to the development of helping relationships.

Empathy

Empatheia is the Greek word that refers to affection plus passion touched by the quality of suffering. In Latin, the word *pathos* is analogous to the Greek *patheia* with the added dimension of "feeling." Through the years, this somewhat vague meaning has evolved into a more comprehensive definition of **empathy**. For example, Brammer (1981) views empathy as the ability to appreciate and understand the client's perspective. More simply, empathy is the ability to see things from another's point of view. Empathy is viewed by many professionals as the most important characteristic in a helping relationship. It serves as a basis for relating and communicating. For example, when clients feel deeply understood, they are generally more willing to risk disclosure of their inner feelings. Carkhuff and Berenson (1967) conclude that "the therapist's ability to communicate at high levels of empathic understanding involves the therapist's ability to allow him or herself to experience or merge in the experience of the client" (p. 109).

Empathy is often viewed as conveying sensitivity to the client and trying to understand what "walking in the other guy's shoes" may feel like. The helper need not necessarily have undergone the experiences of a client in order to understand the client's feelings. Feelings are universal. Different experiences often generate similar feelings. For example, death of a loved one and divorce may both generate feelings of loss and anguish.

For empathy to be constructive and worthwhile, it must be demonstrated, as in the following example.

Client: I just recently lost my father, who had cancer.

Helper: It must be a very painful experience, causing you to feel angry, sad, and abandoned.

Genuineness

Genuineness is the expression of true feelings. To be a genuine helper, one must avoid role playing or feeling one way and acting another. Genuine helpers do not take refuge in any specific role, such as counselor or therapist. Genuineness involves self-disclosure. It implies a willingness to be known to others.

In most types of helping relationships, a certain degree of modeling behavior takes place. The client sometimes tries to emulate the characteristics of the helper. If the helper is genuine, free, and expressive, the client is also free and able to express authentic feelings.

Shulman (1991) adds two dimensions to our examination of this characteristic by introducing parallel elements: "Two words are closely related in explaining the meaning of genuineness—**congruency** (when one's words and actions correspond) and **authenticity** (when one is him- or herself, not a phony)" (p. 307, emphasis added). Being genuine, however, is not free license for the helper to do or say anything to the client on a whim. Helpers are not "free spirits" who inflict themselves on others. Being genuine does not necessarily mean expressing all one's thoughts to the client.

Helpers can be genuine without being hostile or hurtful to the client. For example, a client may ask the helper, "What do you really think of me?" Assuming that the helper has negative feelings at the moment toward the client's behavior, these feelings could be openly expressed in a variety of ways without appearing as a direct attack on the client. The helper might express disappointment at the client's unwillingness to attempt to change his or her behavior. In other words, one can dislike a person's rigidity but can still respect the person as an individual.

Sharing personal experiences with the client can sometimes be helpful. For instance, the counselor may be helping someone come to grips with problems generated by a recent divorce. The helper may have been divorced and can therefore understand the range of the client's feelings on a personal level. In this instance, it may be appropriate to share experiences with the client and disclose how one worked toward resolving and understanding those feelings. Of course, it is possible for the helper to share emotions and feelings without discussing specific events or circumstances in his or her life.

Objective/Subjective Balance

Subjectivity refers to private, personal, and unique ways of experiencing situations. Being subjective means one's experience is unique and not directly observable by another person. It is a private reaction to or feeling about someone or something. This reaction tends to be biased because it only pertains to the individual's experience.

Objectivity emphasizes verifiable aspects of an event. Objectivity involves the noting of facts without distortion by personal feelings or prejudices. It stresses description of what can be seen, heard, touched, and so on. An objective statement based on verifiable evidence might be, "Bill is 5 feet 6 inches tall, weights 145 pounds, and has blue eyes," whereas a subjective statement of these same conditions could be, "Bill is too short, overweight, and has unattractive, weird-looking eyes."

Subjectivity and objectivity represent opposite ends of a continuum. In the helping process, there are disadvantages to each quality when carried to extremes. The helper who is too subjective can become too emotionally involved with the client, as in the case of taking sides in marital counseling. In this sense, the helper can run the risk of losing the ability to make appropriate decisions or judgments.

Pure objectivity alone is also not a desired quality. Objectivity refers to a detachment from one's personal feelings. The purely objective helper can run the risk of being viewed by the client as cold, uncaring, aloof, and uninterested in the client's well-being. This can cause obvious difficulties in communication and build up feelings of resentment on the part of the client.

Either quality, when carried to extremes, can lead to difficulty in understanding people. The quality to be desired is an objective/subjective balance. A helper must have the ability to stand back and view a situation accurately but without becoming detached from personal feelings. Human services helpers need a blend of both qualities.

Self-Awareness

Self-awareness is the quality of knowing oneself. It includes knowledge of one's values, feelings, attitudes and beliefs, fears and desires, and strengths and weaknesses. The self is composed of one's thoughts about oneself. This means that there are literally hundreds of ideas and images that make up the sense of self. One's values, beliefs, ideas, and images become clear when one asks questions such as: What's important to me? What aspects of myself do I like or dislike? The self-concept can be regarded as the inner world in which one lives. In the helping process, the helper often expresses this inner world and makes it visible to the client.

The effective helper must be aware of what messages are being transmitted to the client through both word and action. It is only through self-examination that we can begin to understand what aspects of ourselves would be most beneficial to the helping process. Combs, Avila, and Purkey (1978) stressed the following:

> Professional helpers must be thinking, problem-solving individuals. The primary tool with which they work is themselves. This understanding has been referred to as the self as instrument or self as tool concept. In the human services a helping relationship always involves the use of the helper's self, the unique ways in which helpers are able to combine knowledge and understanding with their own unique ways of putting them into operation. (p. 6)

It is generally accepted among many professionals that if one wants to become more effective as a helper, it is necessary to start with self-awareness. Helpers who aspire to use self in an effective way must be aware of their patterns of personality and their needs. Helpers have a responsibility to be conscious of the ways in which their personalities and behaviors affect others. The helper's beliefs, values, and attitudes can have a powerful effect on the helping process.

Acceptance

Acceptance is demonstrated by viewing the client's feelings, attitudes, and opinions as worthy of consideration. The accepting helper sees each person as having a fundamental right to think, act, and feel differently. From the humanistic perspective, communicating acceptance of the other person is vital to developing and maintaining the helping relationship. Communication of acceptance leads to feelings of psychological safety on the part of the client. In this setting, the client believes that no matter what he or she discloses, the counselor will react in an accepting manner. As an accepting person, the helper recognizes the uniqueness in each human being. Brill (1973) suggested that

> the basis of any relationship is acceptance of the individual's right to existence, importance, and value. . . . Out of acceptance should come freedom to be oneself—to express one's fears, angers, joy, rage, to grow, develop, and change—without concern that doing so will jeopardize the relationship. (p. 48)

A major problem with understanding the quality of acceptance is that one can confuse acceptance of a client with approval of the client's behavior. Accepting a person does not imply that one likes or approves of all the values or behaviors of that person. For example, a counselor may be working with a heroin addict who is attempting to kick the habit. The counselor may accept the client's feelings, experience, and beliefs but not approve of heroin addiction. Thus, when a helper says of a client, "I can accept anyone except a child abuser," the helper is judging the behavior as a total representation of the client. Individuals are made up of numerous values, attitudes, and behaviors. No single value, attitude, or behavior represents the total individual.

Desire to Help

Many proponents of the humanistic perspective believe that effective helpers have a deep interest in other people and a desire to help, which allow them to receive satisfaction in promoting the growth and development of others. The feelings of self-satisfaction derived from seeing others make positive changes in their lives are a basic reward to the helper. This sincere desire to help is displayed and becomes readily observable in the helper's attitude toward his or her work. Just as people respond more favorably to a salesperson who evidences enthusiasm and interest in the product he or she is selling, so clients respond more favorably to a helper who is enthusiastic about and interested in helping. One caution should be noted in this regard: Sometimes the helper's desire to help can extend too far, creating unnecessary client dependence on the helper for various tasks that clients should take care of themselves.

Helpers accept as a social value the belief that people should help one another. When one devotes a considerable amount of time and energy to helping others, it demonstrates a basic belief that those being served do have the fundamental ability to change (Cowen, Leibowitz, & Leibowitz, 1968). Many professionals agree that a desire to help people is a basic value for those who enter the human services field.

Patience

Patience is the ability to wait and be steadfast; it is refraining from acting out of haste or impetuousness. As a helper, one may often feel that it would be beneficial to a client to do a particular thing, confront a situation, and so on. Patience is based on the understanding that different people do things at different times, in different ways, and for different reasons according to their individual capacities.

Frequently, a helper must wait for a client to be ready to take a next step toward resolving a particular problem or toward achieving a desired goal. For example, a helper might be helping a retarded individual to use eating utensils, a task that often involves a lot of repetition over a long period of time. People do not always proceed on a prescribed timetable. Human beings can be awesomely frustrating creatures who often resist change even though the change is recognized as ultimately beneficial. An effective helper must have the patience to allow for the client's development and growth according to the client's needs and abilities.

BASIC HELPING SKILLS

Human services professionals must master certain basic skills to be successful. A skill is an ability to perform a particular task in a competent fashion. Many individual skills make up the helping process.

Individuals are not born with the skills that are essential for relating effectively to other human beings. These skills are learned through training. Some helpers do, however, have more natural abilities than others. Effective helpers continue to acquire additional skills and strive to refine already existing skills. Because each individual is different, each helper must develop his or her own style and way of using these skills, which become the "tools of the trade." In this section, we discuss seven basic helping skills.

Listening

To listen means to pay attention to, to tune in to, or to hear with thoughtful consideration. Skillful listening is as important as talking and acting. It is through listening that the helper begins to learn about the client and how the client sees the world and himself or herself. The helper needs to listen attentively to all messages from the client about such matters as how the client views his or her problems and what the client expects the helper to do about them. Without listening, all forms of potential help may become misguided.

To be effective as a listener, one must become aware of more than just the words that are spoken. There is a basic difference between hearing words and listening for the full meaning and message of the words. It is often not what the client says but how she or he says it that is important. A client's body posture, tone and pitch of voice, silences and pauses, and speech patterns are all significant in understanding what a client is trying to communicate. A phrase spoken in a sarcastic tone means something different from the same phrase spoken in a voice filled with cheer and lightness. You probably often ask friends, "How are you?" When a friend responds "Fine," you can either accept it at face value or suspect that there is something beneath the surface that contradicts the message. In other words, you may sense a negative feeling that contradicts the overt statement. Effective listening requires sensitivity to inconsistencies between a person's words and actions. The client who says "I'm fine" while tears begin to well up in his or her eyes is obviously communicating a contradictory message.

When listening to clients, the helper must recognize both the cognitive and affective content of what is being communicated. Cognitive content refers to thoughts and ideas. Affective content refers to the feeling tone of the message. When we watch a mime perform on stage, no words are spoken, but the mime's actions convey a full range of feelings and behaviors. The affective content sometimes differs from the cognitive content and is often less apparent. Responding accurately to a client's statement depends on the helper's ability to hear and understand what is being said and to perceive the underlying message. Helpers must ask themselves, "Does the client's behavior fit his or her words?" and "What is the client really trying to communicate?"

Another aspect of listening is the concept of selective perception. Selective perception means that individuals sometimes hear only the aspects of another's message that they wish to hear and disregard the rest. For instance, a helper might ignore the message conveyed by a client's tone of voice and respond only to the usual meaning of the words spoken. Johnson (1986) adds the following:

> There is considerable evidence that you will be more sensitive to perceiving messages that are consistent with your opinions and attitudes. You will tend to misperceive or fail to perceive messages that are opposite to your opinions, beliefs, and attitudes. If you expect a person to act unfriendly, you will be sensitive to anything that can be perceived as rejection and unfriendliness. (p. 93)

The helper's beliefs and attitudes can distort the message being received. When listening to others, it is essential to be aware of the possibility of selectivity in what you hear and perceive. Effective helpers are always listening for the full message.

Communicating

Communication is the process of transmitting feelings or thoughts so that they are understood. This process involves conveying information verbally or nonverbally through a variety of means such as body movements, facial expressions, and gestures. To communicate, there must be both a sender and a receiver of a message. Generally speaking, all behavior transmits certain information and may, therefore, be involved in communication.

Many aspects of human services work require the ability to communicate. Communication is an integral part of human services and may take the form of transmitting particular knowledge, information, or skills. For example, when a helper is counseling individuals facing retirement, the content of the communication may focus on financial planning, housing needs, or social or emotional concerns. At the other end of the life cycle, helpers working in children's human services programs may focus the content of their communication upon the development of basic life skills. Com-

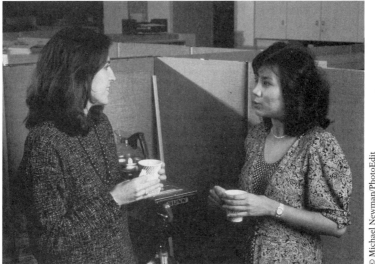

© Michael Newman/PhotoEdit

Communication

municating effectively and responding appropriately are often the key factors in determining the success of any attempt to help.

You can easily understand the complexity of communication by considering the example of the game of passing a single message through a series of individuals. In this game, one person thinks of a message and in turn whispers it to another. The next person attempts to whisper the same message to another person, who does the same, passing it to as many people as possible. When the last person tells the entire group what his or her version of the message is, it is usually very different from the original message. How does a relatively simple message become distorted when conveyed to another person? To understand this, we must look at the various factors involved in communication and understand the obstacles and barriers that can distort even the simplest of messages.

Accurate communication occurs between people when the receiver interprets the sender's message the way the sender intended it. Difficulties in communication arise when the receiver imparts to the message a meaning that was not intended. When the sender attempts to convey a message, the receiver interprets the message before he or she can respond to it. All forms of communication require some degree of interpretation, meaning that an individual must construe, understand, and attach individual meaning to a message. It is through this act of interpretation that communication can become distorted. The process of interpretation is always filtered through our individual biases, expectations, and prejudices. As mentioned previously, when information is transmitted, the listener tends to accept what seems to fit into his or her belief system and sometimes rejects or distorts information that is inconsistent with those beliefs. Also, people are sometimes so positive they know what the other person is going to say that they distort the incoming message to match their expectations. For example, if a man who has very low self-esteem asks his boss for a raise, he may take the boss's statement "I'll have to give it some thought" as a sign of refusal.

A common problem in communication occurs when the receiver understands the words of the message but fails to recognize the sender's underlying meaning. For example, a person might say "Sure is a rainy day" in an attempt to change the subject, but the receiver might assume the person is really concerned about the weather. Another example is the client who sits in the office looking down, arms crossed, slouched deeply in his or her chair, who responds to the question "How do you feel?" by saying "Fine." The client's nonverbal behavior, consisting of posture, eye contact, and facial expression, seems to indicate the opposite. Which message does one respond to? The answer is both. The helper must hear the words but also be aware of additional information conveyed in the communication.

Helpers must have an awareness of their own styles of communication. Becoming aware of style means that you know when you as a helper might be creating difficulty in communication by sending out conflicting verbal and nonverbal messages to the client. To this degree, you can see how the quality of self-awareness enhances the skill of communicating effectively. Inappropriate use of language can also lead to mishaps in communication. The helper should avoid using words the client may not understand or may find objectionable. The helper's vocabulary must be understandable to the client. Since words do not mean the same thing to all people, the helper must sometimes provide clear definitions and examples of meaning. If the client's message is unclear, the worker has the responsibility of helping the client to clarify its meaning.

Giving Feedback

Giving **feedback** is the process of conveying to clients perceptions, feelings, observations, or other information concerning their behavior. Feedback basically represents an individual opinion or evaluation of the client by the worker. It helps clients become aware of how they are perceived by others. Clients can then decide to correct errors in judgment, change undesirable behaviors, and establish goals.

People do not operate in a social vacuum. We often seek out other individuals to give us their evaluation of how well we accomplish a particular task or perform a certain job. For example, actors and actresses often anxiously await the theatrical reviewer's evaluation of their latest performance. In the same manner, a child proudly displays his or her latest work of art to the parents and awaits the parents' comments. Feedback is a basic requirement of human beings in many aspects of life.

For the human services worker, learning how to provide feedback effectively is an essential task. Danish and Haner (1976) stated that "to be helpful, the feedback must be given in such a way that the receiver

(a) understands clearly what is being communicated; and (b) is able to accept the information" (p. 14). Timing is an important factor in the appropriate use of feedback. Is the client receptive to another point of view at this time? Sometimes a client is not receptive because he or she is in a highly emotional state.

The relationship between worker and client is another critical issue in the use of feedback. If one respects and values the opinion of the other, one is more likely to accept what is offered.

The worker has to exercise judgment in regard to clients' abilities to accept feedback concerning their behavior or problems. Consider the example of the client who thinks she has a wonderful sense of humor, yet people tend to shy away from her when she jokes around. Several individuals may already have informed her that her jokes are not funny, but she may ignore these people, claiming they have no sense of humor. If in the worker's judgment the client would be more receptive to feedback from a helper, the worker can point out to the client that her sense of humor tends to be sarcastic and hurtful, and this may be a reason that people shy away from her.

Feedback serves many purposes. It can reaffirm what the client already believes and feels. It can inform clients of aspects of their behavior of which they were not previously aware. It can provide motivation for change and can also be a source of support during difficult times.

Observing

For the purpose of this discussion, we define observing as the process of noting or recognizing an event. An event could be almost anything from the weather to the facial expression of a particular individual. Observing occurs in two stages: receiving sensory input and giving meaning to the information.

The human services worker always looks for any signs or clues to understand more of what is going on with the client. Areas in which clues can be found include the following:

- facial expressions
- vocal quality
- body posture
- gestures
- clothing
- general appearance
- eye contact
- distance between worker and client

Workers usually rely on the sense of sight to provide them with basic information. The sense of hearing is equally important, however. In fact, all the senses receive messages that can supplement, confirm, or negate the initial impression derived from sight.

For example, the worker notes that the client is slouched, apparently at ease. However, as the interview progresses, the worker hears the client's rapid speech and intermittent stuttering, indicating tension. In effect, the worker's initial impression of the client as being relaxed has now been negated by other sensory information. This example also illustrates that an important aspect of observation is interpretation, or attaching individual meaning to an occurrence. Another helper might come up with a different interpretation of the behavioral clues.

Confronting

Confrontation is a word that conjures up fear in some individuals. People often associate the word with some form of attack, anger, or hostile behavior. In the context of the helping profession, the term requires a different understanding. Confrontation can be defined as calling to the attention of the client discrepancies between or among the client's thoughts, attitudes, or behaviors (Ivey, Ivey, & Simek-Downing, 1987). A confrontation is actually an invitation to the client to become more aware of and to examine more fully certain aspects of behavior that seem to the counselor to be harmful or self-defeating for the client. It is through the process of confrontation that clients are made aware of specific obstacles that have impeded or could interfere with reaching their desired goals. Through this process, clients optimally learn to accept responsibility for their behavior.

Confrontation need not focus exclusively upon negative aspects of clients' behavior. It can be used to show clients strengths and resources that they have overlooked. The acknowledgment of strengths can sometimes produce anxiety in clients, however, because then more can be demanded of them. Thus, confrontation involves challenge even when a positive aspect of behavior is pointed out. Before individuals can change, they must perceive a need for change. Confrontation provides one stimulus for change.

Constructively challenging the client can take various forms. Counselors can call attention to the client's self-defeating attitudes, point out discrepancies between what the client says and actually does, focus upon various manipulations or forms of game playing, or as mentioned previously, address unrecognized areas of strength. Following are some examples of the use of confrontation in counseling.

Example A

Client: I am not really interested in a better-paying job. It will probably demand more of my time and I will have to learn new skills and even wear a tie and jacket to work.

Counselor: You say you are not interested in a better job, yet you have spent several sessions talking exclusively about it. Is it possible you really want to go after the better job and are afraid of failing, so you have convinced yourself that you really do not want the job? Are you possibly afraid of new demands that could be placed on you?

This confrontation addresses the client's incongruent behavior.

Example B

Client: I am really concerned about the shape of the world today. People do nothing to change the situation. People are starving. Trash is scattered all over the streets, crime is everywhere, and people do not get out and talk to one another anymore.

Counselor: You say you are a concerned person, but the bulk of your time is spent sitting in front of the television and drinking beer.

This confrontation focuses the client on the discrepancy between what he claims concerns him and what he actually does about it.

The misuse of confrontation can have negative effects on clients. If the client is not ready to accept the challenge of the offered information, the confrontation is not helpful. The counselor must time the confrontation so that it is most helpful.

Clarifying

The basic purpose of clarifying is to make clear what information is being conveyed by the client and how it is being received by the counselor. Sometimes difficult situations and painful emotions can create problems with communication. When the counselor clarifies aspects of the client's message, the client knows how the message has been received. The process of clarifying often involves using the skills of paraphrasing, highlighting, and summarizing.

Paraphrasing.   When the counselor **paraphrases** a client's message, he or she rewords it. In doing so, the counselor attempts to focus the client's attention on the main element of an immediate message. Through the use of paraphrasing, the counselor conveys to the client that the meaning and the feelings of the message have been received and understood. Consider the following example:

Client: Even though I feel I have a lot of friends, I feel as if no one understands me or really wants to. My mother and father don't listen to me. My teachers ignore me, and my girlfriend says I'm no fun to be with anymore.

Counselor: It sounds as if you feel that you have no one you can really talk to.

Client: Yeah, I guess that is how I feel.

In this example, the counselor rewords and restates the client's message and pinpoints the basic feelings. This serves to focus the client on the main areas of concern in addition to conveying to the client that the counselor understands what is being expressed.

Highlighting. Highlighting is very similar to paraphrasing but has a slightly different purpose. Paraphrasing is often done as a response to the client's immediate message. Highlighting, however, is not an immediate response and does not necessarily follow the sequence in which the client is expressing the message. Highlighting is an attempt to capture the recurring theme of messages during a counseling session. In this way, the counselor emphasizes the main aspects of what the client is expressing over a short time. This serves to focus the client's train of thought and draws the client's attention to the main areas of concern being expressed.

Following the previous example, the counselor has just spent 20 minutes listening to the client's appraisal of himself and his many friendships. The counselor is now attempting to highlight the major theme and feelings expressed by the client.

Counselor: Even though you say you have many friends, you still feel that no one really understands you.

The counselor has now identified the major theme of the client's message and is again drawing the client's attention to what he has already expressed as his main concern.

Summarizing. Like paraphrasing and highlighting, **summarizing** is a means of giving back to the client the essence of what he or she has been trying to convey. The distinction concerns the amount of material covered. Paraphrasing and highlighting concentrate on the immediate aspects of client messages during parts of a single counseling session, whereas summarizing involves restating the chief elements of the client's message over one or a series of counseling sessions (Schulman, 1991). When the worker summarizes the major points of information and recurring themes brought forth by the client over several sessions, the client can develop a broader perspective on and deeper understanding of the depth and significance of specific problem areas. This process brings to the attention of the client changes in feelings and attitudes that may have gone unnoticed. It enables clients to develop a frame of reference in which to see where they were, where they are now, and where they would like to be.

Report Writing

Report writing is a means of recording the interactions between clients and events. Most reports concern client behavior and progress. Report writing is not generally perceived as one of the more exciting skills to acquire within the human services field, but nevertheless, it is one of the most practical and valuable. Report writing in one form or another is necessary in many aspects of the human services field. All professionals and institutions require a consistent method of keeping track of what happens to whom, when, and why, although specific methods and styles of report writing vary. Many human services agencies use a standardized form for the various types of reports. Obviously, writing clearly and using language accurately are important. More specifically, reports are usually compiled with two basic objectives in mind: to establish a documented record for future reference and to convey current information regarding a specific case or event (Wicks, 1979).

A counselor working with many clients must keep an accurate report of each one's progress. Clients may be taking medication, which necessitates that a consistent and accurate report be kept on the type of medication, dosage, and consequent reactions. If a client changes counselors, the report of the previous counselor may be requested by the new counselor as a means of gaining background information on the client. In many clinics, it is mandatory to keep reports of patient contacts, diagnoses, and treatments. Very often these reports are monitored by state and federal agencies to ensure a continuous level of compliance with state and federal regulations.

Reports are crucial when professionals evaluate or consult with public or private agencies, institutions, or schools. For instance, a human services specialist might be brought in to evaluate the effectiveness of a specific program or service. The evaluator would rely heavily on the records and reports submitted.

FACTORS THAT INFLUENCE THE USE OF SKILLS

This chapter has so far described a variety of skills and characteristics needed for effective helping. There are a number of factors that can influence the way in which the worker applies these skills and characteristics. These factors are discussed in the following sections.

Values

A person's sense of right and wrong, likes and dislikes, and standards of appropriate behavior are all a part of values. One's personal, professional, and societal values develop through one's experiences with family, peers, and culture. Of immediate relevance is the fact that the individual's values guide behavior in professional or working relationships. How a worker reacts to a particular client, situation, or problem is partly determined by the worker's values. Most workers of the humanistic orientation accept the principle that the helper should not try to impose values on the client but should help the client clarify his or her own values. To be effective, workers must fully understand their own values and respect the client's right to have different values.

Consider the example of a human services worker who has strong personal values against abortion. The worker is asked to counsel a pregnant teenage client who is unsure about having the child. Obviously, the worker's personal values could have a strong influence on the way he or she goes about the helping process. If the worker pressures the client to make a decision in line with the worker's values, the client may later feel that she betrayed her own sense of what was right in this situation.

How can you as a beginning worker avoid placing values on others? It may help to think about the influences that shaped your values and beliefs. This will help you to appreciate the fact that people who come from different backgrounds may have values different from your own. Other people feel that their values are "right" just as your values feel "right" to you.

To begin the process of clarifying your values, you might answer these questions:

+ What values underlie your desire to help others?
+ What social issues do you feel strongly about?
+ Which client behaviors would you have trouble accepting?
+ Which of your values would you like to change?
+ What would you like to accomplish in human services?
+ How do you go about solving personal problems?
+ Do you readily seek help from others when you need it?

Professional Codes of Ethics

The development of professional **codes of ethics** involves the concept of "moral correctness." Deciding what is morally correct for everyone all of the time is a difficult, if not an impossible, task. One needs only to read a newspaper or listen to a TV news report to hear of the major battles fought daily in our elected legislative bodies over such issues as abortion, homosexuality, obscenity, premarital sex, or euthanasia. Certainly, the religions of the world vary in their views toward these and other issues. Even the law of the land varies considerably in different sections of the country regarding each of these issues. In 1973, the U. S. Supreme Court in the case of *Miller* v. *California* stated that local municipalities have the right to set their own standards concerning what is obscene.

Those charged with the responsibility of developing professional codes of ethics face the same difficult challenges. How can a particular set of guidelines or set of principles encompass everyone's varying beliefs? How one personally interprets the individual codes of ethics is yet another issue.

At present there is no single code of ethics that applies to all careers or disciplines in the broad field of human services. Rather, the professional organizations that represent individual careers have established separate codes of ethics to provide guidance and direction for their own members. Some professional organizations that have established such codes are the American Psychological Association (APA), the National Association of Social Workers (NASW), the American Medical Association (AMA), the Council for Standards in Human Service Education (CSHSE), the National Organization for Human Service Education (NOHSE), the American Association for Counseling and Development (AACD), the American Association for Marriage and Family Therapy (AAMFT), and the National Academy of Certified Clinical Mental Health Counselors (NACCMHC).

The general guidelines offered by professional codes of ethics could not possibly instruct the practitioner on what to do or how to behave in all professional situations. Ethical codes do, however, serve various important functions. For example, codes define minimal standards of professional conduct and attempt to ensure that workers meet various standards, requirements, or levels of competency (Corey, Corey, & Callanan, 1993). Ethical codes also define the scope or range of responsibilities for individuals and help to clarify various common issues of major concern within a particular field. Van Hoose and Kottler (1986) cited additional reasons that such codes exist: (a) they are self-imposed as an alternative to having regulations imposed by legislative bodies; (b) they are designed to prevent internal bickering and disagreement within the profession; and (c) they are designed to help protect the practitioner in areas of malpractice.

There are many areas of overlap among the various codes of ethics. The issue of client confidentiality and the right to privacy is one such area. The concept of confidentiality serves to protect the client from any unauthorized use of information by the human services worker without the informed consent of the client. In general, confidentiality can be viewed as a safeguard for clients' rights. Various professional codes offer guidelines articulating what is considered to be appropriate or responsible action for the practitioner in matters pertaining to this issue. For example, should a human services worker always share information concerning his or her client with the court if asked to do so? Is the worker ethically obligated to get the client's consent? The issue of client termination is another example. When is it considered to be ethically appropriate to disengage or terminate your work with a particular client? What responsibilities does the worker have to the community at large when working with dangerous or high-risk clients?

The Code of Ethics of the National Association of Social Workers (1993) addresses the issue of confidentiality in this manner:

H. Confidentiality and Privacy—The social worker should respect the privacy of clients and hold in confidence all information obtained in the course of professional service.

1. The social worker should share with others confidences revealed by clients, without their consent, only for compelling professional reasons.
2. The social worker should inform clients fully about the limits of confidentiality in a given situation, the purposes for which information is obtained, and how it may be used.
3. The social worker should afford clients reasonable access to any official social work records concerning them.

4. When providing clients with access to records, the social worker should take due care to protect the confidences of others contained in those records.
5. The social worker should obtain informed consent of clients before taping, recording, or permitting third party observation of their activities.*

The Ethical Standards of Human Service Workers (1995) also address client confidentiality:

The Human Service Professional's Responsibility to Clients

Statement 1   Human Service professionals negotiate with clients the purpose, goals, and nature of the helping relationship prior to its onset, as well as inform clients of the limitations of the proposed relationship.

Statement 2   Human service professionals respect the integrity and welfare of the client at all times. Each client is treated with respect, acceptance, and dignity.

Statement 3   Human service professionals protect the client's right to privacy and confidentiality except when such confidentiality would cause harm to the client or others, when agency guidelines state otherwise, or under other stated conditions (e.g., local, state, or federal laws). Professionals inform clients of the limits of confidentiality prior to the onset of the helping relationship.

Statement 4   If it is suspected that danger or harm may occur to the client or to others as a result of a client's behavior, the human service professional acts in an appropriate and professional manner to protect the safety of those individuals. This may involve seeking consultation, supervision, and/or breaking the confidentiality of the relationship.

Statement 5   Human service professionals protect the integrity, safety, and security of client records. All written client information that is shared with other professionals, except in the course of professional supervision, must have the client's prior written consent.

Statement 6   Human service professionals are aware that in their relationships with clients power and status are unequal. Therefore they recognize that dual or multiple relationships may increase the risk of harm to, or exploitation of, clients, and may impair their professional judgment. However, in some communities and situations it may not be feasible to avoid social or other nonprofessional contact with clients. Human service professionals support the trust implicit in the helping relationship by avoiding dual relationships that may impair professional judgment, increase the risk of harm to clients, or lead to exploitation.

*Copyright 1993, National Association of Social Workers, Inc. Reprinted with permission from the *Code of Ethics of the National Association of Social Workers,* page 6.

Statement 7   Sexual relationships with current clients are not considered to be in the best interest of the client and are prohibited. Sexual relationships with previous clients are considered dual relationships and are addressed in Statement 6 (above).

Statement 8   The client's right to self-determination is protected by human service professionals. They recognize the client's right to receive or refuse services.

Statement 9   Human service professionals recognize and build on client strengths.*

As we have discussed, in many instances professional codes of ethics can be very helpful to practitioners in their own fields. As with any set of guiding principles, the limitations are also apparent. Mabe and Rollin (1986) point out some of these limitations as follows:

1. Some issues cannot be suitably covered within the context of a code.
2. There are difficulties with the enforcement of codes.
3. There are possible conflicts between two codes, between the practitioners' values and the code requirements, and between the code and institutional practice.
4. There are instances in which issues in the various codes may be in conflict with the results of a court decision.

For additional information concerning the various professional codes of ethics, refer to the listing of professional organizations at the conclusion of Chapter 6. You can write directly to a professional organization and request a copy of their code of ethics.

Physical and Emotional Well-Being

Even such relatively mild physical maladies as a cold, a toothache, or an upset stomach can alter or diminish one's ability and efficiency in attending to others. While experiencing physical discomfort, we tend to be more focused on ourselves than on other people. In addition to distracting us, physical discomfort can distort the accuracy of sensory information we receive. A worker who feels depressed, run-down, or in a state of mental fatigue is also less likely to be as efficient as he or she ordinarily could be. When the worker is aware of these difficulties, he or she might do well to keep in mind how the difficulties can affect interaction with a client.

Environmental Factors

Physical space influences both the worker and the client. For example, arrangement of furniture influences behavior. Barriers placed between individuals, such as a desk separating a worker from a client, create a more formal, businesslike, less personal style of interaction. This physical sepa-

*Reprinted by permission of the National Organization for Human Service Education.

ration of several feet is analogous to keeping someone "at arm's length." Many large organizations serving the public often use barriers such as desks or counters with large plastic windows to create this type of environment. Acting in an intimate, personal, or less formal manner in this type of setting is often considered inappropriate. Removing the barriers and consequently becoming more physically accessible and closer to others create a different set of behavioral expectations. The worker should consider these factors.

Multicultural Awareness

Current demographic projections indicate that by the year 2000, 5 billion of the 6 billion people on Earth will be nonwhite (Hernandez, 1989). In the United States, immigration patterns continue to add to the mosaic of a culturally diverse population in which many different ethnic groups exist side by side. Within the human services field, it is increasingly likely that human services workers and their clients will have cultural backgrounds that differ. Understanding and working with cultural diversity have always been a part of the training of human services workers; however, their importance has become increasingly obvious, as the current population data confirm.

One's culture has a major influence on how one sees and experiences the world. Culture creates and shapes just about every aspect of a person's life, including language, beliefs, values, leisure activities, food consumption habits, clothing preferences, attitudes toward time, eye contact, gestures and body movements, facial expressions, and even attitudes toward life and death. Does a human services worker need a thorough knowledge of every client's cultural background in order to be effective? Current research findings differ somewhat on this question. For example, must all Native American counselors be trained to fully understand Chinese culture in order to work effectively with all Chinese clients? Lewis, Lynch, and Munger (1977) point out that counselor/client ethnic identity may have little relationship to the overall effectiveness of the counselor. On the other hand, Dillard (1987) concludes that to work effectively with clients of different cultures, counselors need to understand the social and psychological forces that affect their clients' verbal and nonverbal behavior. Cultural diversity is a fact of life in today's world. Pedersen (1990a) makes the point that counselors have two choices: to ignore the influence of culture or to attend to it. Either way, culture will still influence both the clients' and counselors' behavior. Pedersen believes that the focus on cultural diversity is the most important development in the counseling profession in the past decade. Although various research studies ascribe different degrees of importance to the need for multicultural awareness, we believe that a sensitivity toward and a knowledge of a client's cultural background can only serve to make the human services worker more effective.

Axelson (1985, p. 17) strongly suggests that all human service workers:

- become knowledgeable in several cultures
- study differences and similarities among people of different groups and their special needs and problems
- gain an understanding of how the individual relates to important events in life; what his or her personal values and morals are, and how they are constructed to form his or her world view

Skilled human services workers must become consciously aware of how their own background influences the application of their skills. Brill (1995, p. 251) stresses that workers must be aware of what they hold in terms of personal attitudes, biases, beliefs, and knowledge about their ethnically different clients that can affect their ability to consider problems objectively, define them accurately, make valid assessments, and present acceptable solutions. They must be particularly aware of the ever-present danger of stereotypes and generalizations as explanations of behavior. They must also consider the impact that conflicting demands have on people of one culture who are trying to adapt to life in another culture. Conflict can arise between family loyalties that may require a person to select a mate from within his or her original cultural group as opposed to the new environment, which offers many other possibilities.

Prior Training

As we indicated in Chapter 4, various theoretical approaches to helping are prevalent in the field. The approach a worker follows can influence how he or she perceives the client and therefore can affect which aspects of behavior he or she notes with particular emphasis. For example, the worker who employs a behavioral approach to helping might be more apt to notice and emphasize the client's overt physical manifestation of symptoms such as insomnia, weight loss, or nervous habits. The behaviorally oriented worker might not pay attention to certain aspects of the client's life history that could indicate an early childhood trauma. The psychoanalytically oriented worker, on the other hand, would be much quicker to notice and emphasize the earlier life experiences of the client. Strict adherence to a specific theoretical approach can limit the scope of one's skills.

HUMAN RIGHTS, THE LAW, AND HUMAN SERVICES

The laws of society affect all areas of human behavior. The law requires the members of a society to learn what is acceptable (i.e., legal behavior) and what is unacceptable (i.e., illegal behavior). It defines the rights of individuals and outlines society's obligations to its members. In many instances, the legal system has a direct influence on the provision of human services. As society becomes more complex, the interaction between the law and the human services system tends to increase. Slovenko (1973) has highlighted several of the more significant areas of concern as follows:

> In some instances, human services have assumed the role of religion explaining the causality of behavior. Behaviors previously viewed as sinful or unlawful may now be attributed to physiological or genetic causes. In this manner, individuals are *not* held responsible for their actions. Our discussion of the medical model in Chapter 4 highlights this point.
>
> Emphasis may be placed upon rehabilitation rather than retribution. The offender should be helped through our human services system rather than punished through our legal system.
>
> The state can intervene in the lives of those considered unable to handle their own affairs and who might present a problem to society. Some persons judged by the courts to be suffering from mental illness might be deprived of their rights.

The law can override the values of a professional code of ethics of a particular profession. This might occur when deemed legally necessary to protect the health, safety, and welfare of the public. For example, one such situation involves client confidentiality. The need for confidentiality is outlined in various professional codes of ethics and considered necessary to ensure the effective treatment of clients. However, the law may require the disclosure of client information in an effort to prevent harm to others. An illustration of this issue would be the California Supreme Court decision in the case of *Tarasoff* v. *Regents of the University of California* (1976). The court supported a "duty to warn" possible victims of clients whose counselors or therapists have such information. In general, the court stated that when therapists determine that a patient presents a serious danger to another, they are obligated to warn the intended victim. They are to apprise the victim of the danger, notify police, and take whatever other steps are reasonably necessary to protect the potential victim. Mehr (1995) expands these issues further when he points out the increased concern with the constitutional rights in regard to such issues as involuntary treatment, incarceration, and protecting the public.

As we have discussed, working within the complexities of our human services system requires a basic knowledge of the law. Specifically important is the relationship of law as it relates to various human rights issues. We now examine some of these more common and controversial issues further.

Voluntary and Involuntary Services

These concepts and their implications have broad meaning within our human services system. As Mehr (1995) suggests, the concept of **voluntary services** generally embraces some of the following guidelines:

1. The client decides that some form of help is needed, and he or she contracts with the service provider for help.

2. The client takes part in creating the objectives and goals of his or her own treatment.
3. The client can discontinue or terminate the treatment if desired.

The concept of **involuntary services** is quite the opposite. Services are assumed to be involuntary based upon these guidelines:

1. An individual or agency other than the client decides that a service is necessary. For example, the police or courts might require a homeless person to leave a public area and go to a shelter.
2. Various authorities (i.e., courts, legal guardian, therapist) require the client to obtain a particular service.
3. Various individuals other than the client set treatment goals.
4. The decision to terminate the service is determined by someone other than the actual client.

These concepts are examined more closely in Chapter 2 in our discussion concerning drug treatment programs.

The Right to Refuse Services

As helping professionals, we assume that our actions toward our clients are intended to be in their best interests. It has sometimes been assumed that we could successfully administer services even if the clients resisted our efforts. The clients' resistance was regarded as a function of their particular disorder, and it was thought that we knew what was best for them. Such actions of the past are no longer valid or legal in certain situations under current law. Recent law now stipulates that clients do have the right to refuse services. A common and often cited example would be the case of a patient within a mental hospital setting who refuses to take a particular medication prescribed by a physician. The courts have stated that it is illegal to force a patient to take the medication. However, if a judge declares the specific patient to be legally incompetent to make such decisions on his or her own behalf, then the patient can be forced to submit to involuntary treatment. Each situation must, of course, be reviewed based upon its own individual circumstances. People may still be committed to hospitals against their will and be required to receive treatment for specified periods of time. This issue is a multifaceted, controversial problem. The limits of the law relating to the extent to which patients can refuse certain types of treatment are currently being reexamined.

Due Process

The Constitution of the United States contains a provision under the 5th and 14th amendments that states if government activities affect an individual in a manner that would deprive the individual of liberty or property, this must be done with **due process** of law. Put quite simply, if you feel that you have been treated unfairly and would like the opportunity to state your position in court and rectify the wrong, you are seeking due process. For example, before a client can be committed for involuntary service for an unspecified period of time, the law provides for a hearing before a judge. Within a school setting, the right to due process may take the form of requiring school administrators to specify in writing various offenses for which a student can be disciplined. They must notify the children and their parents when rules are violated and then conduct a hearing. There can be either full or partial due process procedures. Full due process procedures usually involve representation by a lawyer, a hearing before an impartial judge and jury, the right to present evidence and have witnesses, and the right to a written statement of findings. This type of procedure is most common when a person might be seriously damaged by a particular decision.

In certain situations, when there is less potential for harm, the law provides for partial due process procedures. Partial due process procedures are usually less formal and may involve an administrative hearing rather than trial by jury. In these circumstances, there might be a notice of the charges and some type of assistance given in the preparation of a case. Human services organizations most commonly are involved with partial due process proceedings in disputes with clients. In this instance, the client has a right to appeal an organization's decision. An administrative hearing may be requested in which the client is allowed a legal advocate and an opportunity to state his or her case.

The Least Restrictive Alternative

Clients have the right to treatment in settings that are the **least restrictive** to their personal freedoms and liberties. For example, as Mehr (1995) points out, if clients can receive proper outpatient treatment while residing in a community setting, then they should not be hospitalized because that would deprive them of more personal freedom than necessary. Many individuals, however, remain in institutional settings, such as mental hospitals, mental retardation facilities, or nursing homes, because there may not be a less restrictive alternative available to them in a particular community.

THE WORKER IN GROUP SETTINGS

The responsibilities of a human services worker sometimes involve working with groups. This requires using the skills previously discussed in a somewhat different manner, as well as using additional skills. This section will focus on the basics of group dynamics and the skills necessary to facilitate group work. It is intended as an introduction for the beginning human services student; many additional concepts, skills, and techniques can be acquired through advanced training in group work.

Definition of a Group

There are a variety of ways to define a group, and many types of groups exist. For the purpose of our discussion, we can define a group as a collection of people who share a common purpose and who come together to achieve their goals by working together in some form. The primary characteristics of groups include the following:

- Group members perceive themselves to be a part of a group.
- Members are interdependent in some manner.
- Members strive to achieve goals.
- Members influence each other in some way.

Types of Groups

Because human services workers function in a variety of settings, the variety of groups they may be involved with is large. The following categories illustrate the broad range of types of groups:

- families with problems
- goal-oriented groups: task forces, teams, commissions, and so on
- personal growth groups: assertiveness, sensitivity, encounter, T-groups
- treatment groups: group therapy and group counseling around a wide variety of problems and using a wide variety of approaches such as Gestalt, rational-emotive, and transactional analysis therapies

It should be noted that categories can overlap to some extent. Often groups can have a multiple focus. For example, they may be both therapeutic and educational for members.

Group Leadership Skills

Group leaders share many traits with orchestra conductors (Benjamin, 1978). Both set the pace and the tone for the rest of the group. A worker who leads a group must be aware of the needs and goals of all members. What follows is an examination of basic group leadership skills found to be most useful in and applicable to group settings in the human services field.

Selecting Group Members. In many groups, especially in therapy or counseling groups, the selection of group members is an important consideration. Establishing a balanced group composition is often desirable. The worker might want to provide a varied mix of young and old, male and female, or talkative and quiet. Previous knowledge and information about an individual can help the worker make appropriate decisions concerning a person's suitability to a particular group.

Establishing Goals.   Once the group is established, the leader, together with the group members, must determine the group's objectives and goals. Goals are based on the members' level of functioning. In a group with a low level of functioning, the goals are usually set by the leader. Whether the goals are specific or general, they must be clearly defined and agreed upon by the group members. The leader should normally discuss group goals, suggest procedures, and provide an opportunity for group members to express their views.

Establishing Norms.   Establishing a clear set of group rules at the beginning helps the group to proceed more effectively toward its goals and enables the leader to determine whether or not the group is on the right track. Group rules or guidelines might address the issue of confidentiality by having participants agree to discuss group matters only within the confines of the group itself. Another rule might involve allowing each member to finish talking before another member can interrupt.

Intervening.   The helper **intervenes** by stepping in and attempting to change, modify, or point out something that is occurring in the group. Intervening is not focused exclusively on blocking negative aspects of a client's behavior. It can also be used to point out the positive aspects. For example, a helper may intervene between two clients who are arguing over a particular issue to point out to one of the clients that she is finally standing up for what she believes in. The leader may also intervene when one member violates the established rules of the group.

Sometimes groups get stuck. The leader may intervene in a group discussion when the discussion has reached an impasse. The leader may then suggest additional or alternative ways of viewing the situation or problem. The leader may also intervene by introducing a specific therapeutic technique, such as role playing, to help clarify and bring additional insights to a particular problem that a client or group of clients may be experiencing. Knowing how and when to move in is as important in group work as it is in interviewing.

Promoting Interaction.   By skillfully facilitating, the group leader helps to promote and bring about interaction among the group members. Promoting interaction can lead to the establishing of clear channels of communication among clients. When group members are linked to one another, they begin to work together and relate personally to one another. To be effective as a facilitator, the leader needs to be insightful and sensitive. The leader has to find ways of relating the concerns of one individual to the concerns or struggles of another. This provides further opportunities for mutual support and helps to develop a feeling of interconnectedness and cohesiveness.

The result of this process can be the creation of a climate of safety and acceptance in which members trust one another and are therefore likely to engage in productive interchanges (Corey & Corey, 1987). As a facilitator, the group leader helps the participants to express their problems, provides support as members explore aspects of themselves, and essentially helps group members reach their individual goals through this mutually influencing process.

Appraising/Evaluating.   The group leader must appraise the ongoing process and goals of the group. It is particularly helpful to do this after each group meeting. The leader must reflect on what is happening in the group, the direction it seems to be taking, how it helps certain participants and not others, and the types of interventions that may be helpful in the next group session. Often a leader will suggest that the members become part of this process by sharing their evaluations of what is happening in the group with group members. In this process, group members can become more aware of how they are influenced by others and how others may be influenced by them. As a result of the process, constructive changes or new goals can be implemented to enable the group to fulfill more of each member's stated needs.

Termination in the Group.   The issue of termination emerges in every group in various ways. Workers must know how to end each group session. Sessions can be terminated in a number of ways. The leader can suggest to members how to transfer what they have learned in the group to other life situations or environments. The leader can summarize what happened during a session or can ask the members to think about some point that has emerged. The leader can also end a session by suggesting minigoals for clients to work on.

Workers must know when it is most appropriate for a certain member to leave the group. In this decision, the worker must consider and evaluate all available information that pertains to the client, such as the client's stated goals, his or her past and present abilities to achieve stated goals, and whether the group is still useful for the client's present situation.

A worker must also know when an entire group has completed its work and it is time to disband. Has the group achieved its stated purposes or goals? If the leader has previously highlighted a clear set of group goals, developed constructive group guidelines, and consistently monitored the group's progress, the group is now in a good position to decide about termination.

THE WORKER IN THE COMMUNITY

As human services systems have developed in order to identify and meet human needs, new and diverse activities and functional roles have been created for workers. Workers are spending increasing time in community settings because of the need to locate services for clients, to enlist the aid of

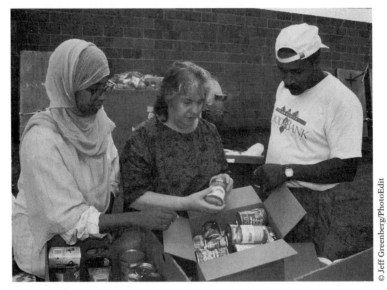

A helping hand from a community outreach worker

various organizations in developing new services, and to provide information that might help to prevent problems. As any system gets larger, workers need additional skills and knowledge to understand and effectively use the resources available within the system. The individual and group skills previously examined in this chapter are, of course, components of all human services activities. As the contemporary worker has become more involved in various aspects and activities of the community, the need for additional knowledge and skills has emerged. Additional skills useful for the community worker are the following:

- ◆ advocating
- ◆ negotiating
- ◆ organizing
- ◆ coordinating
- ◆ educating
- ◆ planning
- ◆ consulting
- ◆ gathering information
- ◆ acting as liaison
- ◆ lobbying
- ◆ reaching out

By examining some of the functional roles and activities most often performed by workers in the community, you can begin to understand why these skills are needed and how they might be used.

Client Advocacy

When functioning as a client advocate, the human services worker represents clients by helping them obtain whatever services they need. The worker attempts to bring community resources to the individual or group. In this context, the worker identifies and assesses the needs of the client or group and matches the available community resources to the client's or group's needs. For example, a client may be entitled to social security or welfare benefits but may be denied these services for improper reasons or because of lack of information. The helper's work then involves educating the client about all available services. The worker may literally act for clients, confronting and negotiating bureaucratic mazes to ensure that clients receive all the governmental services to which they are entitled. Often this work involves coordinating and gathering a substantial amount of information concerning the various programs of service available and the procedures necessary to qualify for the programs.

As the client's representative, the worker actually pleads the client's case to other individuals who represent different services or agencies within the larger system. This can often be extremely frustrating, and it is all too easy to lose one's patience and temper. Negotiating skills are very useful here. Knowing when to be forceful and when to compromise often makes the difference between getting needed services and not getting them.

Community Organizing

As an organizer, the human services worker acts to bring various sections of the community together to create, improve, or maintain programs. Some examples of this organizing function might include the development of a job-training program within a community or setting up an after-school program using already existing playground facilities. An organizer brings together various agencies and programs and uses all available resources to resolve a particular problem.

To accomplish these tasks, the worker must know the community political structure and the various financial realities. Functioning in this capacity often brings the worker into the political arena. Knowing who has the power to accomplish a particular task is very important. It helps if the worker is a skilled and articulate speaker because it is often necessary to plead one's case before groups and committees. Being able to work independently and under pressure is another important attribute of the community organizer.

Community Outreach

Human services workers who perform outreach activities can generally be found working directly in the client's environment. In many instances, a client may be unable or unwilling owing to physical or emotional illness to come to a specific human services center. In this case, the outreach worker actually visits the client's residence and helps with a variety of concerns related to all aspects of daily living. A typical service involving these types of activities is a home-bound elderly program. Elderly individuals can become, through illness or other factors, unable to accomplish certain tasks for themselves. The worker's activities here might involve helping the client to shop for groceries, teaching the client how to budget money more effectively, informing and educating the client about health and nutrition concerns, and actually helping the client to learn or relearn many daily activities that other people take for granted.

Other outreach activities and services focus on the recently discharged psychiatric patient, who may require some form of help to make the transition back into community living. Here, the worker might be involved in teaching a client how to use forms of public transportation, linking clients to other services available in the community, and helping clients to develop a range of personal interests that could enhance their quality of life. It is often the outreach worker who is the primary liaison between clients in the community and available community services.

Coordinating Services

Service coordination is becoming more common and visible in today's human services systems. The service coordinator is responsible for overseeing a certain caseload of clients. The primary task is to make sure the identified clients receive access to a system of coordinated services designed to meet their individual needs. Through personal interviews and by gathering previous reports and evaluations from other workers, the service coordinator determines to which available services it is appropriate to channel the client. For example, a client seeing an outpatient counselor once a week for specific problems may also be unemployed and in need of vocational training. Unemployment and lack of money may have also caused the client to be in need of adequate housing. The service coordinator must evaluate all of this client's needs and try to develop a coordinated treatment plan designed to meet the stated needs.

Often, the service coordinator meets regularly with staff representatives from the various services or programs the client is involved with to discuss and monitor the client's progress and make necessary adjustments. The service coordinator becomes primarily responsible for the client within the context of the services system. The ability to gather information, to plan and coordinate services, and to work effectively with a variety of professionals from different parts of the system are required for this work activity.

Providing Information

One of the major tasks confronting human services is to educate and inform the public. Often, people can prevent small problems from becoming larger ones if they only know who to turn to for help, what legal rights they possess, and what alternatives are available to them. Access to information can actually prevent some prevalent social problems.

To provide information to the community, human services workers are involved with many aspects of our daily lives. For example, workers can be found visiting local high schools to provide current information on such topics as drug abuse, birth control, and alcoholism. In other segments of the community, workers are likely to be involved with civic or church-related groups, providing information concerning social security benefits, welfare procedures, or family planning. Many community mental-health centers have a specific consultation and education department whose designated task is to provide these types of information to a particular community. A more in-depth examination of the role of prevention in the human services field is provided in Chapter 8.

ADDITIONAL READING

Andrews, L. M. (1989). *To thine own self be true.* New York: Doubleday.

Berry, C. R. (1989). *When helping you is hurting me: Escaping the Messiah trap.* San Francisco: Harper & Row.

Devore, W., & Schlesinger, E. G. (1981). *Ethnic-sensitive social work practice.* St. Louis: C. V. Mosby.

Fischer, L., & Sorrenson, G. P. (1985). *School law for counselors, psychologists, and social workers.* New York: Longman.

Johnson, D. W., & Johnson, F. P. (1982). *Joining together: Group theory and group skills* (2nd ed.). Englewood Cliffs, NJ: Prentice Hall.

Knapp, M. L. (1972). *Nonverbal communication in human interaction.* New York: Holt, Rinehart & Winston.

Kottler, J. A. (1983). *Pragmatic group leadership.* Pacific Grove, CA: Brooks/Cole.

Maeder, T. (1990). *Children of psychiatrists and other mental health professionals.* New York: Harper & Row.

Schulman, E. D. (1991). *Intervention in human services: A guide to skills and knowledge* (4th ed.). New York: Macmillan.

REFERENCES

Avila, D. L., Combs, A. W., & Purkey, W. W. (1978). *The helping relationship sourcebook.* Boston: Allyn & Bacon.

Axelson, J. A. (1985). *Counseling and development in a multicultural society.* Pacific Grove, CA: Brooks/Cole.

Benjamin, A. (1978). *Behavior in small groups.* Boston: Houghton Mifflin.

Brammer, L. M. (1981). *The helping relationship—Process and skills* (4th ed.). Englewood Cliffs, NJ: Prentice Hall.

Brill, N. (1973). *Working with people.* Philadelphia: Lippincott.

Brill, N. (1995). *Working with people: The helping process* (5th ed.). New York: Longman.

Carkhuff, R. R., & Berenson, B. G. (1967). *Beyond counseling and therapy.* New York: Holt, Rinehart & Winston.

Combs, A. W., Avila, D. L., & Purkey, W. W. (1978). *Helping relationships.* Boston: Allyn & Bacon.

Corey, G. (1986). *Theory and practice of counseling and psychotherapy* (3rd ed.). Pacific Grove, CA: Brooks/Cole.

Corey, G. (1991). *Theory and practice of counseling and psychotherapy* (4th ed.). Pacific Grove, CA: Brooks/Cole.

Corey, G., & Corey, M. S. (1987). *Groups: Process and practice* (3rd ed.). Pacific Grove, CA: Brooks/Cole.

Corey, G., & Corey, M., & Callanan, P. (1993). *Issues and ethics in the helping professions* (2nd ed.). Pacific Grove, CA: Brooks/Cole.

Cormier, W. H., & Cormier, L. S. (1985). *Interviewing strategies for helpers: Fundamental skills and cognitive behavioral interventions* (2nd ed.). Pacific Grove, CA: Brooks/Cole.

Cowen, E. L., Leibowitz, E., & Leibowitz, G. (1968). Utilization of retired people as mental health aides with children. *American Journal of Orthopsychiatry, 38,* 900–909.

Danish, S. J., & Haner, A. L. (1976). *Helping skills: A basic training program.* New York: Human Services Press.

Dillard, J. M. (1987). *Multicultural counseling.* Chicago: Nelson-Hall.

Ellis, A., & Yeager, R. J. (1989). *Why some therapies don't work.* Buffalo, NY: Prometheus Books.

Green, J. W. (1995). *Cultural awareness in the human services* (2nd ed.). Boston: Allyn & Bacon.

Hernandez, H. (1989). *Multicultural education: A teacher's guide to content and process.* Columbus, OH: Merrill.

Ivey, A. E., Ivey, M. B., & Simek-Downing, L. (1987). *Counseling and psychotherapy: Integrating skills, theory, and practice* (2nd ed.). Englewood Cliffs, NJ: Prentice Hall.

Johnson, D. W. (1986). *Reaching out—Interpersonal effectiveness and self-actualization* (3rd ed.). Englewood Cliffs, NJ: Prentice Hall.

Julia, M. C. (1996). *Multicultural awareness in the health care professions.* Boston: Allyn & Bacon.

Kohut, H. (1984). *How does psycho-analysis cure?* Chicago: University of Chicago Press.

Lewis, M. H., Lynch, M. L., & Munger, P. F. (1977). The influence of ethnicity on the necessary and sufficient conditions of client-centered counseling. *Journal of Non-white Concerns, 5,* 134–142.

Mabe, A. R., & Rollin, S. A. (1986). The rate of a code of ethical standards in counseling. *Journal of Counseling and Development, 64*(5), 294–297.

May, R., & Yalom, I. (1989). Existential psychotherapy. In R. J. Corsini & D. Wedding (Eds.). *Current psychotherapies* (4th ed., pp. 363–402). Itasca, IL: F. E. Peacock.

Mehr, J. (1995). *Human services: Concepts and intervention strategies* (6th ed.). Boston: Allyn & Bacon.

Neukrug, E. (1994). *Theory, practice, and the trends in human services.* Pacific Grove, CA: Brooks/Cole.

Nichols, M. P., & Schwartz, R. C. (1995). *Family therapy concepts and methods* (3rd ed.). Boston: Allyn & Bacon.

Parson, R. D. (1995). *The skills of helping.* Boston: Allyn & Bacon.

Pedersen, P. (1990a). The constructs of complexity and balance in multicultural counseling theory and practice. *Journal of Counseling and Development, 68*(5), 550–554.

Pedersen, P. (1990b). The multicultural perspective on a fourth force in counseling. *Journal of Mental Health Counseling, 12,* 93–95.

Rogers, C. R. (1961). *On becoming a person.* Boston: Houghton Mifflin.

Schulman, E. D. (1991). *Intervention in the human services* (4th ed.). St. Louis: C. V. Mosby.

Shriver, J. M. (1995). *Behavior and the social environment.* Boston: Allyn & Bacon.

Slovenko, R. (1973). *Psychiatry and the law.* Boston: Little, Brown.

Spiegler, M. D. (1983). *Contemporary behavioral theory.* Palo Alto, CA: Mayfield.

Truax, C. B., & Carkhuff, R. R. (1967). *Toward effective counseling and psychotherapy.* Chicago: Aldine.

Van Hoose, W., & Kottler, J. (1986). *Ethical and legal issues in counseling and psychotherapy* (2nd ed.). San Francisco: Jossey-Bass.

Wicks, R. J. (1979). *Helping others: Ways of listening, sharing, and counseling.* New York: Chilton.

Woodside, M., & McClam, T. (1994). *An introduction to human services* (2nd ed.). Pacific Grove, CA: Brooks/Cole.

6

Careers in
Human Services

INTRODUCTION

All human services share the goal of helping people to live healthier and more productive lives. The range of career fields within human services that shares this goal is broad and includes mental health, education, health, social services, vocational rehabilitation, child care, and housing. There are a variety of specific job titles within each of these fields. Considering the wide range of career options, it is not surprising that the beginning worker often feels uncertain about which path to follow. This chapter is intended to provide basic career information to help you make an informed choice.

We have selected for coverage a representative cross section of human services careers, as it is not possible to describe in the space of a chapter all the career options. The emphasis is on career fields that together are attracting the large majority of individuals entering human services today. These are generalist human services work, therapeutic recreation, creative arts therapy, psychiatric nursing, occupational therapy, clinical psychology, social work, and psychiatry. Because psychiatry demands lengthy, difficult, and costly training, this career may not attract the same numbers of students as other career options in the human services field. It is examined in this chapter because the majority of human services workers are likely to come into contact with psychiatrists in their professional work. Some knowledge of the psychiatrist's background and training may therefore be helpful.

You will notice that a great deal of overlap exists among careers in terms of work setting, duties, and levels of responsibility. To help you obtain additional information about each career field described, names and addresses of professional organizations associated with each field are provided at the conclusion of this chapter.

GENERALIST HUMAN SERVICES WORK

Many educators feel that the term **paraprofessional,** widely accepted in the past, no longer accurately reflects the knowledge, abilities, skills, and training of graduates of recognized undergraduate human services programs of today. They feel that graduates of such programs should be considered professional human services workers. Another group of educators believes that the professional label should be reserved for only those who have attained a graduate degree in one of the traditional human services fields, such as psychology or social work. We will use the term **generalist human services worker** and discuss this controversy further in Chapter 9.

Functions

The work roles and functions of generalist human services workers vary greatly. Generalist workers represent the largest number of workers and usually have the most contact with those in need. In some instances, the duties of generalist workers are similar to those of professionals.

The generalist human services worker may perform some of the same duties as the traditional professional, but the extent of decision making, the level of responsibility, and the range and depth of activity are not as great (Schmolling, Burger, & Youkeles, 1981). For example, as a staff member working within a social service agency, a generalist worker might perform preliminary interviews and client screening, make home visits, gather information, perform administrative functions including preparing reports or setting fee schedules, and act as a member of a treatment team. The professional worker might also perform these functions and in addition might make diagnoses, provide short- and long-term psychotherapy, and plan specific courses of treatment or action. Although an overlap of duties may exist, the traditional professional most often acts in a supervisory capacity and is, therefore, given greater responsibility for all work performed.

During the 1960s, the worker shortage in human services greatly spurred the training and use of generalist human services workers. The new workers not only helped alleviate the shortage but also provided services in many ways (Sobey, 1969). However, the influx of generalist workers into the field caused tension and controversy to develop between them and the traditional professionals in many agencies. This tension was caused, in part, by the belief of generalist workers (and certain professionals as well) that advanced graduate or professional training was not always necessary to perform many functions in human services satisfactorily. Others believed that advanced education and/or traditional professional training was essential for many tasks. This controversy (which is discussed further in Chapter 9) continues to the present day.

There are many specific job titles within the broad category of generalist human services work. Different institutions, agencies, and programs use various titles to refer to generalist workers. For example, a state psychiatric hospital may use the job titles of psychiatric aide, mental-health aide, mental-health technician, or mental-health trainee. A social services system might use the job titles of social work aide, social work associate, or community worker. Not only are there a variety of titles, but other designations are also used to refer to a specific level of work and responsibility within a given job title. For example, as a mental-health aide, one might be at level I, II, III, IV, or V. Each higher level usually denotes a greater degree of responsibility and/or supervisory function and also carries with it a higher salary and greater prestige. These various levels indicate a career ladder approach in human services similar to that of the civil service system.

The following examples illustrate more clearly some of the functions of generalist workers. It must be emphasized that these examples represent only a limited portrayal of generalist human services work drawn from a broad range of activities.

Example A: Social Work Assistant III

Ms. G. has a bachelor's degree in psychology and is a generalist human services worker under the job title of Social Work Assistant III in a nursing home. She is a member of a treatment team, along with an MSW, certified social worker, a master's degree-level psychologist, and a psychiatrist. The team meets twice weekly, during which time Ms. G. shares information of social and emotional significance observed during daily interactions with specific clients. The goal of these meetings is to develop and monitor treatment plans that may be required for individual clients. Other aspects of her weekly work activities include a great deal of patient contact, such as leading a weekly discussion group with clients, transporting nonambulatory clients to meals and appointments, and assisting an art therapist who conducts weekly classes for the clients.

Example B: Mental-Health Assistant II

Mr. F. is a generalist human services worker who has an associate of science degree in community mental health and works in a large psychiatric hospital under the job title of Mental Health Assistant II. He already has basic academic and fieldwork experience in the mental-health field, but he is required to participate in a year-long training program conducted by the hospital for all its generalist worker staff. These workshop training programs are designed to familiarize the generalist worker with hospital procedure and to teach specific treatment approaches, methods, and problem-solving techniques. Mr. F.'s primary duties involve working with a professional social worker to conduct daily therapeutic group discussions with the clients, implementing individual treatment programs with clients, attending treatment team meetings with other generalist workers and professional staff, and performing a variety of clerical duties such as ordering various supplies for the ward to which he is assigned. In addition, Mr. F. regularly conducts tours through his ward and provides information for visiting students who are currently enrolled in college mental-health programs.

Example C: Psychiatric Aide III

Ms. C. is a generalist human services worker who has a high school diploma and 1 year of college coursework. She works in the day treatment program of a community mental-health center under the job title of Psychiatric Aide III. Ms. C. works with former long-term institutionalized patients who attend this program as part of their discharge treatment plan from the hospital. She leads various groups with clients on a daily basis. The group topics often include nutrition and health, current events, money management, and basic adult reading and writing. She often organizes and arranges trips with clients to various activities and events in the community. As a member of a treatment team, she works with social workers, psychologists, and psychiatrists to help develop treatment plans for the clients in her program. A great deal of her work involves helping clients with activities of daily living, which include shopping for groceries, getting help with housing problems or welfare problems, buying clothing, and using the public transportation system.

◆

A Day in the Life
of a Generalist Human Services Worker

Amy E. Earned her B.A. degree in applied psychology/mental health at an eastern university. She is presently employed as a milieu therapist in a halfway house serving ten deinstitutionalized mental patients. There are five female and five male residents served by seven staff members consisting of a director, assistant director, and five generalist workers called milieu therapists.

A typical day for Amy might look like this:

9:00–9:30 A.M.: Amy reads the reports of what occurred with the residents during the previous evening and overnight. She notes that John had an intense argument with Dan during the evening and that the anger did not lessen before bedtime. She will keep an eye on both residents and try to help them deal with their anger without hurting each other.

9:30–10:00 A.M.: Amy meets with other staff members to discuss plans for the day. They discuss who will be liaison to job sites and sheltered workshops, who will supervise the making of meals, who will accompany residents to hospital or doctor, and similar assignments.

10:00–11:00 A.M.: Amy meets with John and Dan, whose display of anger is of concern to other residents and the staff. She attempts to help them discuss their feelings toward each other and resolve their differences before they become a risk to themselves and others.

11:00 A.M.–12 noon: Amy attends a case management meeting with the assistant director. They discuss plans for Judy, a resident who is presently able to enter a sheltered workshop on a limited basis and who must also see her therapist regularly.

1:00–2:30 P.M.: Amy calls and/or visits the different job sites and sheltered workshops in which residents are placed. She meets with supervisor to discuss the problems or progress of the residents. On this day there are no particular problems or signs of noticeable progress on the part of any of the workers.

2:30–4:30 P.M.: Amy meets with the residents assigned to the sheltered workshop to discuss the happenings of the day and any problems they may have encountered. Mary tells Amy that she is upset about how the workshop supervisor spoke to her. The group then discusses how Mary might respond to the supervisor.

4:30–5:00 P.M.: Amy writes up her notes on her work with the residents and her perceptions of the residents' progress or problems. These notes are shared with the entire staff to be used in making future plans to help the residents.

It is clear that Amy is very interested and enjoys her work. It is a learning experience and could be even more so if there were more (professional) supervision.* ◆

Training and Education

Training for a generalist human services worker career is usually accomplished by one of two routes. The first route involves formal completion of a 2- or 4-year college or university academic human services program. These degree-granting programs prepare the individual for an entry-level position in the human services field. Completion of a 2-year program gives the individual basic coursework and fieldwork experiences. A typical 2-year community mental-health program leading to an associate degree might include such courses as basic psychology, developmental psychology, behavior pathology, interviewing, and fieldwork. Field-based courses have students work directly in community field sites under the supervision of a college faculty member. This 2-year program is the primary route to a generalist worker career. Completion of a 4-year college program is usually viewed as preparation for a more advanced professional career.

A 4-year program might have class and fieldwork requirements similar to the 2-year program but usually requires more extensive coursework in other areas as well. The 4-year program places greater emphasis on liberal arts studies and offers more advanced coursework in specific types of therapy and additional skills training.

The second route to becoming a generalist human services worker is through training offered by specific institutions such as mental hospitals, social service agencies, or community mental-health centers. These institutions usually have on-the-job or in-service training programs for individuals who lack a formal college degree but desire a generalist worker career. Such programs usually provide basic courses focusing on administrative procedures, patient and staff issues, counseling or treatment methods, medical issues, and other selected topics pertaining to that specific institution. It should be mentioned that there are agencies that hire generalist

*Reprinted with permission from Schmolling, P., Burger, W., & Youkeles, M. (1986), *Careers in Mental Health: A Guide to the Helping Occupations.* Garrett Park, MD: Garrett Park Press.

workers but provide little or no training. This lack of generalist worker training has raised serious questions and concerns.

THERAPEUTIC RECREATION

Therapeutic recreation is the selected use of recreational activities as an aid in the treatment, correction, or rehabilitation of physical or mental disorders. The primary focus of this form of treatment is corrective or rehabilitative. Recreation alone cannot cure a disability or disease. It can help an individual with a temporary disability regain his or her former level of functioning, or it can help an individual with a permanent disability learn to function maximally within the limits set by the specific disability.

Functions

Recreation therapists work in a variety of treatment and nontreatment settings, including nursing homes, hospitals, mental-health centers, rehabilitation institutions, recreation centers, parks, senior citizen centers, and Ys. The recreation therapist is most often part of a treatment team in treatment and/or institutional settings. Such a team may consist of a physician, a psychologist, a social worker, a nurse, or representatives from other fields as necessitated by the individual needs of a patient. Nontreatment settings usually find the recreation therapist working independently. In either setting, this specialist can function with individuals or groups. Recreation can have an educative function in addition to having therapeutic value and providing pleasure. The educative functions are present in many aspects of a recreation therapist's work, but these functions are most clearly evident in nontreatment settings such as YMCAs, park programs, and senior citizen centers.

In nontreatment settings, the recreation therapist designs and implements programs for special populations, such as children with disabilities, individuals with weight problems, or senior citizens who desire a constructive and consistent fitness program. In addition to developing the programs, the specialist spends time instructing individuals in the rudiments of such a program. The specialist often conducts brief classes to explain the benefits of the program, teaches individuals how to use any equipment involved in the program, and monitors individuals' progress toward desired goals.

As previously mentioned, in treatment settings such as mental hospitals, mental-health centers, or rehabilitation centers, the recreation therapist's work activities are usually coordinated with recommendations from the treatment team. Consider the example of a patient in a mental hospital who has a history of aggressive and antisocial behavior. One of the recommendations of the treatment team is that the patient slowly be introduced to recreation activities that might serve as an outlet for pent-up anger and frustration and facilitate the development of a sense of social cooperation. The recreation therapist develops a suitable treatment approach to achieve these goals. The patient is initially introduced to activities that can be performed alone, such as playing basketball, jogging, and swimming. Over a period of weeks and months, the specialist may give the patient some instructions as to the finer points of the activity and possibly do the activity with the patient. After another length of time, the patient may wish to test his or her skill with another patient or staff member. The hope is that the patient will gradually begin to function more constructively with others, using recreation as the vehicle to attain this goal.

The recreation therapist may also perform various other functions in addition to providing direct services to clients. Administrative duties often involve directing recreation training programs in colleges and universities. Many recreation therapists consult with private and public agencies and institutions. Other specialists may work for city, county, or state government agencies designing or planning recreation programs for specific communities.

Training and Education

To become a professional recreation therapist, one must complete a bachelor's degree, with major emphasis in the therapeutic recreation, from an accredited college or university. Such college or university programs usually include coursework in recreational leadership, therapeutic recreation, biology, psychology, physical education, and other relevant areas. Many programs require a practical fieldwork experience in addition to coursework. In this context, the aspiring recreation therapist learns to put theory into practice. It is advisable, although not usually mandatory, for the student to gain proficiency in selected sports or activity areas.

Master's degree programs are also available and are another way to enter the field. Individuals with bachelor's degrees in areas other than therapeutic recreation can pursue a master's degree in the field and enter the field on that level. Of course, pursuing a master's is ordinarily an advantageous way of increasing one's expertise and training in the field, even if one already possesses the bachelor's degree in therapeutic recreation. Coursework in master's programs may include therapeutic recreation for special populations, administration of therapeutic recreation services, and consultation in therapeutic recreation.

CREATIVE ARTS THERAPY

Dance, music, and art therapy constitute what are broadly referred to as **creative arts therapies** or expressive therapies. Creative arts therapists use dance, music, or art in a therapeutic manner to facilitate an individual's insight, self-expression, and social awareness. Creative arts used in a therapeutic manner can provide a means of nonverbal communication in which an individual can express psychological needs. The fields of dance, music, and art therapy share many common characteristics, which will be discussed, but the fields differ regarding specific training and required skills.

Functions

Creative arts therapists are employed in many settings, including public and private hospitals, nursing homes, mental-health clinics, rehabilitation centers, senior citizen centers, public and private schools, and halfway houses. Many interesting and innovative programs using the creative arts have been established in prisons and facilities for the terminally ill. The creative arts have been shown to be a useful form of therapy for a wide range of populations, including the learning disabled, emotionally disturbed, retarded, blind, deaf, and physically disabled.

Many creative arts therapists function as members of therapeutic treatment teams, particularly in agency or institutional settings. The creative arts therapist, as a member of this team, makes recommendations regarding a client's plan of treatment, evaluates a client's progress, and works directly with an individual client, group, or family. Consider the following example.

A creative arts specialist with expertise in art therapy is working with an emotionally troubled child in a residential treatment facility. The child is relatively nonverbal and feels somewhat threatened, unable to talk about her feelings and problems. Psychotherapy, which relies heavily on a person's verbal ability, has thus far been unable to uncover any specifically useful material with which to help the child understand and learn how to cope with her problems. The treatment team recommends art therapy as an appropriate means to facilitate more fruitful insights into this child. The creative arts therapist begins by having the child draw pictures of herself and her family and surroundings. This visual representation of the child's feelings and perceptions reveals a lot about the child's current problems. How the child works with the various art materials, such as oil paints, charcoals, and clay, also indicates and helps release high levels of tension and frustration. The creative arts therapist and the treatment team are not in a more advantageous position from which to evaluate the needs of the child and develop a more complete plan of treatment.

The creative arts therapist with expertise in dance or music can function in a manner similar to the art therapist. Dance therapy focuses on the nonverbal aspects of personality and behavior as represented by an individual's body movement. Music therapy can increase an individual's self-confidence, help develop a sense of accomplishment and personal satisfaction, improve eye-hand coordination, and increase an individual's attention span.

Whereas many creative arts therapists work in institutional settings, others work as consultants and/or maintain private practices in which they work with clients. Some therapists teach in training programs or college or university programs. The creative arts therapist may serve as an administrator in creative arts or expressive therapy departments in virtually all the settings previously described.

Training and Education

As mentioned earlier, training and educational requirements vary somewhat for the different types of creative arts therapists. The professional organization associated with each field develops criteria for professional recognition within the field.

Art.   At present, to be recognized as a creative arts therapist with expertise in art and to be professionally qualified to use the title of art therapist, one must obtain a master's degree in art therapy or complete a graduate-level training program in an institute or clinic that is accredited by the American Art Therapy Association.

Dance.   In the field of dance therapy, the American Dance Therapy Association also considers a master's degree or equivalent graduate-level training to be the minimum for an entry-level position in the field. Successful completion of graduate training qualifies the creative arts therapist with specialization in the field of dance to use the title of dance therapist.

Music.   In the field of music, the National Association for Music Therapy considers the completion of a 4-year undergraduate degree with major emphasis in music therapy to be sufficient for professional recognition as a music therapist.

PSYCHIATRIC NURSING

Psychiatric nursing is the specialization within the broad field of nursing that places emphasis on treatment of the physical and mental well-being of a patient. Psychiatric nursing is directed toward assisting the patient to maintain and restore optimum levels of physical and mental health.

Functions

Psychiatric nurses are employed in a variety of settings, including inpatient and outpatient units of public and private hospitals, community mental-health clinics, rehabilitation centers, and residential mental-health treatment facilities. Psychiatric nurses can also maintain private practices in which they provide consultation, counseling, or psychotherapy services to individuals, families, or groups. Psychiatric nurse specialists can also teach in a variety of training programs in hospital, clinic, and college or university settings. Psychiatric nurses can function as administrators of such programs and pursue specific research interests in any of the many professional settings available.

The specific work activities and functions of the psychiatric nurse vary considerably depending on the setting. Still, there are common work activities and functions that can be discussed. The psychiatric nurse in the psychiatric hospital setting is often a member of a therapeutic treatment team. He or she meets regularly with other team members, who may include a psychiatrist, a psychologist, a social worker, a generalist human services worker, and other professional staff. The psychiatric nurse, as a member of this team, is integrally involved in developing individualized treatment plans for patients, implementing treatment, and evaluating progress.

A major portion of a psychiatric nurse's professional time is spent working directly with patients who have physical as well as mental disorders. He or she is a key figure in establishing and maintaining a therapeutic relationship with the client. The psychiatric nurse often explains to patients specific aspects of their illnesses. If the patient is taking prescribed medication for an illness, the psychiatric nurse can administer the medication and explain what the medication is and does and what to expect. He or she is trained to observe and understand patient behavior. The psychiatric nurse may work as a counselor to patients, helping them to understand and cope with their illness and helping them to regain a higher level of control over their lives. An emotional illness can often interfere with the patient's ability to understand and meet physical health needs. In this case, the psychiatric nurse might teach patients how to take better care of themselves both physically and emotionally.

Training and Education

According to the American Nurses Association and the National League for Nursing, professional recognition as a clinical specialist in psychiatric nursing requires successful completion of an accredited master's degree program in a clinical psychiatric nursing specialty area. Many colleges and universities provide graduate study in child, adolescent, and family psychiatric nursing, which presently constitute the clinical psychiatric nursing specialty areas.

Before attending a master's degree program in psychiatric nursing, one must complete the training required to become a registered nurse. This usually can be accomplished by completing an accredited program of study offered by various hospital nursing programs, 2-year community college programs, or 4-year bachelor's degree programs. A typical bachelor's degree program includes coursework and supervised clinical internships. Undergraduate programs usually emphasize courses in anatomy and physiology but also offer other courses such as nursing the emotionally ill, family-centered maternity nursing, nursing of children, emergency health care, and drug calculations in nursing. The clinical internship offers students practical nursing experience in different settings under the supervision of a faculty member from the student's college or university nursing program.

The American Nurses Association considers a nurse without advanced clinical training (from an accredited master's degree program) to be a general nurse, even if he or she works exclusively in a psychiatric setting. In-service training programs, continuing education programs, and workshops are available for registered nurses who desire more proficiency in psychiatric nursing but are not enrolled in a master's degree program. Nurses at this level can be certified as generalists through the American Nurses Association rather than as clinical psychiatric nurses.

One can apply to the American Nurses Association for professional recognition and certification as a clinical psychiatric nurse upon completion of the master's degree program of study. There are no current universal state certification requirements for psychiatric nursing. Some states require certification for psychiatric nurses, whereas other states, such as New York, presently have no such requirement. Various doctoral programs are available for psychiatric nurses wishing further training and professional recognition beyond the master's level.

OCCUPATIONAL THERAPY

Occupational therapy is the selective and purposeful therapeutic use of activities to aid in the treatment of physical or mental disorders. Occupational therapy can serve as one part of an individual's overall treatment plan (along with other therapeutic approaches such as psychotherapy or physical therapy) or can be the sole therapeutic approach used to aid an individual. The range of uses of occupational therapy is enormous. It has proved a useful treatment for problems such as physical disabilities, emotional or developmental disorders, and injuries due to accidents. It is particularly useful in the teaching of daily living skills. All programs of treatment are designed for a client's specific needs and may consist of a single activity or a combination of activities. Activities can be educational, recreational, or social in nature and can include prevocational testing and training, personal care activities, and the use of creative arts.

Functions

Occupational therapists are employed in a variety of settings, including but not limited to hospitals, mental-health clinics, nursing homes, rehabilitation centers, day care centers, sheltered workshops, home health care agencies, and public and private schools. The majority of occupational

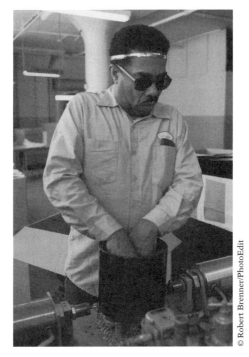

A visually impaired client engaged in occupational therapy.

therapists have positions in hospitals, and the majority of clients served fall into the physically and emotionally disabled target populations. Of course, the everyday activities of an occupational therapist vary according to the setting and target population.

The occupational therapist very often functions as a member of a therapeutic treatment team. Other members of this team might include a psychologist, a psychiatrist, a social worker, or a nurse. As a member of this team, the occupational therapist is the specialist most often called upon to design and implement a program of activities to reduce specific disabilities and develop an atmosphere in which to promote restoration of ability. The treatment approach used most often to accomplish this involves three phases: assessment, treatment, and evaluation. Initially, assessment is needed to determine the individual's ability level. Based on the assessment, a treatment program is developed. At the final stages of treatment, an evaluation is done to judge the effectiveness of the program.

Consider the example of an individual who is a stroke victim and has spent considerable time in the hospital. As a result of this illness, the individual must relearn basic skills such as feeding, dressing, walking, and speaking. The illness has also made his former employment difficult, if not impossible, and he must develop new interests and possibly a new career.

Once the individual's level of abilities is assessed, a treatment program might include the following:

- teaching the patient to use equipment (e.g., a wheelchair, prosthetic device, crutches, or braces) to aid with eating, walking, speaking, and general mobility
- working with creative materials (e.g., paints or clay) to improve coordination, build confidence, and provide a source of exercise
- working with progressively more difficult materials (e.g., leatherwork, ceramics, or printmaking) to refine motor coordination, build strength, and increase work tolerance
- prevocational testing to assess the individual's abilities and skills and to explore other talents
- prevocational training to give an individual practical experience in specific jobs

The individual's progress is consistently monitored throughout treatment, and an overall evaluation is done at the conclusion of the program. This determines whether additional treatment is needed or if the individual is ready to resume activities of daily living. A patient may return to visit the occupational therapist periodically to discuss any problems that may arise. Treatment may be simple or complicated, depending on the client's needs. Highly experienced and talented occupational therapists actually design innovative therapeutic devices to meet the needs of a given situation.

Although most occupational therapists are involved in direct patient care, many perform a variety of other duties. A certain percentage of occupational therapists teach in college or university programs. Many perform administrative functions as directors of occupational therapy programs in hospitals or clinics. Still others maintain private practices and act as consultants to various programs and agencies.

Training and Education

The field of occupational therapy contains two forms of classification. One can either be a certified occupational therapy assistant (COTA) or a registered occupational therapist (OTR). Each requires a different form of preparation.

A certified occupational therapy assistant is one who completes an approved 2-year associate degree program in occupational therapy from an accredited junior or community college. There are also various educational institutions that have 1-year certificate-granting programs. Most programs require a combination of coursework and fieldwork training. A certified occupational therapy assistant most often works under the supervision of a registered occupational therapist.

The registered occupational therapist is required to complete a 4-year course of study in a approved college or university program. The individual is then awarded a bachelor of arts or sciences degree in occupational therapy. A passing grade on a national certification exam administered by the American Occupational Therapy Association is required to be considered professionally competent for employment. Graduates of approved 4-year programs are immediately eligible to take this certification examination. In certain situations, certified occupational therapy assistants can become eligible to take this exam (through an accumulation of a minimum of 4 years of job-related experience). Upon successful completion of the exam, the assistant can become a registered occupational therapist. A variety of master's degree programs in occupational therapy exist for those individuals who seek more advanced training in specific areas of the field.

CLINICAL PSYCHOLOGY

Clinical psychology is the specialization within the broad field of general psychology that focuses on the diagnosis and treatment of mental and emotional disorders. Of specific interest to clinical psychologists are the causes of abnormal behavior. Clinical psychologists use all applicable scientific methods in their investigation of behavior. These methods may include psychological testing, controlled experiments, and direct observation.

Functions

Clinical psychologists engage in a wide variety of work activities, including research, testing, counseling, psychotherapy, teaching, supervising, and consulting. This range of work activities may be performed in psychiatric hospitals, mental-health clinics, hospitals, training institutes, public and private schools, research centers, colleges and universities, and federal, state, and local government programs. The type of setting often defines the clinical psychologist's primary work activities and the range of his or her responsibilities. To illustrate this diversity of settings and work activities, consider the following examples.

Setting A: Psychiatric Hospital

The clinical psychologist conducts individual and group psychotherapy sessions with patients. As a member of the ward treatment team, he or she helps to develop and monitor the individual treatment plans for patients. A clinical psychologist often administers a battery of psychological tests to a patient in an effort to better determine the nature and scope of the client's problems. This specialist may conduct a group ward meeting with all the patients twice weekly to discuss problems or grievances, disseminate new information that may affect patients, and help patients adjust to the ward environment.

The clinical psychologist may be called upon to conduct a staff workshop in his or her own particular area of expertise as part of the hospital's ongoing staff development program. As a member of the senior clinical staff, he or she can also supervise the work of various generalist human services workers and other staff members. As a representative of the hospital, the clinical psychologist often consults with other hospitals, agencies, programs, or the court system in reference to specific patients, program development, or treatment issues. The clinical psychologist may also maintain a private practice with individuals or groups in addition to these primary work responsibilities.

Setting B: Public or Private School

In a school setting, the clinical psychologist is most often involved with counseling children to help promote their social and intellectual development. Students who are most often in need of the services of a clinical psychologist might include those with learning disabilities, maladaptive behavior problems, or those experiencing temporary crisis situations. The clinical psychologist often administers standardized psychological tests to help determine the nature of a student's present problems.

The clinical psychologist frequently consults with teachers concerning the specific needs of students. He or she may, in cooperation with teachers, develop special programs of instruction for students whose disabilities require such individualized programs.

Setting C: Community Mental-Health Center

The majority of clinical psychologists functioning in community mental-health centers serve as clinical members of outpatient treatment programs. Other primary work activities vary according to the nature and scope of the clinic. For example, whereas some clinics may be organized solely for outpatient services, others may provide additional services such as day treatment programs, social programs, medical services, prevocational training, and residential services. The clinical psychologist may be involved in any or all such available services, depending on interest and expertise. In the outpatient setting, the clinical psychologist usually maintains a caseload of clients. The number of patients in a given caseload varies depending on the size of the clinic, number of other staff members, and number of clients being served. An average number of clients being treated by a single clinical psychologist per week might be 25. The methods of treatment used by clinical psychologists vary greatly. The treatment method often depends on which psychological theory or theories the particular clinical psychologist believes to be most effective. The treatment approaches most often practiced are derived from the psychoanalytic, humanistic, or behavioristic models, described in Chapter 4. The outpatient clinician conducts individual and/or group or family sessions with his or her clients to treat specific problems. The clinical psychologist works in a treatment team, with the help of other staff members, to design and monitor individual client treatment plans. As a supervisor, the clinical psychologist oversees the training and quality of work of generalist human services workers and other staff.

The growth of community psychology approach to mental illness means community mental-health clinics maintain close ties with other people and agencies in the community. The clinical psychologist may become involved with helping to plan and establish community service and prevention programs such as after-school programs for troubled youth, services and workshops on drug prevention or teenage sexuality, or social programs for the elderly.

◆

A Day in the Life
of a Clinical Psychologist

Sam G. is a clinical psychologist who was recently awarded a Ph.D. by the graduate school of a large university in the Midwest. He is employed by a state mental hospital located near the capital city of his home state as a staff psychologist on an cute admissions ward. The patients are all males who have recently suffered serious breakdowns involving some loss of contact with reality. Many of the patients on this ward are confused, agitated, and highly emotional.

What follows is a brief description of a typical day in Sam's professional life.

9:00–9:30 A.M.: As usual, Sam begins his day with a visit to the nursing station. He talks to the charge nurse about several incidents that took place during the night. One patient was assaulted by another during an argument about stolen money. No serious injury was involved. Since Sam is not treating either patient, no intervention on his part is needed.

9:35–10:25 A.M.: Sam attends the staff meeting with the team leader of the ward, who happens to be a senior psychologist. Also present is the psychiatrist who is primarily responsible for medication of patients on this and another ward, a social worker, a psychiatric nurse, and two mental health therapy aides. Discussion focuses on a 38-year-old male schizophrenic who feels strongly that he is ready for discharge. Various members of the team express doubts about the patient's readiness to go back to the community. Sam is asked to administer a battery of psychological tests to judge the patient's degree of contact with reality.

10:30–11:20 A.M.: Psychotherapy. The patient is a young, street-wise, male patient with a history of multiple substance abuse. During this session, Sam focuses on the patient's hostile attitudes toward various members of his family. Unless there is some reduction in these negative feelings, it seems unlikely that the patient will be able to live at home again.

11:30 A.M.–1:00 P.M.: Supervision of two psychology interns who are learning the rudiments of testing under Sam's direction.

2:00–3:00 P.M.: After lunch, Sam administers an intelligence test to the patient discussed at the earlier meeting. He plans to administer personality tests including the Rorschach inkblot test on the following day.

3:00–4:10 P.M.: As usual, Sam reserves the later part of the afternoon for his written work. He puts the finishing touches on his report on a patient tested several days ago. Then he makes some notes on his therapy patients.

4:15–5:00 P.M.: Sam confers informally with the senior psychologist about a research project on which they will collaborate. Essentially, it is a continuation of Sam's thesis research on thinking processes of schizophrenic patients.

It goes without saying that Sam is involved in informal contacts with patients and staff at various times during the day, and that he has occasional phone conversations with other professionals. Basically, Sam likes his position at the hospital. However, he believes that there is an overemphasis on medication at the hospital. He would like to see more in the way of group and individual therapy with increased time spent in therapeutic activities. In general, he feels the patients spend too much time sitting around watching inane daytime TV programs.* ◆

Training and Education

Training for a career in the field of clinical psychology begins with the attainment of the bachelor's degree with a major emphasis in psychology. This degree alone does not qualify an individual to become a psychologist; further graduate-level preparation is required. Many individuals pursue a master's degree in psychology as their final degree, whereas others consider the master's-level training an intermediate step before entering a doctoral program in clinical psychology. Individuals can enter a PhD program in clinical psychology directly after attaining the BA degree.

One can become a master's-level psychologist and function in the field. Job opportunities and salaries are, however, generally less than those available to the PhD-level psychologist. The doctoral-level training most widely accepted is a PhD program approved by the American Psychological Association. Most PhD programs require 5 years of graduate study, during which time the student completes a range of coursework and clinical internship of approximately 1 year's duration. The student is placed in a setting such as a psychiatric hospital to fulfill his or her internship requirement. The student intern is supervised in performing a variety of tasks in

*Reprinted with permission from Schmolling, P., Burger, W., and Youkeles, M. (1986), *Careers in Mental Health: A Guide to the Helping Occupations.* Garrett Park, MD: Garrett Park Press.

which he or she could be involved after the completion of graduate study. Internships usually provide a good experience for the student to learn first-hand what it is actually like to perform the duties of a psychologist. The last phase of graduate study, after all coursework and internship requirements have been met, involves writing a formal dissertation. The dissertation is an original piece of research conducted by the student under the supervision of a committee of selected faculty members. The student is awarded the PhD upon successful completion of his or her dissertation.

A new type of doctoral program, granting a PsyD degree, recently has been approved by the American Psychological Association. A number of graduate schools are offering this new degree. A doctoral dissertation is not required, as the major focus of the training is the development of clinical skills. This type of program is designed to appeal to those individuals more interested in clinical psychology than research or academics.

Most states have some form of licensing and/or certification require-ments, including a written examination, that must be fulfilled by clinical psychologists. In certain states, licensing law restricts the use of the title psychologist to those individuals who have met the requirements of that state. These laws are designed to stop unqualified individuals from practic-ing therapy.

SOCIAL WORK

The field of **social work** focuses on helping individuals to realize their po-tential in order to live as fully and successfully as possible. The practice of social work addresses itself to the full range of human problems that con-fronts individuals in almost all areas of life. Social workers help individu-als, families, and groups to cope with personal problems and also try to help shape society to be more sensitive and responsive to human needs. Because human problems frequently overlap professional boundaries, so-cial workers often function within the many allied human services fields such as health, criminal justice, community service, or education.

Functions

As previously described, social workers function in a variety of settings with a variety of duties and responsibilities. Some examples of social work settings are mental-health clinics, public and private hospitals, nursing homes, rehabilitation centers, health care agencies, public and private schools, social service agencies, correctional institutions, senior citizen centers, or colleges and universities. When one refers to different kinds of social workers, one is usually referring to the setting in which the social worker is employed rather than to basic differences in training or social work practice (Schmolling et al., 1981).

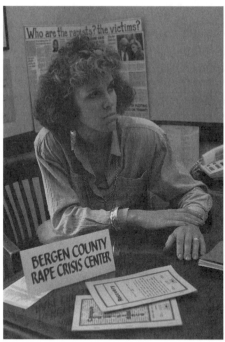

A social worker in a rape crisis center.

Although individual functions and activities vary among social workers, there are common work activities. One such activity involves face-to-face contact with clients or those receiving services, this personal contact is referred to as direct practice. Direct practice can be performed in most settings. For example, the social worker employed by a psychiatric facility (psychiatric social worker) might work with individuals or groups to help them solve their specific emotional problems. The social worker employed by a school system (school social worker) might counsel individual students concerning specific school or social problems. The social worker might work directly with families in social service or family agencies. A series of therapeutic sessions might be used to help the family improve communication and solve specific family problems. The social worker employed by a community agency might function as a community organizer and have direct contact with many elements of the community. The social worker in this role usually helps individuals to improve conditions and services in their neighborhood. Many social workers also maintain private practices in which they offer a range of psychotherapy services to individuals, families, or group.

Many social workers provide supervision to other professional and nonprofessional staff. A more experienced social worker might supervise the work of others by providing advice about developing individual client treatment programs and alternative treatment approaches or by offering suggestions concerning how workers can improve their professional competence.

Another common work activity in the social work field is administration. The amount and extent of administrative responsibility vary according to the experience and training of the individual as well as with the type of employment setting. For example, the duties of a senior administrator of an agency or facility might include designing specific programs of service, developing and monitoring budgets, supervising personnel, and evaluating the effectiveness of programs. In general, a senior administrator is responsible for making sure the various programs fulfill their stated missions or purposes.

The social worker may work closely with various agencies, facilities, or branches of government as a consultant. For example, he or she may be requested by the court system to give a professional opinion or provide specific information regarding a client who is accused or convicted of a crime. Consultants may also help an agency develop or reorganize a particular department or program.

Many social workers engage in research or education activities. Experienced social workers can function as teachers or professors in social work training programs at colleges and universities. Social workers involved in research may investigate programs, develop theories, or gather data concerning who needs help, where and what type of help is needed, or how a service may be improved.

◆

A Day in the Life
of a Social Worker

Gary is a licensed certified social worker with an M.S.W. degree. He works in a settlement house located in a poor urban neighborhood of a large city. Gary was promoted to the position of supervisor of the teenage division, serving boys and girls between the ages of 13 and 17. He supervises two licensed and certified social workers, a dozen generalist human services worker club and activity leaders, and three graduate students of social work. Gary and his staff work in the afternoons and evenings.

A typical day for Gary might look like this:

1:00–2:00 P.M.: Gary meets with his supervisor, the program director of the agency, to discuss the plans of the teenage division, problems and progress of the staff, teenagers and their groups, and budget issues. For example, Gary is concerned about one of his professional staff members who is having personal problems that are affecting the quality of his work.

2:00–3:00 P.M.: Gary chairs the teen division staff meeting. The staff and Gary bring up problems they are having in their work with the teenagers. They explore ways of dealing with the problems and how they might improve the entire program. One of the things they talk about is the importance of sharing information on individuals and groups that are having behavior problems so that all the staff can pool their knowledge and be more effective in helping those with problems.

3:00–4:00 P.M.: Gary has a supervisory conference with one of the graduate social work students to discuss the student's efforts in helping his group members to limit their aggressive behavior in the agency and on the street.

4:15–5:45 P.M.: Gary meets with a coed group of older teenagers who are dating and are concerned about intimacy, sexuality, and parenting.

7:00–8:00 P.M.: After dinner, Gary meets with a group of parents concerned about the possibility of their teenage children becoming drug users.

8:00–9:30 P.M.: Gary meets with the teenage council made up of representatives of the teenage clubs in the agency to listen to their plans, problems, and feelings about the teenage programs. Gary tries to help the council resolve its problems as well as develop and carry out its plans.

9:30–10:00 P.M.: Gary makes notes on the meetings of the groups he led directly.

Gary is kept busy as supervisor of a large program. He enjoys working with teenagers, even though at times they are prone to impulsive behavior and resist any authority.* ◆

Training and Education

The National Association of Social Work, the governing body in this field, determines the criteria for the professional social worker. Currently, the minimum requirement set forth for acceptance as a professional social worker is satisfactory completion of a bachelor's degree program in social work and acceptance for membership status in the National Association of Social Work. The college program must be accredited by the Council on Social Work Education.

Bachelor's degree programs in social work (BSW) prepare individuals for entry-level positions in the field. Coursework stresses different aspects of the field, which might include the history of social work and the practice of social work in different settings. In addition to coursework emphasizing social work, the student is exposed to a broad liberal arts background. All accredited programs require the student to complete 300 hours of supervised fieldwork. The student is placed in a selected social work field site

*Reprinted with permission from Schmolling, P., Burger, W., and Youkeles, M. (1986), *Careers in Mental Health: A Guide to the Helping Occupations.* Garrett Park, MD: Garrett Park Press.

and, under the supervision of a professional social worker, gains experience working directly with clients.

Traditionally, the only route available to becoming a professional social worker has been to attain a master's degree in social work (MSW). This requires completion of a graduate program (usually 2 years of full-time study). The recent development of BSW programs means the MSW is not the only route to social work; however, the master's degree is often necessary for advancement in the field. In fact, many professional social work agencies, institutions, and facilities set the MSW as a requirement for supervisory positions.

One does not necessarily have to possess a BSW degree to gain acceptance into an MSW degree program. Individuals possessing undergraduate degrees in other fields, such as psychology or sociology, may be accepted for graduate study, provided they meet other criteria established by individual schools.

MSW training requires 2 years of supervised fieldwork. The coursework, for the most part, pertains exclusively to the profession of social work, with many schools emphasizing the common elements of direct practice and increasing the student's knowledge of the field. MSW degree-granting programs, like all BSW programs, must be accredited by the Council on Social Work Education.

In recent years, doctor of social work (DSW) programs have been established in various colleges and universities. This doctoral-level program seems to attract social workers whose primary interests are in pursuing advanced-level training in the areas of teaching, administration, and social policy. A doctor of social work program, like many other doctoral programs, usually takes an average of 4 years to complete and includes a program of required coursework and the successful completion of a doctoral dissertation.

PSYCHIATRY

Psychiatry is the medical specialty that investigates, diagnoses, and treats mental, emotional, or behavioral disorders. Psychiatrists are initially trained as medical doctors. As such, they are the only category of human services professionals legally authorized to prescribe medicine.

Functions

Psychiatrists, because of their extensive training and preparation, generally occupy positions of elevated status within the human services field. This is reflected by their high salaries and the scope and depth of their responsibilities. For example, within a therapeutic team composed of other human services workers, the psychiatrist often functions in a leadership or supervisory capacity. The majority of psychiatrists maintain some type of private practice, but few contribute all their professional time to treating patients in a private setting. The psychiatrist may also work in a clinic or hospital setting, perform consultations, conduct research, teach, or occupy an administrative position. A psychiatrist's specific function varies according to the setting in which he or she is working, but all licensed psychiatrists can prescribe medication.

The psychiatrist who works in a psychiatric hospital is involved in many activities. For example, he or she normally carries a specified caseload of patients. As mentioned earlier, the psychiatrist is most likely also a member of a hospital team in which patient treatment plans are developed and monitored and the possible discharge of improved patients is discussed. The psychiatrist is often called upon to consult with other workers in the hospital concerning specific cases in which a psychiatric opinion is requested. Psychiatrists also act as expert consultants to courts, prisons, and other public and private institutions.

Many psychiatrists engage in work that is primarily administrative, such as directing a psychiatric hospital staff or program, directing a mental-health clinic, or overseeing a governmental program such as the National Institute of Mental Health. The psychiatrist serving in this capacity is largely involved in the development of programs, budget preparation and monitoring, and staff management. As an administrator, the psychiatrist establishes the framework within which other professionals work.

Research and training are other possible career areas for the psychiatrist. Research opportunities and interests are varied, and the range of possible research subjects is enormous. For example, the psychiatrist might study the effect of a certain drug on a specific disorder, the impact that maternal stress has on a newborn child, or the effects of a new treatment approach. As a teacher, the psychiatrist may be found in medical schools, institutes, and colleges and universities.

An additional area of specialization now emerging for the psychiatrist is that of community psychiatry. Community psychiatry is based on the belief that the community should play a more vital role in preventing and treating mental illness. Prevention and treatment are accomplished by means of a variety of community programs. The psychiatrist involved in this field is most likely employed by a **community mental-health** center. In this context, he or she might be involved with designing such community programs as residential centers for exinstitutionalized patients, working with schools to establish programs for troubled youth, or designing social programs for senior citizens.

Training and Education

The training of a psychiatrist is lengthy and demanding. Many individuals do not realize that preparation for such a career actually begins as early as high school with attainment of excellent grades. A solid aptitude for science and mathematics is necessary because a great deal of required coursework is in these areas. The aspiring psychiatrist usually majors in a premedical course of study in undergraduate school. A premed program frequently includes courses in inorganic and organic chemistry, physics, biology, and advanced mathematics.

Application to medical school is made after the student has been granted a bachelor's degree. Medical school is a highly demanding 4-year course of study. During these 4 years, the student learns the practice of medicine and is considered a full-fledged physician upon graduation from medical school.

Following medical school, the new physician must enroll in another course of study called the residency. It is during this 4-year program that the physician specializes in the field of psychiatry. The training may take place in one of several settings, including university medical centers, accredited psychiatric hospitals, or psychiatric divisions of general hospitals. The coursework and practice are devoted exclusively to psychiatry, and it is within this framework that the physician sharpens his or her clinical skills.

The psychiatrist is able to take an examination certifying competence in the field upon satisfactory completion of his or her residency training. He or she is now awarded a certificate in the specialty of psychiatry until passing the national exam administered by the American Board of Psychiatry and Neurology. This certification is not a legal requirement for a physician to practice psychiatry, but the board-certified psychiatrist normally has more career opportunities and enjoys greater acceptance in the medical community.

PROFESSIONAL ORGANIZATIONS

For more information about the career areas discussed in this chapter, you can write to any of the organizations listed on the following pages.

Generalist Human Services Work

> National Organization for Human Services Education
> Franklyn M. Rother
> President
> Human Services Program
> Brookdale Community College
> Newman Springs Road
> Lincroft, NJ 07738–1597
>
> Dr. Douglas A. Whyte
> Membership Coordinator
> Mental Health/Social Service
> Community College of Philadelphia
> 1700 Spring Garden Street
> Philadelphia, PA 19130–3991

Council for Standards in Human Services Education
Mary DiGiovanni
President
Northern Essex Community College
Elliott Way
Haverhill, MA 01830–2399

National Association of Human Service Technologists
1127 Eleventh Street, Main Floor
Sacramento, CA 95814

Therapeutic Recreation

The National Therapeutic Recreation Society
1601 N. Kent Street
Arlington, VA 22209

Creative Arts Therapy (Art, Dance, and Music)

American Art Therapy Association
427 E. Preston Street
Baltimore, MD 21202

American Dance Therapy Association
Suite 230, 2000 Century Plaza
Columbia, MD 21044

National Association for Music Therapy Inc.
PO Box 610
Lawrence, KS 66044

Psychiatric Nursing

National League for Nursing
10 Columbus Circle
New York, NY 10019

Occupational Therapy

American Occupational Therapy Association
6000 Executive Boulevard
Rockville, MD 20852

Clinical Psychology

American Psychological Association
1200 Seventeenth Street NW
Washington, DC 20036

Social Work

>   Council on Social Work Education
>   111 Eighth Avenue
>   New York, NY 10011
>
>   National Association of Social Workers
>   1425 H Street NW, Suite 600
>   Washington, DC 20005

Psychiatry

>   American Medical Association
>   535 N. Dearborn Street
>   Chicago, IL 60610
>
>   American Psychiatric Association
>   1700 Eighteenth Street NW
>   Washington, DC 20009

ADDITIONAL READING

Baron, R. A. (1996). *Essentials of psychology.* Boston: Allyn & Bacon

Barton, W. E., & Sanborn, C. J. (Eds.). (1978). *Law and the mental health professions: Friction at the interface.* New York: International Universities Press.

Duignan, P., & Rabushka, A. (Eds.). (1980). *The United States in the 1980s.* Stanford, CA: Hoover Institution.

Ellis, A., & Yeager, R. J. (1989). *Why some therapies don't work.* Buffalo, NY: Prometheus Books.

Gustafson, K. E., & McNamara, J. R. (1987). Confidentiality with minor clients: Issues and guidelines for therapists. *Professional Psychology: Research and Practice, 18*(5) 503–508.

Haaga, D. A., & Davison, G. C. (1986). Cognitive change methods. In F. H. Kanfer & A. P. Goldstein (Eds.), *Helping people change* (3rd ed., pp. 236–282). New York: Pergamon Press.

Huhn, R. P., Zimpfer, D. B., Waltman, D. E., & Williamson, S. K. (1985). A survey of programs of professional preparation for group counseling. *The Journal for Specialists in Group Work, 10*(3), 124–133.

Human Resources Development Center. (1980). *Paraprofessionals in deinstitutionalized settings: A systematic study of effective use and potential.* New York: National Child Labor Committee.

Jaffe, D. T. (1986). *The inner strain of healing work: Therapy and self-renewal for health care professionals.* New York: Brunner/Mazel.

Levine, D. V., & Havighurst, R. J. (1984). *Society and education* (6th ed.). Boston: Allyn & Bacon.

Monohan, J. (Ed.). (1976). *Community mental health and the criminal justice system.* Elmsford, NY: Pergamon Press.

Morse, S. J., & Watson, R. I., Jr. (1977). *Psychotherapies: A comparative casebook.* New York: Holt, Rinehart & Winston.

Porter, R. A., Peters, J. A., & Headry, H. R. (1982). Using community development for prevention in Appalachia. *Social Work, 27,* 302–307.

Posthuma, B. W. (1996). *Small groups in counseling and theory: Process and leadership* (2nd ed.). Boston: Allyn & Bacon.

Walsh, J. A. (1982). Prevention in mental health: Organizational and ideological perspectives. *Social Work, 27,* 298–301.

Whittington, H. G. (1972). *Clinical practice in community mental health centers.* New York: International Universities Press.

REFERENCES

Bugental, J. F. T. (1987). *The art of the psychotherapist.* New York: Norton.

Corey, G. (1990). *Theory and practice of group counseling* (3rd ed.). Pacific Grove, CA: Brooks/Cole.

Corey, G. (1991). *Case approach to counseling and psychotherapy* (3rd ed.). Pacific Grove, CA: Brooks/Cole.

Corey, G., & Corey, M. (1990). *I never knew I had a choice* (4th ed.). Pacific Grove, CA: Brooks/Cole.

Corey M., & Corey, G. (1989). *Becoming a helper.* Pacific Grove, CA: Brooks/Cole.

Holloway, E. L., & Rochike, H. J. (1987). Internship: The applied training of a counseling psychologist. *The Counseling Psychologist, 15*(2), 205–260.

National Organization of Human Services. (Fall, 1982). Newsletter.

Santrock, J. W. (1991). *The science of mind and behavior.* New York: William C. Brown.

Schmolling, P., Burger, W., & Youkeles, M. (1981). *Helping people: A guide to careers in mental health.* Englewood Cliffs, NJ: Prentice Hall.

Siegel, B. (1988). *Love, medicine, and miracles.* New York: Harper & Row.

Sobey, F. (1969, November). *Nonprofessional personnel in mental health programs: A summary report based on a study of projected support by the National Institute under contract #PL4366–967* (No. 5028). Washington, DC: National Clearinghouse for Mental Health Information.

Social Policy

INTRODUCTION

Social policy, a topic usually discussed in advanced courses, is considered by many to be too complex to be included in introductory courses. We, however, believe that social policy is a most appropriate topic for introductory courses in human services. Without an understanding of social policy, the human services worker cannot appreciate the significant impact it has on the design and delivery of services. We will try to show some ways, direct and indirect, in which social policies affect the human services worker and the consumer of human services.

The first section of this chapter provides a general description of social policies with regard to what they do and who they affect. The remaining sections focus on making and implementing social policies.

Throughout the chapter, we try to show the relevance of social policy to the individual human services worker. In one section, there is a discussion of the role of the human services worker in introducing or initiating policy proposals. This is followed by a discussion of when and how the worker might influence the formulation or the final form of social policy. Finally, examples are given of how the human services worker affects existing policy and how policy affects the worker. The general focus is on the connections between social policy, the human services worker, and the delivery of human services. For you to understand these connections, a discussion of definitions, development, and implementation of social policies is required. Definitions of social policy are discussed first.

WHAT IS SOCIAL POLICY?

A policy, according to the *Random House Dictionary* (1978), is "a guiding principle or course of action adopted toward an objective or objectives." The word *social,* according to the same dictionary, refers to "the life, welfare, and relations of human beings in a community." Gil (1981) summed it up very well when he wrote that "social policies are a special type of policies, namely, policies which deliberately pertain to the quality of life and to the circumstances of living in society, and to intra-societal relationships among individuals, groups, and society as a whole" (p. 13).

Titmus (1974) made it clear that the study of social policy includes an understanding of the political, social, and economic forces in society. Although such an understanding is beyond the scope of this text, it is certainly worth mentioning. Titmus claimed that "social policy can be seen as a positive instrument for change; as . . . part of the whole political process" (p. 26). Another definition is that of Huttman (1981), who saw social policies as "plans of action and strategies for providing services" (p. 2). She added that social policies have the goal of sound human relations. Another definition, dealing with a particular kind of social policy, and one of the more than passing interest to human services workers, namely **social welfare** policy, is the one given by Prigmore and Atherton (1979): "Social welfare policy is a generic term for the guidelines used for decision making on social welfare programs and issues" (p. 8).

Although there are many definitions of social policy, they all seem to agree that social policy is characterized by the following aspects:

♦ Social policy is problem oriented—that is, it seeks to improve an existing or anticipated condition.
♦ Social policy is action oriented—that is, it outlines or describes programs that seek to affect change.
♦ Social policy is focused on individuals or groups, such as the target populations described in Chapter 2.
♦ Making social policy involves making choices regarding the kind and/ or extent of changes to be made.

Although there are many other aspects of social policy, for the purpose of this discussion these four will be highlighted.

What impels a society, or a group or individuals for that matter, to expend hard-earned and limited resources to help those in need? Is such behavior a demonstration of democratic values, religious beliefs, or a matter of survival for society? There appears to be no single answer. In the past, all of these factors have played a significant part in the efforts to help those in need. We now take a brief look at past social policies.

Social Policy in the Past

Social policies in **preliterate societies** were not perceived as such. They were plans for survival that assured food, shelter, and protection against predators, hostile groups, and hostile environments. Physical survival was the goal. The success of the plans depended on the mutual efforts of the family or tribe. Without these efforts, individual survival was jeopardized.

As families or tribes settled in one place and developed villages of relative permanence, and as populations increased, more of the support necessary for survival was provided by the **extended family.** In these different circumstances, those without a family were still able to survive, if only marginally. When communities grew even larger and more complex, organized religion began to provide aid to those who had no family or whose family did not have the resources or ability to provide the needed support. Caring for the mentally ill, homeless children, the physically disabled, and the hungry became a major concern of organized religion. These humanitarian efforts seemed to prevent the turmoil and conflict that often result from threats to survival. Keep in mind the important fact that efforts and plans designed to improve the life of those in need also eliminated a threat to the existing power structure. Large numbers of hungry, desperate people were frequently candidates for riot and rebellion.

Social Policy in Modern Times

The rapid and significant changes that typify modern industrial society caused organized religion, private organizations, and individuals to increase their efforts to help those in need. The loosening of family bonds, the increase in crime, and the increase in the numbers of mentally ill, elderly poor and disabled, and persons living in poverty made it impossible for existing institutions to provide the necessary support for those in need. Their values, plans, and policies did not undergo basic changes; they just did not have the resources in the form of funds, workers, or material to provide the needed help. It is important to note and remember that morality is supposedly a basis for social (welfare) policies, but this value is always in competition with other political and economic values (Beverly & McSweeney, 1987). An example of this competition is what occurred during the 1995–1996 struggle between conservatives and liberals when trying to agree on a bill to balance the U. S. budget by the year 2002. We refer to this issue in more detail later.

As problems grew in size, number, and complexity, governments had to step in to develop and implement programs to prevent starvation and to provide opportunities for gaining resources for an adequate life. An underlying purpose was to reduce dissatisfaction with the existing political or power structure. When one looks at the bottom line, it is obvious that social policies do not stem from humanitarian values alone but also derive from the desire of those in power to remain in control of society's wealth and resources. This is why governments focus on social policies that deal with basic needs such as food, shelter, clothing, and medical care.

Private human services agencies also deal with these kinds of problems, but on a much smaller scale. In addition, they focus on providing help in meeting higher-level needs, such as belonging and self-actualization (described in Chapter 1).

Some human services workers believe that the best way to help is through working for social and economic policies that provide for a more equitable distribution of economic resources and power among the haves and the have-nots. Two basic types of effort have been the mainstay of this approach to date. The first type is the government subsidy (i.e., welfare), which attempts to provide decent food, shelter, clothing, and other necessities of life to families and individuals who for one legitimate reason or another cannot accept employment. The second type of effort is the attempt to provide training and jobs for those who are able to work so that they can pay for decent food, shelter, clothing, and the other necessities of life. So far, and for a variety of economic and social reasons, these efforts seem to satisfy few. Here, too, competition of social, economic, and political values takes place. For example, unofficial or unstated economic policy requires that a *minimum* of 5%, or approximately 7 million people (U. S. Bureau of Labor Statistics, 1993), just remain unemployed in order to prevent inflation. Baker (1995) calls these people "those vital paupers." Yet the struggle

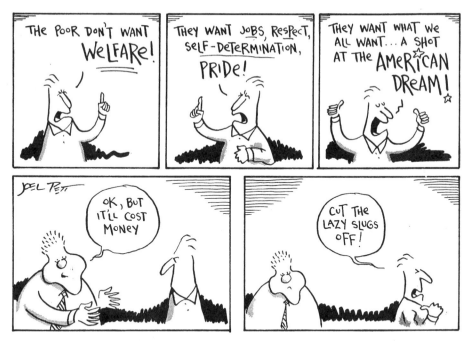

Copyright © 1995 Joel Pett, Lexington Herald-Leader. All rights reserved.

to develop policies aimed at creating jobs, job training, low-cost housing, and comprehensive welfare reform that are acceptable to policymakers and the public is now in progress. A substantial part of this struggle is based upon the ambivalent feelings of much of the population as depicted in the comic strip above.

Meanwhile, human services agencies for the most part try to help people adjust to the existing social and economic situation. Agencies, in effect, seek to maintain the **status quo.** Regardless of the basic motives behind social policy, it seems clear that unless and until more successful or satisfying programs are devised to provide for the basic needs of people who are unable to provide for themselves, much suffering, turmoil, and conflict will result.

PURPOSE AND TYPES OF SOCIAL POLICY

The purpose of social policy today, put simply, is to improve the lives of people. Most often, policy is designed to meet the needs of selected populations, such as those mentioned in Chapter 2. Accordingly, there are many different types of social policies. The most familiar type is social welfare policy, mentioned earlier. Other types of social policies include housing policy, mental-health policy, child welfare policy, and unemployment policy.

Within each of these general categories, there are more specific plans or policies. For example, in the case of housing policy, the focus might be on housing for the elderly or perhaps housing for the poor or for migrants. Mental-health policy could include policies dealing with aftercare services, outpatient clinics, or prevention programs. So although the common purpose of social policy is to meet needs, it is important to recognize that there are many kinds of policies that affect almost all human needs. We recommend that you read Huttman (1981) for a more detailed understanding of this subject.

THE SCOPE OF SOCIAL POLICY

Social policy affects most, if not all, people in society, from the cradle to the grave. For example, there are social policies that deal with abortion, birth control, child care, child abuse, teenage drinking, young adult drug abuse, marriage, divorce, as well as policies relating to older adults, and yes—even death. The number and kinds of policies and programs implemented and/ or proposed by federal, state, local, and private agencies are indeed impressive. It should be noted that because of the sheer number of programs implemented, one can find inconsistencies in purposes and goals.

Not only do social policies affect us throughout our life span, they also affect us in almost every aspect of our lives. Most certainly, they affect us in regard to Maslow's hierarchy of needs described in Chapter 1. For example, policies dealing with basic physiological or survival needs such as hunger and thirst try to prevent malnutrition and eliminate starvation in our society. The food stamp program is one example of such a policy. Safety needs are met through housing and law enforcement policies, to name just a few. An example is a program to provide shelter for the homeless population in New York City. Other kinds of safety needs are met by programs focusing on automobile safety, food and drug monitoring, and public transportation. Programs dealing with these and other needs are often influenced by other kinds of government policies.

Other kinds of government policies include foreign policies, economic policies, educational policies, transportation policies, and defense policies. It is important to recognize that social policies are not the only policies focused on improving society in one way or another. For example, economic policy also attempts to improve society. One might define economic policy as the decisions of those in power concerning money matters. The tax policy described in the first chapter provides a clear picture of how an economic policy might help improve society by creating new jobs. Miller (1985) believes that the goals of economic policies and social policies should be the same—essentially a pro-employment, pro-poor policy. He further claims that, although it might not be apparent, in actual practice "economic policy is about children and families, as much, if not more so, than is social policy" (p. 62). This becomes very clear in the struggle over the effort to balance the budget by the year 2002. The attempt to achieve the goal centers around the size of the reduction in the present rate of expenditures for helping children, poor families, the elderly, and disabled, among others, and methods for achieving that reduction. The claim of both conservative and liberal lawmakers and others is that the goal must be reached so that our children would not be burdened by having to pay off our debt if the budget were not balanced.

When one considers all the different types of policies, at least two things become quite clear. First, there are a tremendous number of policies and programs dealing with issues in every aspect of our lives. Second, there is a need to decide the relative importance of different policies. For example, the need to distribute surplus food to the poor is seen by some in power as less important than increasing the number of submarines. The "guns or butter" issue is still alive, even though more funds are presently being spent on social programs. Witness the additional billions of dollars proposed in the 1996 budget for the acquisition of another atomic submarine, which the military establishment claims it does not need or want, at the cost of $2.4 billion (Priest & Mintz, 1995). Add to that the proposed figure of $1.4 billion for each of the several more B-2 bombers that the military does not need or want either. These funds as well as others could be used for social programs, or at least not be cut from social programs to pay for unwanted, unneeded weapons. There is also a hierarchy of importance in the various social policies. Some people claim that providing funds for the AFDC program is more important than providing outpatient services in the community for released mental-health patients. Regardless of how one determines which policy is more important than the others, it is inevitable that policies are in competition with each other.

This competition is resolved sometimes through compromise and very often through the exercise of raw power. It is rare for everyone to agree on which social policies to promote or on which policies are more important. Gilbert and Specht (1974) state clearly that "different choice preferences will be registered by different policy planners, depending upon the values, theories, and assumptions given the most worth and credence" (p. 49). It's important for human service workers to know who these policy planners are. The concept that compromise and power provide the means for resolving the competition between social policies is discussed in the following sections.

THE MAKING OF SOCIAL POLICY

As indicated earlier, one aspect of social policy is that it is problem oriented. Another way of putting it is that social policy attempts to improve the lives of people who need help in meeting certain needs. If people were able to meet their needs through their own efforts, society would not need to develop programs to help them. It is when the needs cannot be met by the individual that social policies and programs are brought to bear.

As noted earlier, there are often very serious differences and controversies regarding the kind and extent of help required, how the help should be provided, and who deserves or needs the help. How, then, is social policy made? Because it is problem oriented, it begins by focusing on unmet needs.

Identifying Unmet Needs

The first step in social policy formulation is to identify unmet needs. On the surface, this seems to be a very simple task. However, there are some problems even here. In this tremendously complex society of ours, there are so many unmet needs that it is difficult to select those that demand a social policy and program. Could there be, should there be, policies and programs that meet *all* the unmet needs of *all* the people *all* the time? If not, the questions arise: Whose needs and which needs should we attempt to meet? Shall we be concerned about the unmet needs of the wealthy or concentrate on the needs of the poor? If, as most people might agree, we should focus primarily on survival or life-sustaining needs such as adequate food, what direction shall we go from there? What about other unmet needs? Should we be concerned only about the unmet needs that are beyond the control of the individual, or should we also help people who contribute to their own difficulties because of ignorance, poor judgment, or foolishness? Other questions need to be asked: Should social policies be based on the number of people affected? If so, how many people constitute the required number to merit the introduction of a policy and program?

Another major problem in regard to policy formulation is that society is in a constant state of change. And not only is society changing, but individuals, workers, planners, and organizers are changing with society. Alinsky (1971) made the point about an organizer that "truth to him is relative and changing; everything to him is relative and changing" (p. 11). The same holds true for the social planner. Change is not an easy or comfortable process to undergo. It is a process that often, if not always, brings on conflict with oneself or with others, for people change at different rates and in different directions. Another question comes to mind: Don't social problems change without intervention in a changing society? For example, not long ago, unmarried couples living together were not only frowned upon but actively discouraged and prohibited. Today, in an ever-increasing number of states and jurisdictions, unmarried couples living together are permitted and recognized legally in many ways. A changing society in effect has eliminated a problem and the affected social policies. Aren't some problems temporary, and how can one know if they are or not or how temporary they are?

A final question: Who answers all the questions just posed and how?

Who Identifies Social Problems?

Who has the power to determine which issue should be identified as a social problem that requires the formulation of a social policy for its resolution? Power in this context refers to the ability to influence, sway, and somehow persuade a significant number of individuals to recognize and declare that an unmet need is a social problem. According to Alinsky (1971), it is this kind of power that begets even greater power. In other words, the more people one influences, the more influence one can exert. Such power, however, is not easily come by. In fact, many professionals in the human services field, such as Meyer (1983), feel that "politicians control the power to define. Who is to be defined as poor, sick, unemployed, homeless, or uncared for . . . ?" (p. 99). She went on to state unequivocally that "the criteria used to define these conditions are political and economic." Setting poverty levels and acceptable unemployment rates is a political decision based mainly on economic factors. For example, the minimally acceptable unemployment rate, presently 5%, is generally recognized as the point at which a lower rate would lead to inflation.

Private citizens, regardless of their economic status, can also be instrumental in identifying social problems. A layperson may not identify the problem as Maslow or other professionals might, but that does not mean that the identification is any less accurate. In fact, problems are often more clearly and accurately identified by laypeople. For example, one of the largest and most powerful advocacy groups that focuses on the problems and needs of the mentally ill is the National Alliance for the Mentally Ill. It was started by two mothers. The organization presently has over 1000 chapters in 50 states and about 140,000 members, mostly parents of adults who suffer from mental illness. (Foderaro, 1995). This is an excellent example of how a social problem was identified by a private citizen. Usually, however, an individual's problem does not become identified as a social problem just because it is known by the individual. As indicated earlier, numbers are essential when trying to identify a problem as a social problem. In most instances, however, private individuals need the help of human services experts and others to have a problem recognized and established as a social problem.

The human services worker, when working with a population to meet certain needs, often becomes aware of other needs that are not being met. For example, in the mid-1940s in New York City, workers helping older adults with public assistance recognized that these people were also very lonely. The workers then influenced others to provide the older persons with a place to meet other older adults. The facility became a recreation center for the older adults in the community. Additional services were added as other problems, such as those involving nutrition and health, were recognized. From this modest beginning and others like it, the senior center movement was born.

The objective of the worker is to try to obtain the appropriate services for those in need. Human services workers can be, and often are, instrumental in determining unmet needs and in influencing policy. To accomplish this task, the worker must assess the number of individuals involved and the kind and degree of disadvantage involved. Furthermore, the reasons for the lack of services must also be established, for they will have a direct bearing on decisions the worker must make in an attempt to rectify the problem.

Among the many reasons for a lack of needed services in a community, four seem to be prevalent. First, there might not be any resources in the community (or anywhere else, for that matter) to provide the needed service. Second, the resources might be available in the community, but the individuals in need might not be aware of their existence. Third, even if the resources are known, those in need might not know how to use such resources. Fourth, those in need might not be eligible for the services—that is, they might not meet age, sex, racial, income-level, neighborhood, or other criteria determined by the providers of the services. In the instances where a lack of knowledge of existing resources or how to use such resources is the major stumbling block, the worker's major role might be to supply the needed information to those seeking the services. Where there are no resources or where eligibility requirements are not met, the worker may be required to enter the realm of social policy in order to meet the needs of clients.

Austin, Skelding, and Smith (1977) pointed out that risks are involved when fighting for the rights of those in need and attempting to affect policy. Advocating, they rightly claimed, often means speaking out, confronting agencies, and risking one's job. This raises the question that all human services workers ask themselves at one time or another: Should you try to defend the consumer's right to service, or should you keep quiet and accept things as they are? Increasingly, human services workers and agencies are standing up and being counted when the need arises. Unfortunately, this does not occur as often as one might wish. Azarnoff and Seliger (1982) indicated clearly that "advocacy has risks which impede action for many staff people. Dismissal or loss of advancement must be considered as a realistic threat" (p. 209). Whether or not one is successful in obtaining the needed services is often a function of how one goes about the attempt. The worker must exercise tact, skill, and a judicial use of power to win support for new programs.

Initiating Social Policy

Once a problem has been identified as a social problem, the next step might be to inform others about the situation. Informing and educating other workers and clients are some of the necessary steps in the process. The human services worker, usually a member of an agency staff, might inform his or her co-workers and/or supervisor of an unmet need. The worker might then try to enlist their aid in an attempt to meet the need. By informing other clients, the worker makes others aware of the problem and thus may arouse additional interest and support. The hope and intent are to mobilize as much strength as possible in the effort to obtain the needed service.

This kind of an approach often leads to contacts with individuals and groups who have the influence and resources to help resolve the problem. These influential persons include politicians, professionals and their organizations, and government officials who might initiate an investigation in order to determine the breadth and depth of a particular problem. The results of the investigation are then examined and presented to those who make the decisions regarding programs and policies.

Who Are the Decision Makers?

The decision makers include board members of voluntary agencies and local, county, state, or federal legislators. The majority of the local, county, and state legislators are, according to Lynn (1980), only "political amateurs." Even today, for the most part, they are part-time legislators (see box on page 286). The board members of voluntary agencies are generally part-time volunteers. How these part-time "political amateurs" affect the human services and the making of social policies will be discussed in the section on pressure and lobbying.

Sometimes it is the client population together with human services workers who initiate the move toward the introduction of new programs and policies. Many years ago on the lower east side of New York City, the director of a summer sleep-away camp of a sectarian agency was approached by community residents of various faiths and races to discuss providing camping services of their children. The community members pointed out the desperate need for these services that could not be met by other agencies in the community. They also pointed out that many children attending the director's camp did not live in the community. The director agreed to accept some of the children in question. Within a relatively short period of time, the agency served all those who desired service, with the understanding that the agency would maintain its sectarian nature and goals. Community members in this example used their power to influence policy of a community agency. Until recently, it was the agencies that determined their policies, and the recipients of services did not have the power to change or affect them significantly.

Baker and Northman (1981) suggested that citizen involvement in policy determination is really a form of redistribution of power that previously did not allow for such sharing. Dobelstein (1980), on the other hand, asserted that "even in the present consumer-oriented society, those who are the principal recipients of welfare policies are rarely involved in making welfare decisions" (p. 30). Although one might agree with the latter point of view, we believe that it may be a mistake to underestimate the power of the consumer and/or the human services worker to affect policy. It is sometimes impossible to tell in advance if one will be able to affect programs and policies, and to what extent. Actually, one may be able to affect such

COMPARISON

The Diversity of State Legislatures

State legislatures across the country vary greatly in many respects, such as in the time that they meet and in the compensation given to their representatives. The National Conference of State Legislatures grouped them into three types based on their length of session, salaries, and staff size.

Types of Legislatures

TYPE 1	TYPE 2		TYPE 3	
Full time	**In-between hybrid**		**Part time**	
High pay			**Low pay**	
Large staff			**Small staff**	
California	Alabama	Minnesota	Arkansas	Utah
Illinois	Alaska	Mississippi	Georgia	Vermont
Massachusetts	Arizona	Missouri	Idaho	West Virginia
Michigan	Colorado	Nebraska	Indiana	Wyoming
New Jersey	Connecticut	North Carolina	Maine	
New York	Delaware	Oklahoma	Montana	
Ohio	Florida	Oregon	Nevada	
Pennsylvania	Hawaii	South Carolina	New Hampshire	
Wisconsin	Iowa	Tennessee	New Mexico	
	Kansas	Texas	North Dakota	
	Kentucky	Virginia	Rhode Island	
	Louisiana	Washington	South Dakota	
	Maryland			

Length of Session

Average number of months in session for 2 years (some legislatures meet every other year), 1990 to 1991, for each type of legislature. In that time, Congress met for 22 months.

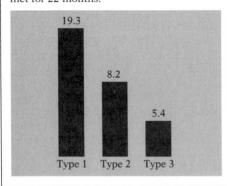

Legislator Compensation

Average compensation in 1991, including salaries and other reimbursements that are taxable. Congressional compensation averaged $125,100.

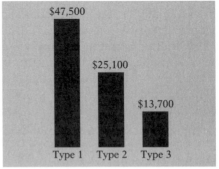

Source: "With Power Shift, State Lawmakers See New Demands," by S. H. Verhover, *New York Times*, September 24, 1995, pp. 1, 24. Copyright © 1995 by The New York Times Co. Reprinted by permission.

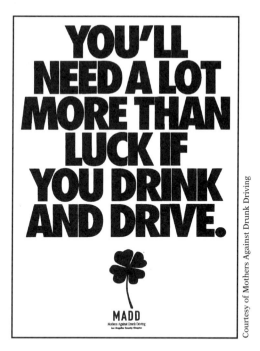

An example of how laypeople affect social
policy

decisions more than one might imagine. As far as the individual worker is
concerned, opportunities for initiating programs occur more frequently on
the local than on the state or federal levels. As an ancient Chinese philoso-
pher was reported to have said, "A journey of a thousand miles starts with a
single step."

FACTORS IN ESTABLISHING POLICY

Azarnoff and Seliger (1982) affirmed that the president and Congress pass
the laws and formulate policies based on their perceptions of what the public wants and needs. What is the basis of their perceptions? Often it is the
results of research or the pressure of groups and individuals lobbying for or
against a certain policy. We look at these factors in this section.

Research

The basic sources of information used in deciding policy are studies, surveys, experiments, reports, and records. Data gathered from these sources
are examined, interpreted, discussed, and presented to the president and

Congress for their consideration. This process also takes place on the state and local levels and involves the legislatures and executives of each jurisdiction. Voluntary agencies formulate their policies and programs in essentially the same manner. Data are gathered, examined, interpreted, discussed, and presented to the executive and board of directors for their decisions. It is rare indeed that agencies, governmental or voluntary, devise policies or programs without going through this process. Sound research and its application, although not guarantees of perfect policies or programs, are extremely useful tools in developing sound social policies and programs.

The Community Mental Health Centers Act of 1963 is an excellent example of how research can be used to develop policies and programs to help the mentally ill. In this instance, it was a presidential commission that gathered data on the increasing numbers of people in need of mental-health services. The lack of trained personnel, facilities, and resources was highlighted in the report of the commission. Congress adopted legislation that provided funds to set up community mental-health centers throughout the country. In addition, funds for training more personnel were made available. The intent was to reduce the number of people needing long-term hospitalization. Much was accomplished but, as with almost any complex problem, solutions were only partially achieved and other problems were created. Unfortunately, the research in this instance did not provide enough data to avoid some of the problems that developed. Some problems are not the fault of the research. In too many instances, the information asked for is limited to specific and existing problems rather than also focusing on predicting and preventing future problems.

It has sometimes happened that research, surveys, and studies have been devised to prove a point rather than to gather data and let the chips fall where they may. Other situations have occurred in which the individuals conducting the research (often human services workers themselves) have had little knowledge of acceptable methods of gathering and interpreting **valid** and **reliable data.** Anecdotal records and similarly limited types of studies have all too frequently been the basis for program policy changes. These approaches are at best questionable. There have also been instances when agencies have ignored or discarded data that did not enhance the image or viability of the agency. Capoccia and Googins (1982) suggested that in an environment of limited choice of policy decisions or limited funding, mobilization of interested groups and the exercise of power become more important than research in assessing needs. They added that the more limited the choices, the less the chances are for determining need through an objective or rational process. Social policy decisions may be determined not by objective analysis of the issues, but rather by emotional and general descriptions, all too frequently provided by the media (Miringoff & Opdyke, 1986). We shall discuss the media's effect on social policy shortly.

The results of biased or inadequate research have sometimes led to poorly planned policies and programs. Such policies might be considered politically practical, but they might also be useless and destructive to those they are intended to serve. Witness the **deinstitutionalization** policy and program of the 1970s for the mentally disabled. The title of a report to the Congress in 1977 by the Comptroller of the United States gives an idea of the results of this policy: *Returning the Mentally Disabled to the Community: Government Needs to Do More*. The report refers both to the positive aspects of the various programs and to the many problems resulting from a lack of facilities and services, as well as to the inadequacy of follow-up for those returned to the community. Mechanic (1980) was more specific in this regard. He stated that "large numbers of mental patients were released from hospitals into the community without adequate preparation, . . . appropriate services, or consideration of the social costs" (p. 83). He added, significantly, that whereas the thrust for such programs came from many sources, a major one was the economic pressures on state governments. He pointed out that the programs were generally supported by mental-health professionals who held overly optimistic views of anticipated results. What did result in many instances was patient "dumping," leading to community fears and resistance and the victimization of patients by the unscrupulous as a result of the lack of support services. More adequate research regarding the needed criteria for facilities for patients, the number of patients involved, and the level of support services might have led to more successful programs.

Pressure and Lobbying

When one studies the development of social policies on the federal level, one becomes awed by the pressure brought to bear on Congress and the president to influence the development and purposes of social policies and programs before a final decision is made. White (1982) confirmed this view in his description of the rapid growth in the number of lobbyists who try to affect legislation. He wrote that in the first half of 1981, over 1000 new lobbyists registered in Washington. His report on a recent survey told about the existence of more than 50 lobbies for minorities. more than 30 for social agencies, more than 30 for women's groups, and many others. This does not include the offices of almost 30 states and 70 cities that are in Washington trying to obtain their share of the pie as well as to influence programs and policies that could help their constituents. Clymer (1995) described the growth in the number of lobbyists. He tells us that "about 6,000 lobbyists are currently registered; perhaps 3 to 10 times as many will now have to [register]" (p. 36). He also points out that the definition of lobbyists has been expanded from its current narrow range of those who spend the majority of their time with members of Congress to include those part-timers who also work with the staff of Congress or executive branch agencies. When one adds the countless individuals and groups, including many

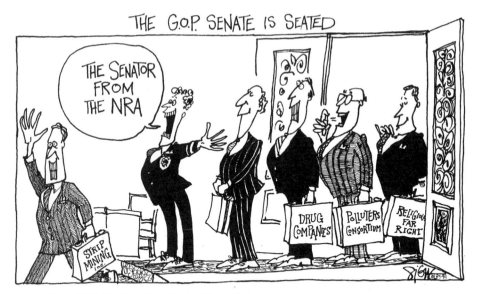

By Signe for the Philadelphia Daily News. Reprinted by permission.

human services worker organizations, that march, testify, send letters, make calls, and otherwise attempt to influence the lawmakers, it becomes clear that the pressures on Congress and the president are awesome.

The question then is: How does all this constant pressure affect their perception and decisions regarding policies and programs? One example of pressure and lobbying is that of corporate welfare. Pianin (1995) discussed the power of the corporate lobbies and how they obtained $51 billion in direct subsides to industries and $53 billion in tax loopholes. Huff and Johnson (1993) give what they believe is a conservative annual projection of over $170 billion in support of what they call "the phantom welfare state." In addition, Lancelot and De Gennaro (1995) describe corporate welfare that has a more direct impact on people. The federal subsidy to the sugar industry doubles the price of sugar and increases the cost of products that use sugar. It becomes quite apparent that regardless of what decisions are made, not everyone will be happy. The same pressures exist on state and local levels of government and within voluntary or private agencies, although on a smaller scale. The general outcome is that the decision makers try to give important groups, those with clout (or money) at least some of what they want.

One of the problems in trying to affect policy on the state and local levels, according to Lynn (1980), is that most state and local lawmakers are overworked and underpaid (see box on page 286). Because much social policy legislation is new and unfamiliar to them, they generally listen to those who can have the greatest effect on their political lives. Consequently, they are very responsive to the power groups in their local and state communities. These groups include businesspeople, developers, unions, reli-

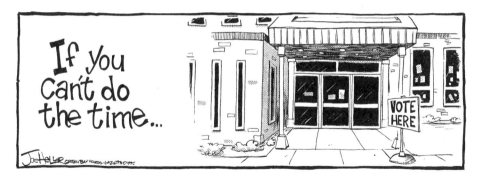

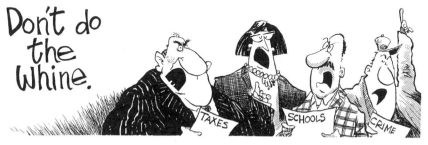

Reprinted with permission of Joe Heller, Green Bay Press-Gazette.

gious groups, homeowners, and the media, among other interest groups. According to Dye (1987), public opinion has a limited effect on the decision makers. Most ordinary people do not write or talk to their legislators. Unfortunately, most eligible voters do not even vote, thus allowing powerful lobbyists of large corporations and those with sources of huge sums of money to become much more effective.

Human services agencies and their constituents, usually the poor and minority groups who do not vote in large numbers, often do not compete effectively with the power of the groups mentioned earlier. Human services agencies have the best chance of being heard when an issue raises a great deal of compassion and costs very little to resolve. In difficult economic times, such as during the 1991–1992 recession, however, human services agencies are among the first to feel the economic pinch. Teltsch (1991) noted that federal cutbacks and the recession caused further reductions in government funding for nonprofit organizations, and fund-raising efforts and foundation gifts cannot make up for those cuts. She claims that government money is the major source of income for nonprofit human services agencies. There are times, however, as in 1995, when the economy was quite strong, and still funds for social programs and agencies were significantly cut.

The boards of directors of nonprofit human services agencies consist primarily of affluent, well-meaning, dedicated, and frequently knowledgeable part-time volunteers whose major functions are to raise money and determine policies for their own organizations. Their familiarity with and knowledge of how best to serve their constituents are secondhand and quite limited, coming most often from the administrators they hire and from the media. Their major concern is raising funds, for it is money that significantly affects the policies they develop and the programs they provide.

The Media

When we read newspapers and magazines, watch TV, or listen to the radio, we may not be fully aware of attempts to influence our views of social policy. This may be done by selecting which stories to highlight and by "slanting" them in either a liberal or conservative direction. When politicians or lobbyists discuss the details of policy matters in the media, we frequently do not take sides or think that the issues are important enough to affect us. However, when the media cover issues that obviously affect a large portion of a population directly (regarding their health and pocketbook), people listen and policies are often affected. A recent example of this phenomenon was the coverage of the 1993–1994 struggle over the health care issue. A most recent example is the struggle to "end welfare as we know it," which was discussed in Chapter 1. With regard to the ending of welfare as we know it, however, other questions come to mind. Who, for example, are the "we"? How much do we know about all, or any, welfare programs and what they do, whom they serve, and what criteria are used? Do we know the strengths as well as the weakness of specific programs? One wonders how many politicians and human service workers, much less the general population, really know the welfare system in order to ethically support, much less vote to change, something so complex.

Politicians, lobbyists, all types of organizations, and all types of groups know how important it is to use the media to achieve their goals. It is only through the media that some segments of the general population become aware and/or somewhat knowledgeable of issues and make their opinions known. Polls run by or reported by the media are also used to sway the opinions and votes of people. It is important to know who took the surveys, what questions were asked, who interpreted the raw data, and so on before accepting the polls as gospel.

One must also be careful, however, when listening and/or reading about issues. We must be aware of the sources of information, the accuracy of the material, and the pros and cons of the issues. Politicians, for example, will frequently make general statements that are at best exaggerated and at worst false to sway opinions. Examples have occurred almost everyday in the battles over the budget, welfare, and medical coverage in 1994–1995 when politicians used the phrase "the American people want . . . " or "the American people believe . . . " One must remember that in 1994 a little over one-third of eligible voters voted. Of that group, a little over one-half decided who was to represent them. Yet on the national level, politicians claim "the American people want" this, that, etc. These kinds of statements, often used by politicians, their supporters, and lobbyists, are examples of techniques described in the critical thinking activity, Recognizing Deceptive Arguments, located at the end of this chapter.

Human service workers need to learn how to use the media to help gain support for their work and point of view. The amount and kind of support they obtain will be in large measure dependent on their ability and skill in the use of the media. Furthermore, in order to be effective advocates and helpers, human service workers must be able to distinguish fact from opinion, provable statements from unprovable statements, and recognize deceptive arguments. They must also be able to recognize stereotypes, evaluate sources of information, and distinguish between bias and reason if they are to be effective workers and professionals. To help develop these skills, critical thinking activities taken from those used and described in detail in the Opposing Viewpoints and Current Controversies series of the Greenhaven Press of San Diego, CA, can be very useful. Examples of these activities are at the end of this chapter.

Opposition

Opposition refers to efforts to defeat proposed policies or to changes in existing policies or programs. These efforts play an important role in determining the final form of accepted policies and programs. Sometimes there is little change in the original proposal as a result of opposition, but in some instances, one might have some trouble recognizing the original idea. The degree of transformation is related to the strength of the opposition and the nature of the compromise reached by the opposing groups. Compromises might be in philosophy, funding, resources, politics, or a combination of these factors. For example, the struggle for ending welfare as we know it by conservatives and some fiscally conservative liberals has engendered a great deal of opposition by most liberals. Although welfare reform legislation has finally been enacted, it required significant compromises on the part of Congress and the Clinton administration. It did not, however, really satisfy conservatives or liberals.

Opposition is frequently based not upon moral, political, or philosophical issues, but rather on self-serving economic factors. The survival of an agency or program has been known to be a major obstacle to new policies or policy changes. Jobs of human services workers are often at stake, and this factor, as difficult as it might be to acknowledge, has been known to be a major obstacle to eliminating or changing an obsolete or ineffective agency or program.

THE IMPLEMENTATION OF SOCIAL POLICY

Once a policy has been decided on, regardless of its purpose or limits, a program must be devised and carried out if the policy is to have any impact. Remember, a policy is a plan or guide: It tells us what to do, not how to do it. For example, there is a policy stating that child abuse should be eliminated and prevented. This policy has been established by many organizations, public and private, concerned with child welfare. These agencies often make funds available to help in the effort. There are many ways one could approach the problem. Some agencies might focus on working with young parents who were victims of child abuse themselves. Others might provide information and education through the media. Yet another approach would be to attempt to discover the causes of child abuse through research and then develop a program to deal with those causes. In an actual program, any one or a combination of these approaches is considered an effort to implement the policy of preventing child abuse.

The discussion that follows provides some idea of what is involved in developing programs to implement social policy. It includes additional insights regarding opportunities for human services workers to affect programs and policies. The purpose is to introduce you to some of the factors at work in the **implementation** of social policy.

Funding

Money! Money makes the world go 'round! Money talks! Money isn't everything! There seems to be some truth in all those comments. With regard to social policies, it is almost certain that the availability of funds determines whether or not a policy is established or implemented. Money also determines the degree to which a policy is implemented. For example, the policy of most states is to provide adequate treatment and living facilities for patients in mental hospitals. In practice, however, there are too many institutions that provide little or no treatment along with minimal custodial care. Unfortunately, the same holds true with regard to many institutions serving the aged, the retarded, and juvenile offenders. In most cases, the excuse given for these conditions is lack of funds. This is very frequently the case. What is also true, however, is that how one uses available funds is a factor in determining the degree to which a policy is implemented and the degree of effectiveness of a program. On the other hand, it should be understood that while ample funds do not guarantee the effective implementation of policies, insufficient funds do guarantee ineffective implementation of policies.

Another problem of funding social policies occurs when a policy is decided on and no funds are appropriated to carry out the policy. In some cases, monies are appropriated but are not permitted to be spent (Fill, 1974). An example of this type of problem came about when the policy of busing children from one area to another to integrate schools was proclaimed by the courts. Funding to provide the buses to carry out the mandated policy was sometimes not forthcoming from other branches of government. Federal, state, and local governments have often mandated programs without providing sufficient funds to implement them effectively. Obviously, funds are vital to the process of implementing policy.

It is clear that funding affects policies and policies affect funding. It is also clear that human services workers are seriously affected in their efforts to carry out policies depending upon the level of funding available to them.

Interpretation of Policy

A second factor that has a significant impact on policy implementation is the way policy is interpreted. Interpreting policy means more than just explaining policy. According to the *Random House Dictionary* (1978), interpretation is "construing or understanding in a particular way." It involves an understanding or conception of another's words or deeds. The question here, of course, is how social policies are interpreted. It is useful, at this point, to make a distinction between general policy and operational policy. For example, the elimination of poverty is a general policy. How one goes about eliminating poverty—for example, through welfare programs or government work programs—involves operational policy (Huttman, 1981). In other words, a general policy states a broad objective, whereas operational policy is concerned with the methods and procedures used to meet the objective.

There is usually little controversy regarding the interpretation of general policies. Few would argue with the policy of trying to eliminate poverty. Problems arise, however, on the operational level when it becomes necessary to determine the income at which a person or family is considered to be living in poverty. Further questions then arise. To what extent should people be helped, under what conditions, and for how long? Different states, **jurisdictions,** and agencies have different criteria for resolving such questions.

For example, Congress at one time tightened eligibility rules for the social security disability program. It was felt that the government was providing funds to people with disabilities who were able to work. It was subsequently reported ("U. S. Agency Calls," 1983) that decisions to stop disability payments were being based on an extremely hard-line interpretation. It was reported that an examiner said that unless a claimant was "flat on his back in an institution, comatose, or in a catatonic state," he or she would not meet the criteria for continued payment. The policy was thus being interpreted to mean that if one could walk, one could work and would therefore no longer be eligible for disability payments. This interpretation of a general policy eliminated claimants whose disabilities were serious enough to prevent them from working in a competitive society. Furthermore, the decisions were based on written records. There were no face-to-face interviews that would have helped to provide a more accurate basis on which to make a decision. This would have prevented some of the obviously destructive decisions that were made. The stopping of payments on the basis of written records alone is an example of interpretation of an operational policy.

It is apparent that policies can be significantly affected when interpreted differently by those who determine policy and those who implement policy. To complicate matters, both the target population and the general public also become involved in interpreting policy. For example, in discussions in 1982 and 1983 on proposed modification of the social security program, many of those receiving benefits interpreted the planned change as an attempt to reduce their benefits. Many others of the general public shared this view. Some younger people, for instance, interpreted the suggested change as an attempt to reduce future benefits through changing the retirement age from 65 to 68 over the years. When conflicts arise around the interpretation of policy that cannot be resolved by the parties involved, the courts are sometimes called upon to settle the issues.

Who Implements Policy?

A third significant factor in implementing policies is the question of who implements them. Human services workers are usually the ones who actually deliver or provide the services to those in need. These workers include those described in Chapter 6 and others, such as vocational counselors, community developers, and the police. Human services workers are instrumental in the successful implementation of policies and programs. The degree of success of these policies and programs is determined by the amount and kind of training the worker has received. Some time ago, we attended a conference of human services workers and researchers concerned with providing psychotherapeutic services to minority groups. It became very clear, in the papers presented and the discussions that followed, that the training of those providing services to minority populations was not adequate to assure success of such programs. A lack of sensitivity and a lack of knowledge regarding the needs of minority group members were major obstacles to successful interventions.

It is clear that training of human services workers, regardless of the type or level of service, is critical to the successful implementation of programs and policies. The increasing trend toward registration, licensing, and testing of human services workers attests to the importance of training and competence in the view of consumers of human services and employers of human services workers. Improved competency and training not only increase the chances of successful implementation of programs, but also increase the abilities and credibility of workers in their efforts to identify the needs of people and to develop new social policies or improve old ones.

CRITICAL THINKING ACTIVITIES*

Recognizing Deceptive Arguments

People who feel strongly about an issue use many techniques to persuade others to agree with them. Some of these techniques appeal to the intellect, some to the emotions. Many of them distract the reader or listener from the real issues.

A few common examples of argumentation tactics are listed below. Most of them can be used either to advance an argument in an honest, reasonable way or to deceive or distract from the real issues. It is important for a critical reader to recognize these tactics in order to rationally evaluate an author's ideas.

   a. *bandwagon*—the idea that "everybody" does this or believes this
   b. *categorical statements*—stating something in a way that implies there can be no argument or disagreement on the issue
   c. *personal attack*—criticizing an opponent personally instead of rationally debating his or her ideas
   d. *testimonial*—quoting or paraphrasing an authority or celebrity to support one's own viewpoint

The following activity can help you sharpen your skills in recognizing deceptive reasoning. The statements below are derived from the viewpoints in this chapter. *Beside each one, mark the letter of the type of deceptive appeal being used. More than one type of tactic may be applicable. If you believe the statement is not any of the listed appeals, write N.*

   1. The Supreme Court has a greater obligation to protect the rights of victims than those of criminals.
   2. It is clear to every intelligent person that the Eighth Amendment to the U. S. Constitution, protection against cruel and unusual punishment, does not bar the use of victim impact statements.
   3. Victim reforms will destroy the constitutional rights of the accused.
   4. The conservative, prejudiced Supreme Court judges are too stupid to recognize the rights of the accused.
   5. Every decent lawyer believes the harm a victim suffered because of a defendant should be considered when determining punishment.
   6. Victims have absolutely no rights at all.
   7. Everyone agrees that victim reforms are false promises made by legislators seeking to please voters worried about crime.

*The following critical thinking activities are taken from *Opposing Viewpoint Series.* Copyright © Greenhaven Press Inc. Reprinted by permission.

8. The victims' rights movement developed because victims of crime felt they had no rights in the criminal justice system.
9. Thurgood Marshall, a pro-criminal, bleeding-heart liberal, considers the harm a victim suffered irrelevant in a criminal trial.
10. As Justice John Paul Stevens correctly points out, the defendant should have more rights than the state in a criminal trial.
11. Victim impact statements force juries to base their decisions on emotion rather than on objective facts.
12. As Deborah Kelly, chair of the American Bar Association's Victims' Committee, accurately concludes, victims' satisfaction with the criminal justice system depends more on how they were treated than how severely their assailants were punished.
13. Everyone knows that judges let criminals off too easily.
14. Intelligent people agree that victims' rights deny the accused the right to a fair and impartial trial.
15. As the Chief Justice of the U. S. Supreme Court, William H. Rehnquist, states, there is no constitutional rule that excludes victim impact statements.

Defining Poverty

Much of the debate . . . over how serious poverty is in America revolves around how poverty is defined. There are two general methods of defining poverty. One is to use a *relative* definition—measuring the wealth and income of a certain population, and finding out who has the least *relative* to the others. This process does have limitations. For instance, most people would argue that the men in the foreground of the cartoon are still poor, even if there are people worse off than they are. Conversely, in a country populated by millionaires, a person with only a half-million dollars would be considered poor.

Another method of defining and measuring poverty is to use an *absolute* definition. This method sets a minimum standard of income and/or wealth, regardless of how many people are above or below the standard. One example of an absolute definition is the official US poverty line, which defines as poor any couple who earned less than $7132 a year in 1986. A major drawback to absolute definitions is that they don't consider other factors, like differences in cost of living. The couple making $7132 a year will live more comfortably in rural Iowa than in New York City.

In this exercise you will create your own definition of poverty. Consider again the men in the cartoon. Most people would consider a person who does not live in some sort of home or shelter as poor. By this definition the men in the cartoon are poor. But most people would not consider poor a person who couldn't afford a cabin cruiser. Most people view cabin cruisers as luxuries, not one of life's essentials.

What does it mean to be poor?

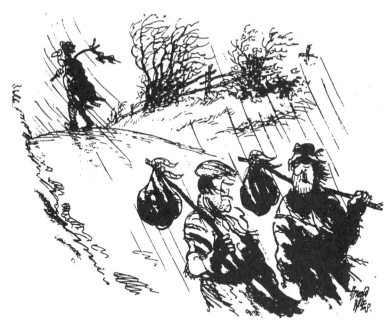

"There's Always Someone Worse Off Than Yourself."

© Wiles/Rothco.

STEP 1

Working in small groups, discuss the items listed below. Mark *E* for essential items—things you believe people must have. Mark *N* for nonessential items—items that are luxuries a person could live without.

three meals a day
shelter
housing with at least one private room
enough money for occasional snacks, trips to movies, cigarettes
indoor running water
private hot shower
one "good" outfit of clothing
more than five changes of clothing
heating
air-conditioning
health care or insurance
annual dental and eye checkups
a washer and dryer
a job
a car
a television set
a VCR

electricity
a warm coat
a refrigerator
meal at fast-food restaurant once a week
high school education
post-high school education (college or vocational school)
a stereo
a radio
a telephone
a personal computer

If necessary, add other items you believe are essential.

STEP 2

Discuss the following questions with your class or group.

1) Examine your list of *essential* items. Which ones are actually essential to survival and which are essential to a "humane" existence—a level above bare survival?
2) Write an item-based definition of poverty: "A person suffers from poverty if he/she lacks these items: _____, _____, _____ . . ."
3) How absolute is your group's definition? If a person lacked only *one* of your essentials, is he/she still poor? If a person has several non-essentials but lacks some essentials, is he/she still poor?
4) Do you think your definition of poverty is better or worse than the two described in the introduction of this activity? Why? What drawbacks does your definition have?

Evaluating Sources of Information

A critical thinker must always question sources of information. Historians, for example distinguish between *primary sources* ("firsthand" or eyewitness account from personal letters, documents, or speeches, etc.) and *secondary sources* (a "secondhand" account usually based upon a "firsthand" account and possibly appearing in a newspaper or encyclopedia). A published diary of a welfare mother is an example of a primary source. A book review of the mother's diary is an example of a secondary source.

Interpretation and/or point of view also play a role when dealing with primary and secondary sources. For example, the welfare mother might strongly believe that any form of welfare is degrading. Her personal experience affects her view of the welfare system. The secondary source, too, should be questioned as to interpretation or underlying motive. The book reviewer might have strong feelings regarding the necessity of welfare, and criticize the diary because of his personal bias. It is up to the researcher to keep in mind the potential biases of his/her sources.

This activity is designed to test your skill in evaluating sources of information. Imagine you are writing a report to the governor on how to reform the state welfare system. You decide to include an equal number of primary and secondary sources. Listed below are a number of sources which may be useful for your report. Carefully evaluate each of them. Then, *place a P next to those descriptions you believe are primary sources.* Second, *rank the primary sources* assigning the number (1) to what appears to be the most accurate primary source, the number (2) to the next most accurate, and so on until the ranking is finished. *Repeat the entire procedure, this time placing an S next to the descriptions you feel would serve as secondary sources and then ranking them.*

If you are doing this activity as a member of a class or group, compare your answers with those of other class or group members. Be able to defend your answers. You may discover that others will come to different conclusions than you. Listening to the reasons others present for their answers may give you valuable insights in evaluating sources of information.

P or S		*Rank in Importance*
_____	1. copies of the forms people fill out to receive welfare	_____
_____	2. interviews with children growing up on welfare	_____
_____	3. a book on poor Americans and welfare programs from 1900 to 1950	_____
_____	4. an article by a social scientist who compares state-by-state welfare benefits and poverty statistics	_____
_____	5. a local television news feature about a pastor who works with poor families in her neighborhood	_____
_____	6. a statewide poll on how people feel about welfare	_____
_____	7. a novel based on the author's childhood growing up under welfare	_____
_____	8. a magazine article about a company which hires people on welfare	_____
_____	9. a speech by a US senator on welfare cheats	_____
_____	10. a pamphlet published by a conservative organization titled "How Welfare Exploits the Poor"	_____
_____	11. a pamphlet published by a leftist organization titled "How Welfare Exploits the Poor"	_____
_____	12. welfare mothers speaking as guests on the Oprah Winfrey show	_____

Recognizing Stereotypes

A stereotype is an oversimplified or exaggerated description of people or things. Stereotyping can be favorable. However, most stereotyping tends to be highly uncomplimentary, and, at times, degrading.

Stereotyping grows out of our prejudices. When we stereotype someone, we are prejudging him or her. Consider the following example: Mr. Smith believes all poor people are lazy. Whenever he sees a homeless person on the street or on television he asks himself, "Why won't that person look for a job?" He disregards any other possible reason why that person is homeless. Why? He has prejudged all poor people and will keep his stereotype consistent with his prejudice.

. . . Consider [the following statements] carefully. *Mark S for any statement that is an example of stereotyping. Mark N for any statement that is not an example of stereotyping. Mark U if you are undecided about any statement.*

If you are doing this activity as a member of a class or group, compare your answers with those of other class or group members. Be able to defend your answers. You may discover that others will come to different conclusions than you. Listening to the reasons others present for their answers may give you valuable insights in recognizing stereotypes.

S = stereotype
N = not a stereotype
U = undecided

1. Many Jews have succeeded economically despite anti-Semitism.
2. Jews have a way with money.
3. Two out of three poor adults are women.
4. Most people on welfare are lazy.
5. Many black youths do not have jobs.
6. Many black youths don't want to work.
7. Divorced men are chauvinists who refuse to pay child support.
8. Mothers do not make good workers.
9. Many poor people live in single-parent households.
10. Most Hispanics are illegal immigrants.
11. Women are more likely than men to quit work to raise their children.
12. All white businessmen discriminate against women and minorities.
13. In cities across the country millions of blacks live in poverty.
14. Many women have babies in order to go on welfare.
15. All people who want to cut welfare are racists.
16. The poor are different from the rest of us.
17. Most feminists are social radicals.
18. The median income of Japanese-Americans is higher than that of Anglo-Saxons.

ADDITIONAL READING

Bell, W. (1987). *Contemporary social welfare* (2nd ed.). New York: Macmillan.

Feagin, S. R. (1975). *Subordinating the poor: Welfare and American beliefs.* Englewood Cliffs, NJ: Prentice Hall.

Galper, J. H. (1975). *The politics of social services.* Englewood Cliffs, NJ: Prentice Hall.

Johnson, W. H. (Ed.). (1980). *Rural human services: A book of readings.* Itasca, IL: F. E. Peacock.

Mills, C. W. (1959). *The power elite.* New York: Oxford University Press.

Parenti, M. (1978). *Power and the powerless.* New York: St. Martin's Press.

Piven, F. F., & Cloward, R. A. (1971). *Regulating the poor: The functions of public welfare.* New York: Vintage.

Richan, W. C. (1988). *Beyond altruism: Social policy in American society.* New York: Haworth Press.

Schenk, Q. F., & Schenk, E. L. (1981). *Welfare, society, and the helping professions: An introduction.* New York: Macmillan.

REFERENCES

Alinsky, S. D. (1971). *Rules for radicals.* New York: Vintage Books.

Austin, M. J., Skelding, A. H., & Smith, P. L. (1977). *Delivering human services: An introductory programmed text.* New York: Harper & Row.

Azarnoff, R. S., & Seliger, J. S. (1982). *Delivering human services.* Englewood Cliffs, NJ: Prentice Hall.

Baker, F., & Northman, J. E. (1981). *Helping: Human services for the 80s.* St. Louis: C. V. Mosby.

Baker R. (1995, January 17). Those vital paupers. *The New York Times,* p. A19.

Beverly D. P., & McSweeney, E. A. (1987). *Social welfare and social justice.* Englewood Cliffs, NJ: Prentice Hall.

Capoccia, V. A., & Googins, B. (1982). Social planning in an environment of limited choice. *New England Journal of Human Services, 2,* 31–36.

Clymer, A. (1995, December 16). Congress sends lobbying overhall to Clinton. *The New York Times,* p. 26.

Dobelstein, A. W. (1980). *Politics, economics, and public welfare.* Englewood Cliffs, NJ: Prentice Hall.

Dye, T. R. (1987). *Understanding public policy* (6th ed.). Englewood Cliffs, NJ: Prentice Hall.

Fill, H. J. (1974). *The mental breakdown of a nation.* New York: New Viewpoints.

Foderaro, L. W. (1995, October 14). Mentally ill gaining new rights, with the ill as their own lobby. *The New York Times,* pp. A1, 24.

Gil, D. G. (1981). *Unravelling social policy: Theory, analysis, and political action towards social equality* (3rd ed.). Cambridge, MA: Schenkman.

Gilbert N., & Specht, H. (1974). *Dimensions of social welfare policy.* Englewood Cliffs, NJ: Prentice Hall.

Huff, D. D., & Johnson, D. A. (1993 May). Phantom Welfare: Public Relief for Corporate America. *Social Work, 38*(3), 311–315.

Huttman, E. D. (1981). *Introduction to social policy.* New York: McGraw-Hill.

Lancelot, J., & De Gennaro, R. (1995, January 31). Green Scissors snip $33 billion. *The New York Times,* p. A21.

Lynn, L. E. (1980). *The state and human services: Organizational change in a political context.* Cambridge. MA: MIT Press.

Mechanic, D. (1980). *Mental health and social policy* (2nd ed.). Englewood Cliffs, NJ: Prentice Hall.

Meyer, C. H. (1983). The power to define problems. *Social Work, 28,* 99.

Miller, S. M. (1985, Winter). Reforming the welfare state. *New York, Social Policy, 15*(3), 62–64.

Miringoff, M. L., & Opdyke, S. (1986). *American social welfare policy: Reassessment and reform.* Englewood Cliffs, NJ: Prentice Hall.

Pianin, E. (1995, August 28–September 3). Welfare as they know and love it. *The Washington Post National Weekly Edition,* p. 13.

Priest, D., & Mintz, J. (1995, October 23–29). The unsinkable Seawolf. *The Washington Post National Weekly Edition,* p. 33.

Prigmore, C. S., & Atherton, C. R. (1979). *Social welfare policy: Analysis and formulation.* Lexington, MA: D. C. Heath.

Teltsch, K. (1991, December 24). Government's cuts to private groups threaten the charities of last resort. *The New York Times,* p. 24.

Titmus, R. M. (1974). *Social policy: An introduction.* New York: Pantheon.

U. S. agency calls cuts in disability pay improper. (1983, April 7). *The New York Times,* p. B14.

U. S. Bureau of Labor Statistics. (1993). *The 1995 world almanac.* Mahwah, NJ: Funk and Wagnall.

Verhover, S. H. (1995, September 24). With power shift, state lawmakers see new demands. *The New York Times,* pp. 1, 24.

White, T. H. (1982). *America in search of itself: The making of the president 1956–1980.* New York: Harper & Row.

Prevention in Human Services

INTRODUCTION

"No major disorder in a population has ever been eliminated by providing one-to-one treatment," stated the report of the Task Panel on Prevention (1978, p. 214) of the President's Commission on Mental Health. Does this mean that treatment of major disorders is of no use? Not at all! Treatment and rehabilitation are essential methods of working with patients. They are, however, not the only effective tools of human services. What this statement does mean is that other approaches are needed if society hopes to successfully cope with the increasing number of individuals who are **dysfunctional**. One such approach is preventing disorders from developing in the first place.

Although prevention in the human services is not a new idea, it is rarely addressed in introductory human services texts. When it *is* discussed in such texts, it is most often covered only briefly. We applaud the recent growth of prevention programs in the human services and are convinced of the great potential of these programs. For this reason, we feel that it is essential to introduce the subject of prevention to those planning to enter the field of human services. It should be clear to you that human services are not limited to the repairing or patching up of dysfunctional persons through treatment and rehabilitation. Furthermore, by introducing the concept of prevention in an introductory text, we hope that human services training programs will be encouraged to begin covering prevention with the same thoroughness now given to treatment and rehabilitation. Adequate information on prevention programs also offers the human services student another option regarding career choice.

The first part of the chapter focuses on what prevention is and what it is one seeks to prevent. A brief history of prevention efforts follows. The remainder of the chapter includes a discussion of the different levels of prevention and the rationale for the importance of prevention efforts. The chapter ends with an examination of current prevention programs and obstacles or barriers to the development of prevention programs.

DEFINING PREVENTION AND ITS TARGETS

To *prevent* means to keep something from happening. In the field of medicine, it is quite clear what one attempts to prevent. Illness, injury, and premature or unnecessary death are the three major targets of prevention programs in medicine. In the human services—not including medicine—the major targets are not so clearly defined or identified. The Task Panel on Prevention (1978) of the President's Commission on Mental Health felt strongly that efforts should focus on the prevention of "persistent, destructive, maladaptive behaviors" (p. 219). These behaviors include child abuse, drug abuse, criminal activities, and desertion of family, among many others.

The panel also stated that disorders should be the target of prevention programs. It is clear that there are many stressful situations, such as puberty, illness, and death, that cannot be kept from occurring, particularly by those faced with the problems. The goal, then, would be to prevent the situation from causing the kind of psychological and social disorders that have been mentioned. For example, during the deep recession of the early 1980s, millions of people were put out of work, and downsizing in the 1990s has had the same effects on those downsized as those unemployed during the deep recession of the 1980s. Unemployment led to the loss of homes for some, the loss of medical benefits for others, the need for some to apply for welfare, and general fear and uncertainty for all. These misfortunes led to increased family disorganization, alcoholism, depression, and similar disorders for millions of individuals and families. These individuals had neither the resources nor the skills to cope with the loss of their jobs and incomes. How to keep disorders caused by loss of income from occurring or how to prevent them from becoming severe enough so that "normal" functioning is impaired is the focus of prevention efforts in the human services. One might consider the unemployment insurance program, for example, as an effort to prevent the breakdown of the jobless. Job training and/or retraining is an additional effort to prevent the impairment of the unemployed. It at least temporarily reduces the stresses associated with unemployment.

PREVENTION IN THE PAST

In this section, we focus on the history of prevention efforts in the human services. Because it is impossible to separate the history of prevention programs from the history of human services, some of the material discussed here will necessarily overlap material in Chapter 3.

Preliterate and Ancient Civilizations

People have always tried to find ways to prevent hunger, injury, illness, and death. In preliterate civilizations, rituals, prayer, and sacrifices were used in the hope of preventing such catastrophes. These preventive rituals focused not only on hostile animals, environments, and people, but also on the weather and other natural phenomena that influenced the supply of food and shelter.

Ancient civilizations also used many of the "preventive" methods of preliterate groups such as prayer and ritual. However, a movement away from the priest, shaman, or religious healer slowly developed. There was an increasing awareness that in many cases illness and death were due to natural rather than supernatural phenomena. In fact, some early efforts at prevention were successful, even though the actual causes of the disease were not known. In ancient Greece, for example, Hippocrates noted that a particular disease, now thought to be malaria, developed and spread near swamps. When people avoided these areas or when the swamps were filled in, the disease abated (M. Bloom, 1981). Ancient Rome also contributed to the prevention of disease, even though the Romans might not have been aware of doing so. Their sewers and aqueducts were built to overcome unpleasant living conditions brought on by waste products and poor-tasting water. In effect, they prevented illness caused by poor sanitation and contaminated water.

The Dark Ages and the Renaissance

With the coming of the Dark Ages, medical practices reverted to an emphasis on prayer and rituals. According to Catalano (1979), medicine in Europe at that time become more of a combination of pagan myth and Christian prayer, then considered the best protection against illnesses of any kind. (This change is described in more detail in Chapter 3.) Prevention efforts related to illness, hunger, and poverty made little headway during the Middle Ages. The Church did, however, provide care and food to many in need, which prevented hunger and the accompanying stress-related problems.

The Renaissance and the Age of Reason saw a return to acceptance of more scientific medical practices. Quarantines were used to prevent the spread of disease. Inoculation against smallpox was developed. This was a powerful preventive measure, for it kept a specific disease from occurring. New drugs were found to be useful in treating and preventing diseases. During the 17th and 18th centuries, other practices and discoveries prevented some diseases. Sanitation projects were improved, general cleanliness was promoted, and a beginning understanding of contagion all helped in prevention of diseases. The lack of knowledge of causes of specific illnesses was not always an obstacle. Scurvy, for example, was practically eliminated without an understanding of vitamin deficiency or of how a diet that included fresh fruit and vegetables prevented it from occurring. Most prevention efforts were made in relation to physical illness. Mental illness was perceived in a different way by most medical doctors and the public at large. The treatment of the mentally ill was influenced by religious beliefs. During this time, the prevention of mental illness was, therefore, based upon a belief in prayer, ritual, and living a life free of sin.

The 19th and 20th Centuries

The 19th and 20th centuries saw even greater advances in medicine. Pasteur introduced the germ theory of disease. Ehrlich introduced the idea of a chemical "magic bullet" against specific diseases, the idea that a single medication could cure or prevent a particular disease. Clinical laboratory diagnosis and specialization became the trend. In the field of mental illness, advances were also being made but at a slower rate. Haindorf, in the early 19th century, introduced the concept that emotional conflicts that disturb the normal functioning of the body result in mental illness. Groos, before Freud, believed that humans are affected by physical forces they are not aware of and that these forces determine their behavior (Alexander & Selesnick, 1966).

Some significant, though rudimentary, efforts to prevent mental illness were made in the latter part of the 19th century and the early 20th century. For example, the **settlement house movement** represented a major attempt to help people deal with the perils and pressures of poverty, hunger, crime, poor education, sweatshops, and filthy living conditions. The primary focus was not on the prevention of mental illness, but rather on helping the millions of immigrants coming to America to establish themselves in their new homeland. Exploitation of these people, many of whom did not even know the language, was the rule. Human services workers of that era were convinced that this exploitation and its attendant hardships contributed to high rates of juvenile delinquency, crime, alcoholism, and poor health. Efforts to prevent these conditions from occurring were a major focus of the settlement house movement. Settlement house workers attempted to help the exploited overcome their poverty through education. Some progressive politicians also tried to alleviate the plight of the poor, and their attempts continued over many years. However, the settlement house movement and cooperating politicians did not have the political power to make significant changes in the distribution of resources to reduce or eliminate the stress brought on by poverty. They did, however, help sensitize the general public to the plight of poor immigrants.

The movement that probably attained the greatest success in preventing the exploitation of the poor was the **union movement.** Unions were formed and supported by exploited workers. Their efforts were supported by the settlement houses, other institutions, and liberal political leaders. The unions not only prevented exploitation of their members through the **collective bargaining** process, but also initiated the actively promoted legislation that increased opportunities for the poor to break the cycle of poverty and its accompanying disorders. The minimum wage laws and unemployment insurance are examples of such legislation. The unions, in effect, brought about a significant increase of resources for their members and millions of others entering or already in the work force. Although the workers did not suddenly become rich, they were much better off financially than before the advent of unions. Economic pressures, one of the avowed causes of emotional stress, was significantly reduced for many. Unions today are very often seen as the cause of economic problems such as high prices and inflation. Whether or not such a view is accurate or justified, there is no question that the union movement was, and still is according to some, a powerful force in enhancing the lives of union members and working people in general.

The latter part of the 19th century and early part of the 20th century also saw movement in determining the relationship between some physical and behavioral problems. There was a recognition that syphilis in its later stages caused many behavioral problems such as impulsive and bizarre actions. During the first 20 years of the 20th century, the mental hygiene movement, one of the most significant reform movements, was initiated by Clifford Beers and his associates. The main impetus for this movement was the autobiography of Beers, a former institutionalized mental patient. His book *A Mind That Found Itself* helped establish the National Committee for Mental Hygiene. One of the stated aims of the committee was the prevention of mental disorders. An article in the first issue of the committee's journal, *Mental Hygiene*, stated that "a healthy life-style could save people from insanity, hence the importance of educating the public as a means of preventing mental illness" (Dain, 1980, p. 103).

Most prevention programs in this country prior to the 1960s were aimed at physical diseases and were carried out largely by the Public Health Service. It was not until the 1960s that prevention efforts related to disabling behaviors were again seriously considered. Federal laws were passed that had an impact on prevention efforts in mental health and behavioral disorders. Some of the more familiar pieces of legislation were the following:

* the Community Mental Health Centers Act of 1963
* the Economic Opportunities Act of 1964—the war on poverty
* the Comprehensive Alcohol Abuse and Alcoholism Prevention, Treatment, and Rehabilitation Act of 1970
* the Child Abuse Prevention and Treatment Act of 1974
* the Juvenile Justice and Delinquency Prevention Act of 1974
* the establishment of an Office of Prevention within the National Institute of Mental Health in 1982

It should be noted that four of the acts listed specifically include "prevention" in their titles. The other two, although not specifying prevention in their titles, most certainly had prevention efforts as an integral part of their programs. In addition, Congress began to earmark funds for research in prevention activities. On the state level since 1974, approximately 12 states have established or are organizing statewide prevention units focused on the prevention of behavioral disorders. Initially, 8 of the 12 were financed by state funds alone. Some of the programs are more advanced than others; a few are still in the final planning stages (Johnston, 1980). In other states, efforts are being made to establish similar programs. In New York state, for example, the New York City Coalition for Prevention in Mental Health, a group made up of consumers, human services workers, and educators representing themselves and different agencies, urged the state for years to establish an office of prevention. Unfortunately, that organization no longer exists, and the effort to have the state establish an office of prevention has dissipated. Heller et al. (1984) noted that with the reduction of funds for human services programs as of 1980, federal and state policies once again emphasized treatment efforts over prevention programs "even though the help offered might only be palliative" (pp. 177–178).

A significant development in the field of prevention was the convening of the first national colloquium on Professional Education in Prevention in

1988. The focus of the conference was on training prevention professionals. There was also discussion of credentialing, evaluating, and testing various prevention models and programs. Sponsors of the conference include the National Prevention Network, the Illinois Department of Alcoholism and Drug Abuse, the Illinois Certification Boards, Inc., and the National College of Education. Although the sponsors are for the most part involved with alcohol and drug abuse causes and programs, the concept of prevention professionals is one that is most welcome and long overdue. We sincerely hope that the idea and practice of training prevention professionals are expanded to include areas such as mental health, child abuse, suicide, and teenage pregnancy, among others.

A program now in the process of being developed appears to be a major primary prevention effort, although it does not use the word *prevention* in its descriptive material. It is called The Family Development and Credentialing Program (FDC) and was initiated by the New York State Department of State, Division of Community Services. The response, in part, to the question raised in their material—Why is the FDC necessary—is:

> . . . For too long, services have been available only when a family is in crisis or about to disintegrate. Public interventions have focused on "rescuing and fixing" families rather than helping families develop their capacity to solve problems and achieve long-lasting self-reliance.
>
> Now on both the state and national levels, families, service providers and policy makers are joining together to reorient the way services are delivered toward a more family-focused and strengths-based approach. . . . ("Some Questions and Answers")

We would hope that other institutions and jurisdictions become involved in similar projects.

LEVELS OF PREVENTION

The various state and federal prevention programs that have been mentioned focus their efforts on different levels of prevention. The concept of levels originated with the Public Health Service and includes primary, secondary, and tertiary levels of prevention. Before discussing these levels, it must be made clear that there are controversies within the field of human services regarding the definition of each level. These differences will be described after a definition and example of each of the three levels of prevention.

Primary Prevention

Primary prevention in the human services is designed to prevent a disorder, disability, or dysfunction from occurring in the first place. An example of primary prevention might be a program to help the unemployed learn new skills and use support networks. Such a program might help prevent depression, alcoholism, and other psychological disorders. In the medical field, the shots given to prevent polio, the flu, or tetanus are examples of primary prevention at work.

Primary prevention is seen by Price, Bader, and Ketterer (1980), Cowen (1980), and the Task Panel on Prevention (1978) as being principally concerned with the reduction of new cases of disorders in a community. If, for example, families with severely retarded children were helped to learn new ways of dealing with their children and how to use all the resources provided for such problems, it might well prevent the onset of family strife or any other disorder that would further keep the retarded individual (or members of the family) from functioning at their potential. Stemming the ever-increasing number of disorders that develop among families facing different problems is one goal of primary prevention. Another example is one involving child abuse. Studies have indicated that people who were abused as children are more likely to become child abusers, delinquents, and prone to various kinds of societal violence. If such individuals are identified, they can be helped to learn other ways of dealing with their children prior to becoming parents. This approach might well prevent that type of destructive and maladaptive behavior from occurring at all.

The Task Panel on Prevention (1978) claims that "primary prevention involves building the strengths, resources, and competence in individuals, families, and communities that can reduce the flow of a variety of unfortunate outcomes—each characterized by enormous human and societal costs" (p. 213). In other words, primary prevention involves providing education and training programs to help the families of severely retarded children and the potential child abusers learn different ways of interacting with their children. When one looks at the "flow of unfortunate outcomes," such as divorce, desertion, delinquency, and depression brought on by these or other problems, one can clearly imagine "the enormous human and societal costs" and thus the need for primary prevention programs.

An additional but critical aspect of primary prevention efforts, according to Cowen (1982), is that they must be group- or mass-oriented. This does not mean that primary prevention programs may not deal with individuals, but rather that the major focus must be on large and/or specific populations. These populations are referred to as target populations, high-risk groups, or the general population. Although these groups may not be demonstrating any disorders, their circumstances, as described earlier, are such that many of them are probably vulnerable or open to such disorders. These groups function, live in the community, and show no signs of disorder.

Secondary Prevention

Secondary prevention can be defined as the early detection and treatment of dysfunction. If, for example, parents noticed that their teenage child was beginning to use alcohol and do poorly in school, and if they sought and obtained help for their child, that would be secondary prevention. In such an instance, the aim would be to help the youngster refrain from using alcohol and to improve in schoolwork, Secondary prevention in medicine is similar. An individual, for example, goes to the doctor with the complaints of headache and slight fever and is diagnosed as having a touch of the flu. The treatment is then focused on eliminating the symptoms and helping the patient get well.

Secondary prevention, according to Goodstein and Calhoun (1982), "involves early diagnosis and treatment of a disorder at a stage when problems may be nipped in the bud" (p. 499). Price et al. (1980) see the goal of secondary prevention somewhat differently as an attempt "to shorten the duration of the disorder by early and prompt treatment" (p. 10). If, for example, a young child of an alcoholic parent began to show signs of withdrawal and the nonalcoholic parent took the youngster for help, this would be considered by many to be secondary prevention. It would include diagnosis and treatment in an attempt to "nip the problem in the bud," or at least to shorten the duration of the problem.

There are those, however, who would claim that this is treatment of an existing disorder. The maladaptive behavior (i.e., withdrawal) has already begun; it has not been prevented or kept from occurring. What, then, if anything, has been prevented? Those who claim that early and prompt treatment is secondary prevention assert that if the intervention or treatment is successful, the signs of withdrawal are reduced or eliminated. In effect, intervention has prevented increased or continued withdrawal and therefore should be considered to be a significant prevention effort. One could argue either way as to whether one should call this example treatment or prevention.

In our view, the very existence of a disorder takes the effort out of the realm of prevention and places it in the category of treatment. Although it is true that prevention efforts could focus on an individual, the major thrust of prevention is toward reaching groups at risk, target populations, or the general population. This may be a technical point, but it does have significance as an obstacle to the development of primary prevention programs. This point is discussed more fully later in the chapter.

Tertiary Prevention

Tertiary prevention is generally defined in terms of efforts to rehabilitate and return to the community those afflicted with severe mental disorders. For example, there are mental patients who suffer from delusions—that is, they believe they are someone else, such as Napoleon, God, or Superman. They even try to behave as such figures, and it is this behavior that keeps them from functioning successfully in society. In many cases, these people are placed in institutions. They remain there until they are able to regain enough of a hold on reality to return to the community. A medical example might be an individual who lost a leg, was fitted with an artificial one, and was taught to walk with the new leg. Tertiary prevention, according to Price et al. (1980), is an attempt "to reduce the severity and disability associated with a particular disorder" (p. 10). Goodstein and Calhoun (1982) describe tertiary prevention in more detail. From their point of view, "tertiary prevention includes efforts to reduce the overall damaging effect of a disorder, to shorten its duration, and to rehabilitate those afflicted for reentry into the community" (p. 499). What seems to come through in both these perceptions is that the focus is on working to overcome a disorder that has developed to the point where it keeps the individual from functioning appropriately or effectively in the community.

If those delusional individuals referred to earlier were treated in an institution and were again able to live and function in the community, this would be considered tertiary prevention by many in the human services. Here again, one might ask what is being prevented. From one point of view, permanent disability or continued institutionalization is the prevention target. Another point of view—one to which we subscribe—states that the tertiary prevention is actually rehabilitation. That is, it restores the individual(s) to better health. It should be noted that most tertiary prevention programs are not focused on a mass of people or on large groups of people but rather on individuals and/or small groups.

WHY AN EMPHASIS ON PRIMARY PREVENTION IS CRUCIAL

What is so important about the idea of primary prevention in the human services? Four major reasons have been put forward to support primary prevention as a top priority. One reason was provided at the very beginning of this chapter: According to the Task Panel on Prevention (1978) and others in the Public Health Service and in private practice, there has never been a major disease or disorder eliminated through treatment alone. If this is so, it becomes clear that treatment and rehabilitation efforts cannot hope to completely eliminate serious disorders. Furthermore, treatment and rehabilitation have been practiced for years, and it is clear that both processes have not been able to stem the growing tide of disorders in our society.

The second reason is that there are not enough human services personnel to treat or rehabilitate all those in need. Although it is true that human services is a rapidly growing field, human services educators recognize that the training of personnel cannot keep up with the increasing numbers of people in need of treatment. This is true in spite of the fact that the primary focus of training has been, and still is, on treatment and rehabilitation. To make things more difficult, the economic policies of the early 1990s have caused a reduction not only in the number of individuals being trained, but also in the number of personnel who are already providing the needed services. This decrease in workers has occurred in spite of an increase in the number of people in need of support and help due to problems of unemployment, people living longer and becoming more dependent, more families breaking up, and increasing child abuse.

Other problems, such as battering of women—the leading cause of injury to women (Faludi, 1991)—suicides, school dropouts, crime, and AIDS, are not getting the attention they need. Further evidence of a shortage of trained workers was provided by the National Academy of Sciences; it was found that of the estimated 7.5 million mentally ill children in 1985, only 2.5 million received treatment and 5 million did not get any type of intervention at all. A recent study by the Institute of Medicine estimated that there are as many as 14 million children who may have mental illness (Gore, 1993). Gore further stated that only one in five receive care. B. L. Bloom (1981) pointed out that in the late 1970s, an estimated 10% of the U. S. population needed help with emotional problems. Almost 4 years ago, we (the authors) indicated that the estimate of those in need of such support was up to 15%. Judd (1990) suggests that 20% of the population will have some mental or emotional problems in their lifetime that will need some support. There is reason to suspect that this figure has increased. According to a survey of junior and senior high school students from the 7th to the 12th grade, over 10.5 million use and abuse alcohol (U. S. Department of Education, 1993). Furthermore, 8 million drink weekly, 6.9 million buy alcohol in stores, 5.4 million have binged at least once, 3 million binged in the last month (of the survey), and 454,000 binge once a week. Binge drinking means having five or more drinks in a row. The survey reports that 8.7 million students say they drink to have fun, 5.5 million say they drink because their friends drink, and 6 million drink to be social (U.S Department of Education, 1993).

This situation reminds one of the story of a man fishing off the bank of a wide and fast-flowing stream. While fishing, he sees a person being swept along with the current. He quickly throws the person a line and pulls him to safety. Before he can do anything more, he spots another person being swept downstream and he pulls them out also. Just as he does this, he sees a few more people struggling in the current. He calls for help as he pulls someone else out of the surging water. Others come to help as still more people are caught in the current. However, it soon becomes impossible to pull everyone out of danger. There are too many victims and not enough helpers. As more and more people float downstream, more and more are lost. It finally dawns on someone to head upstream and try to keep people from falling into the stream in the first place. Many feel that human services workers had best head upstream before they too become less and less effective.

The third reason that primary prevention should be a priority is that society pays a huge cost for disorders that are not prevented. The Task Panel on Prevention (1978), for example, puts its emphasis on the prevention of disorders, each of which is "characterized by enormous human and society costs" (p. 213). According to the Seventh Special Report to the U. S.

Congress on Alcohol and Health, the estimated cost of alcoholism and alcohol abuse was more than $136 billion in 1990 and about $150 billion in 1995 (Secretary of Health and Human Services, 1990). The National Institute of Mental Health (NIMH) estimates that mental illness alone costs our nation over $129 billion a year. Califano (1994) points out that substance abuse costs an additional $200 billion a year (p. 94). He further states that "Congress and Presidents have slashed funds for programs such as childhood immunization, pre-natal care for poor women and early treatment of tuberculosis in order to reduce the immediate year's budget, even though they know such actions will increase costs in future years" (pp. 55–56). The 1995–1996 struggle to try to reach a balanced budget by the year 2002 appears to maintain this practice.

The fourth reason for the promotion of primary prevention is that emotional and behavioral disorders exact an enormous human cost. Human costs have to do with personal pain and suffering. Perhaps the only way to truly realize these costs is for us to try to personalize them. Everyone has had to face, at some time or another, a painful or terrible experience. Some remember the fear of being left behind when parents separated. Some remember the shame of having a "drunkard" in the family. Others who have had a mentally ill person living in the same house can still feel the anxiety, fear, and frustration in that situation. The guilt, shame, and apprehension of having a retarded child still affect many others. The anger and fear of living with a drug addict are still with many. The terror after being abused, mugged, or raped does not leave victims or their loved ones.

How many can recall the gut-wrenching pain and sense of helplessness of watching a loved one suffer and die due to illness? How many remember the rage and bitterness they felt when their disabled child, or they themselves, were made fun of or denied an opportunity to go to school? There is also the feeling of desperation, frustration, and rage known by African Americans, Latinos, or other minority group members when they or their children are abused and denied the opportunity to grow and prosper. The enormous human costs are the tremendous assaults on the emotions and strength of those affected directly and indirectly. Some of the effects radically change the lives of those who, without help, cannot cope successfully with such traumas and too often become alcoholics, abusers, addicts, mentally ill, or develop some other disorder, thus increasing the number of people needing treatment and rehabilitation.

A brief description of what happens when the type of stress just described leads, for example, to alcoholism will bring the issue into sharp focus.

- About 200,000 deaths a year are attributed to the misuse of alcohol (Rice, 1987).
- About 33,000 deaths a year are due to cirrhosis of the liver (Zastrow, 1986).
- Approximately 10,000 murders a year are alcohol related.

- Over 25,000 deaths in automobile accidents are alcohol related.
- A third of all suicides each year are alcohol involved.
- A third of all arrests each year are alcohol related.
- Some experts feel that 65% of child abuse and 80% of wife beating are related to alcohol abuse (Gallagher, 1987).
- It is reported that 10% of all adults are alcoholics and 7% or 8% are alcohol abusers (Kolata, 1987).

The Department of Health and Human Services estimated that 15.1 million adults suffer from alcoholism or alcohol dependence. That is more than 5 times the government estimate of regular cocaine or crack users and more than 30 times the estimated number of heroin addicts (Isikoff, 1990).

Remember, this listing is only a sample of the data on the effects of alcoholism. It does not include data on preteen and teenage alcohol abuse described earlier, death and injuries in the house or workplace, or injuries in auto accidents. Left out are the data on physical and mental illness and disabilities, forcible rape, family disintegration, and many other problems related to alcoholism and alcohol abuse. Still, there is not a significant sustained federal alcohol abuse prevention program in place. A nationwide federal alcohol abuse prevention program might include approaches such as these:

- mandating the listing of health hazards of alcohol on all alcohol containers (the government has mandated a very limited warning regarding the health hazards of alcohol to be placed on all forms of liquor containers)
- mandating the clear presentation of health hazards of alcohol in advertising in the print, television, and radio media
- raising the federal excise tax on alcohol and particularly on beer, the tax on beer being less than 3 cents per 12-oz. container since 1951 (Sessel, 1988)
- enforcing the 21-year-old drinking limit on college campuses, where three-quarters of the students are under the legal drinking age and the massive marketing of alcohol is still continuing (Sessel, 1988)

A 1993 survey discussed by Lipsyte (1995) describes binge drinking at college that includes 18-year-old freshmen. The survey points out that 68% of freshmen will have abused alcohol during their first semester. In discussing the same study, Lipsyte focused on the heavy drinking patterns of athletes, the "role models" on campus. Furthermore, most college presidents have stated that alcohol abuse is the number 1 campus-life problem.

There are many state and local alcohol prevention programs in progress. They include, among others, raising the drinking age to 21, significantly raising the tax on liquor products, limiting the availability of alcohol purchases to specific outlets, strict enforcement of DWI (driving while intoxicated) and similar laws, and initiating education programs in schools and communities.

Primary prevention programs are geared to help people learn how to deal positively and successfully with their problems and stress. If such programs prevent people from developing any of the disorders that have been described, the human cost will have been reduced. We believe that a greater number of prevention programs make possible a greater reduction in human and societal costs.

The acknowledged inability of treatment and rehabilitation programs alone to stem the tide of people in need of human services makes increased primary prevention efforts almost mandatory. A brief look at the two types of strategies used in primary prevention programs will provide a clearer picture of how these programs are developed and how they work.

PRIMARY PREVENTION STRATEGIES

Both active and passive prevention strategies are used in the development of prevention programs (Gilchrist & Schinke, 1985). Passive strategies refer to broad informational-type approaches, such as warnings on cigarette packages or television programs discussing and describing ways to prevent AIDS. Active strategies involve working directly with the target populations in developing skills that enable individuals to deal successfully with pressures and problems that might lead to dysfunction. This is referred to as the life skills model. Such skills include problem solving, making thoughtful and helpful decisions, and recognizing consequences of behavior (Gilchrist & Schinke, 1985). Other skills include identifying behavior options, examining the advantages and disadvantages of the various options, and communication and listening skills (Snow, 1985). The various skills of active strategies are best described by Briar (1985) when he points out that they essentially contain "cognitive and behavioral elements that are aimed not only to help people prevent social and health problems but also to help people promote personal competence and adaptive functioning" (p. 8). A brief look at a sample of primary prevention programs and a listing of major areas in desperate need of primary prevention programs will be helpful at this point.

A SAMPLE OF PRIMARY PREVENTION PROGRAMS

A brief look at different kinds of primary prevention programs will give you a sense of the scope of such efforts and a clear idea of the goals of primary prevention programs. Primary prevention programs have been growing in number since the mid-1970s. Many of them have been short-term, research, experimental, or demonstration programs limited in terms of time and funding. Much of the data derived from these programs indicate positive results in improving individuals' abilities to cope with stress. These data and results can be and have been used to develop additional theories and programs focused on long-term results. There are programs, although too few from the point of view of proponents of primary prevention, that are ongoing. In any case, it should be noted that the final results of these long-term programs are not yet available, for it is impossible to tell whether or not the targeted disorders have been prevented for the entire life span of those in the various programs.

One program aimed at reducing teenage pregnancies by Girls Inc. included 750 girls 12–17 years of age. They were all at high risk of becoming pregnant. The program consisted of a mother-daughter workshop, an assertive training workshop, and educational and career planning workshop, and sessions on sexuality that also provided contraceptive services.

It was reported that the number of pregnancies were reduced by 50% among the girls 15–17 years of age. The number of girls aged 12–14 years who subsequently began having sexual intercourse was also reduced by 50% (Brody, 1991). The results showed that the high-risk characteristics (e.g., being welfare dependent, from a single-parent, female-headed household, living in an urban environment, and having peers and relatives who were pregnant teenagers) were not insurmountable obstacles to a well-planned prevention program. The director of the program pointed out that the cost of the program per year per girl was $116. The director estimated that delaying a single pregnancy until after teenage years could save society $8500 (Brody, 1991); one assumes these savings would be made in a range of welfare benefits.

Tableman, Marceniak, Johnson, and Rodgers (1982) described a pilot program of stress management training involving women on public assistance who were generally isolated and subjected to more than average stress in their lives. None of the women were in crisis, nor did they display maladaptive behaviors that required treatment. The women took part in ten sessions during which they learned skills and methods of reducing stress that helped them change their perceptions of their situations. The program resulted in significant change in the lives of the participants. They were no longer isolated and were able to function more effectively with less stress, thus preventing the kinds of behavioral disorders discussed earlier. The program has been further tested and used with different populations living under stressful conditions.

Another primary prevention program was developed by the Catholic church because of the tremendous increase in the number of divorces. Couples wishing to be married in the church now go through a series of group meetings, led by a member of the clergy, to discuss the responsibilities, joys, and strains of marriage. Childbirth, child-rearing, sex, and other aspects of marriage are among the many topics discussed. The goal is to prevent many of the problems occurring in marriages from becoming serious enough to cause behavioral disorders, family disintegration, and divorce.

The last primary prevention program to be described here centers on promoting mental health in rural areas through informal helping (D'Augelli & Vallance, 1981). Provision of human services in rural areas is more difficult than in urban areas. For example, because of the smaller populations living in rural areas, isolation is usually greater and transportation is not readily available. Many rural residents have close family and community ties, and asking for help from "outsiders" is not looked upon with much favor. Some rural communities have an informal system of helpers. The project under discussion was designed not only to encourage such a system but also to teach members of the community to train those residents who make up this informal system. The focus is to build on the existing strengths of the community by training the local helpers to become more efficient in helping residents deal with personal problems, job loss, sudden illness or injury, and other problems in living. This approach permits local residents to teach other local residents skills in the helping process, and thus they do not have to share problems with or ask for help from outsiders. This method also increases the number of helpers and provides increased sources of support to those who are faced with problems in living before maladaptive behaviors are developed. This particular prevention program is an ongoing one staffed by local volunteers.

We could continue to describe primary prevention programs, but we believe that it will be more enlightening at this point to list just a few areas in which primary prevention programs can make a significant difference. They need no description or further comment.

mental illness
crime
alcoholism
child abuse
teenage pregnancies
rising juvenile crime
violence
battered women
AIDS
increased teenage drug abuse
physical illness
immunization of children
lack of pre- and post-natal care for poor women

Community mental-health centers develop prevention programs as well as provide treatment services. One such center, The Center for Preventive Psychiatry in White Plains, NY, states as its mission " . . . to promote positive mental health attitudes and prevent the onset of mental illness, or reduce its impact, through programs of early identification and treatment, community education, professional training, consultation and research." Unfortunately, there are not sufficient community mental-health centers to provide the needed services that we have described.

OBSTACLES TO THE DEVELOPMENT
OF PRIMARY PREVENTION PROGRAMS

Although there are a growing number of primary prevention programs operating throughout the country, funding for such programs is quite limited in comparison to the funds available for treatment and/or rehabilitation programs. What is frightening is that this is true even in life-and-death situations such as the growing AIDS epidemic. That no one would object to the elimination or significant reduction of the disorders described earlier seems certain. Why, then, the persistent resistance to funding and development of primary prevention programs in the human services field? There seem to be three major categories of obstacles to funding and development: professional, political, and economic. An examination of just a sampling of these obstacles will give you a greater understanding of the problems surrounding the introduction of primary prevention programs. Note that these problems are very closely interrelated.

Professional Issues

Professional issues that create problems regarding the growth of primary prevention programs include the training, practice, philosophy, and ethics of human services workers and human services professions. Very few 2- or 4-year training programs for human services workers discuss, much less focus on, primary prevention theory or skills. Few, if any at all, train workers for careers in the field of primary prevention. Graduate school training is equally limited in terms of primary prevention. For the most part, the training of human services workers is focused on treatment and/or rehabilitation theories and skills. This training leads, naturally, to practice concentrated on treatment and rehabilitation. These services are, in addition, the major services of most agencies in which human services workers are employed.

From a theoretical or philosophical perspective, the fact that primary prevention is not seen the same way by all human services workers creates an additional obstacle to the growth of primary prevention programs. There is no *one* definition of primary prevention acceptable among human services workers. Furthermore, a group of mental-health professionals in a report to the New York State Commission of Mental Health (Prevost, 1982) stated that "the distinctions among primary, secondary, and tertiary prevention do not provide meaningful guidance for the formulation of programs and policies" (p. 3). The group added that the concepts have triggered more arguments than action. For example, when a particular disorder, such as drug abuse, is *treated* successfully, it might be claimed by some that the successful treatment actually *prevented* a potential crime, and thus is really primary prevention. This perception does not include the element of intent, considered to be an essential aspect of primary prevention in mental health

(Cowen, 1980). The intent in the example is to stop the drug abuse and not to stop a crime.

Another issue that causes hesitation and confusion centers around whether primary prevention efforts should concentrate on the causes of disorders or the "trigger" or "spark" that sets off a disorder. To add to the dilemma, the question of whether to approach disorders with a biological, psychological, or sociological emphasis is raised. In a biological approach, disorders are thought to be caused by physical problems such as brain damage, chemical imbalances, pollution, physical disability, or other similar difficulties. In a psychological approach, disorders are thought to be caused by a lack of knowledge or an inability to cope with emotional stress. In a sociological approach, disorders are thought to be caused by institutions or systems that do little to eliminate racism, unemployment, crime, poverty, hunger, poor housing, and similar societal ills.

Ethical questions regarding primary prevention programs also arise from the point of view of some human services workers. Some workers claim that if primary prevention programs were aimed at high-risk groups, unforeseen and unfortunate consequences could occur. High-risk groups, for example, could include children from broken homes or children with alcoholic parents. The children would have to be identified as such, and this could lead to additional problems and violations of privacy. The children would have little or no voice in this matter, yet they might be adversely affected. Another ethical issue raised by some is that if primary prevention programs are aimed at entire communities or populations, what responsibility do providers have to those in the community who feel no need or want no part of the programs?

Another issue, as Califano (1994) describes it, is that "Doctors are not trained or paid to seek or counsel patients about disease prevention or health prevention, and among those that do, instruction comes to only a few hours" (p. 145). Sadly, this is also true in the training of most human service workers.

These and other professional problems cause many to be hesitant and reluctant to expend their resources and efforts on primary prevention to any degree similar to those given for treatment and rehabilitation programs.

Political Issues

Political issues are also obstacles to the development of primary prevention programs. For example, ours is a crisis-oriented society. That is, our society does not usually act or react to problems unless they become great enough to affect and bad enough to frighten large numbers of people. It is at those times that the storm of protest or concern becomes large enough to move legislators and legislatures to attempt to deal with the problem. This is usually done through the rapid passage of legislation and funding. Witness the recent public outcry, programs, legislation, and publicity that have developed around the problem of crime. The unanimity of support for a crackdown on this problem made it comparatively simple for the various jurisdictions to pass legislation and develop programs to deal with the problem.

The more recent outcry regarding the AIDS epidemic is an even clearer example of how a crisis affects the political system. Initially, there was a great deal of resistance to doing much about the issue because AIDS was considered a "gay" or homosexual problem. The political reversal was abrupt and powerful when politicians realized that the epidemic was spreading to the heterosexual community. The lack of a sense of crisis in the view of the public and many human services workers in addition to the lack of unanimity among politicians and professionals regarding the efficacy of primary prevention programs provides little impetus for the political system to press for the development and funding of such programs. Furthermore, how can one justify the use of limited resources to prevent disorders that only *might* occur?

Califano (1994) points out that "As long big bucks are in treatment and the projects are in sick care, that's where members of Congress and influential lobbyists will center their efforts; there are precious few political contributions to be found in health promotion and disease prevention" (p. 245). Unfortunately, here too the same holds true for the human services field.

Economic Obstacles

Economic obstacles to primary prevention efforts pointed out by the Task Panel on Prevention (1978) include limited resources and present funding practices. Limited funding of human services also limits the development of new and uncertain or unproven programs. To take increasingly scarce resources away from treatment and rehabilitation programs and from people who are in immediate need of assistance to fund new and, in the eyes of many, questionable primary prevention programs is not acceptable to many in the human service field. According to Califano (1994), "Perhaps the biggest deterrent to health promotion and disease prevention efforts is the fact that the big bucks are in promoting unhealthy habits and treating poor health" (p. 145). He points out that prevention costs money up front and saves money later, which is an obstacle that lawmakers seem unable to overcome. Once again, these factors hold true in the human services field as well as in the medical professions. Furthermore, the cost of primary prevention programs serving large populations is very high, even though the cost per person is much less than the cost of treatment and rehabilitation of one person. In addition, most hospitals and other human services institutions are not prepared or geared for primary prevention programs, but are certainly dependent on the income derived from their treatment and rehabilitation services. Primary prevention programs might well affect that income adversely. The same threat to income faces those human services workers in private practice. Recipients of third-party payments through their clients' medical insurance could also be affected financially.

CONCLUSION

We believe that these and other obstacles to primary prevention can be overcome. Our strong bias in favor of primary prevention programs has been made obvious purposefully. We just do not believe that the human services profession needs to, or can afford to, stand still regarding the development of primary prevention programs until critics are satisfied and all questions are answered. We do believe that there has been sufficient research to warrant significant increases in funding of primary prevention programs and continued research in this area. The old cliché "an ounce of prevention is worth a pound of cure" is particularly appropriate here. From an economic, social, professional, and moral perspective, it is clear to us that the human services must become more than a "repair shop" for individuals and society.

We are heartened by the increasing awareness that human services educators and professional have of the vital importance of prevention. This is evidenced by the inclusion of prevention courses in schools of social work and by programs of preventive psychology. In the field of psychology, there now are programs to train psychologists in prevention practices (Price, 1983). Primary prevention programs are essential in the fight against dysfunctions, disorders, and disabilities.

ADDITIONAL READING

Addams, J. (1969). *A centennial reader.* New York: Macmillan.

Anletta, K. (1982). *The underclass.* New York: Random House.

Aronowitz, E. (Ed.). (1982). *Prevention strategies for mental health.* New York: Prodist.

McConville, B. J. (1982, December). Secondary prevention in child psychiatry: An overview with ideas for action. *Canada's Mental Health, 30*(4), 4–7.

Plant, T. F. A. (1980). Prevention policy: The federal perspective. In R. H. Price, F. Ketterer, B. C. Bader, & J. Monahan (Eds.), *Prevention in mental health: Research, policy, and practice* (Vol. 1). Newbury Park, CA: Sage.

Porter, R. A., Peters, J. A., & Headry, H. R. (1982, July). Using community development for prevention in Appalachia. *Social Work, 27,* 302–307.

Swift, M., & Weirich, T. (1987). Prevention planning as social and organizational change. In J. Hermalin & J. A. Morell (Eds.), *Prevention planning in mental health. Sage Studies in Community Mental Health* (Vol. 9). Newbury Park, CA: Sage.

Walsh, J. A. (1982, July). Prevention in mental health: Organizational and ideological perspectives. *Social Work, 27,* 298–301.

REFERENCES

Alexander, F. G., & Selesnick, S T. (1966). *The history of psychiatry: An evaluation of psychiatric practice from prehistoric time to the present.* New York: Harper & Row.

Bloom, B. L. (1981, December). The logic and urgency of primary prevention. *Hospital and Community Psychiatry, 23,* 839–843.

Bloom, M. (1981). *Primary prevention: The possible science.* Englewood Cliffs, NJ: Prentice Hall.

Briar, S. (1985). Foreword. In L. D. Gilchrist & S. P. Schinke (Eds.), *Preventing social and health problems through life skills training.* Seattle: University of Washington School of Social Work.

Brody, J. E. (1991, October 8). Helping teen-agers avoid pregnancy. *The New York Times,* p. A14.

Califano, J. A. (1994). *Radical surgery: What's next for american health care.* New York: Times/Random House.

Catalano, R. (1979). *Health, behavior and the community. An ecological perspective.* New York: Pergamon Press.

Committee of the National Academy of Sciences. (1989, June 18). Most mentally ill children don't get help, report says. *St. Louis Dispatch,* p. 12A.

Cowen, E. L. (1980). The wooing of primary prevention. *American Journal of Community Psychology, 8,* 258–284.

Cowen, E. L. (1982, Spring). Primary prevention research: Barriers, needs and opportunities. *Journal of Primary Prevention,* 131–137.

Dain, N. (1980). *Clifford W. Beers: Advocate for the insane.* Pittsburgh, PA: University of Pittsburgh Press.

D'Augelli, A. R., & Vallance, T. R. (1981). The helping community: Promoting mental health in rural areas through informal helping. *Journal of Rural Community Psychology.*

Faludi, S. (1991, September/October). Blame it on feminism: What's wrong with women today? Too much equality. *Mother Jones,* pp. 24–29.

Gallagher, B. J. (1987). *The sociology of mental illness* (2nd ed.). Englewood Cliffs, NJ: Prentice Hall.

Gilchrist, L. D., & Schinke, S. P. (1985). Prevention of social and health problems. In L. D. Gilchrist & S. P. Schinke (Eds.), *Preventing social and health problems through life skills training.* Seattle: University of Washington School of Social Work.

Goodstein, L. D., & Calhoun, J. F. (1982). *Understanding abnormal behavior: Description, explanation, management.* Reading, MA: Addison-Wesley.

Gore, T. (1993). Children and mental illness. Reprinted from the National Forum: The Phi Kappa Phi Journal Vol. Lxx111 No.1. in the Social Issues Resources Series on Mental Health Vol. 4 Article No. 81.

Heller, K., Price, R. H., Reinharz, S., Riger, S., Wandersman, A., & D'Aunno, T. A. (1984). *Psychology and community change: Challenges of the future* (2nd ed.). Pacific Grove, CA: Brooks/Cole.

Isikoff, J. (1990, April 8–15). The nation's alcohol problem is falling through the crack: Some officials question the government's priorities. *Washington Post National Weekly Edition,* pp. 30–31.

Johnston, J. E. (1980, September). *The role of the state mental health authority in prevention* (Mental Health Policy Monograph Series No. 6). Nashville, TN: Vanderbilt Institute for Public Policy Studies, Center for the Study of Families and Children.

Judd, L. L. (1990, February). Putting mental health on the nation's agenda. *Hospital and Community Psychiatry, 41.*

Kolata, G. (1987, December 13). Alcoholism: The judgment of science is pending. *The New York Times,* p. 26E.

Lipsyte, R. (1995, November 26). The college sport of getting smashed. *The New York Times,* Sport Section, p. 7.

New York State Family Development Training and Credentialing Program (FDC). (1995). "Some questions and answers" [Brochure].

Prevost, J. A. (1982, March). *Policy framework for preventive services.* New York: New York State Office of Mental Health.

Price, R. H. (1983). The education of a preventive psychologist. In R. D. Felner, L. A. Jason, J. N. Moritsugu, & S. S. Farber (Eds.), *Preventive psychology: Theory, research and practice.* New York: Pergamon Press.

Price, R. H., Bader, B. C., & Ketterer, R. F. (1980). Prevention in community mental health—The state of the art. In R. H. Price, F. Ketterer, B. C. Bader, & J. Monahan (Eds.), *Prevention in mental health: Research, policy, and practice* (Vol. 1). Newbury Park, CA: Sage.

Rice, P. L. (1987). *Stress and health: Principles and practice for coping and wellness.* Pacific Grove, CA: Brooks/Cole.

Secretary of Health and Human Services. (1990). *Seventh special report to the U. S. Congress on alcohol and health.* Rockville, MD: U. S. Department of Health and Human Services.

Sessel, T. V. (1988, January 1). Two ways to reduce underage drinking. *The New York Times,* p. 30.

Snow, W. H. (1985). Skills training for coping with life changes. In L. D. Gilchrist & S. P. Schinke (Eds.), *Preventing social and health problems through life skills training.* Seattle: University of Washington School of Social Work.

Tableman, B., Marceniak, D., Johnson, D., & Rodgers, R. (1982). Stress management training for women on public assistance. *American Journal of Community Psychology, 10,* 357–367.

Task Panel on Prevention. (1978). *Report.* Washington, DC: President's Commission on Mental Health.

U. S. Department of Education. (1993). Drinking habits, access, attitudes, and knowledge: A national survey. Reprinted from Youth and Alcohol. In *Social Issues Resource Series on Alcohol,* Vol. 5, Article 21.

Warning sought on liquor bottles. (1987, December 27). *The New York Times,* p. 25.

Zastrow, C. (1986). *Introduction to social welfare institutions: Social problems, services, and current issues* (3rd ed.). Belmont, CA: Wadsworth.

Current Controversies
and Issues

INTRODUCTION

You may have gathered by now that the human services field is quite complex. Complete agreement regarding philosophies, methods, goals, services, funding, or anything else just does not exist nor, from our point of view, should it. There are times when controversies and differences are stimulating, healthy, valid, and lead to creative solutions. At other times, they are repetitious, meaningless, and destructive. Too frequently they consume time, energy, and resources that might better be used providing needed services. To this end, we highly recommend that students become familiar with the books in the Opposing Viewpoints series, published by the Greenhaven Press, that deal with issues of concern to human services workers.

The purpose of this chapter is to present a sampling of basic controversies and issues in the field of human services that have not yet been resolved and may never be resolved to everyone's satisfaction. The questions raised in this chapter influence all human services workers. Some issues affect the human services worker more directly than others, but they all impact on the worker and the services provided. Prior knowledge of these and other controversies helps workers know what they might expect from colleagues, politicians, consumers of human services, and the general public. This knowledge can be instrumental in helping the worker provide more effective services.

We do not attempt to resolve these issues here. Our views are often implied by the way we present issues. Furthermore, we do not expect you to come to any specific conclusions or agree with any particular point of view. Whereas issues change, conditions change, and people change, many old issues reemerge that give the appearance of new issues. These so-called new issues have in all probability been with us in one way or another, to one degree or another, for as long as the human services profession has existed. Some examples are discussed in this chapter. The idea is to examine them and understand their significance to human services workers and to the provision of human services, for they very frequently raise questions regarding one's personal and professional values and ethics.

THE CLASH OF VALUES IN SOCIAL POLICIES

At the outset, it is worth repeating that complete agreement about social policies in the human services rarely occurs. Social policies are supposedly based on morals and values; however, there is no consensus about what is morally right. Jansson (1988) identifies five moral issues involved with social welfare policies. In discussing them, it will become quite clear that they are all closely related and overlap each other in many ways. Following are the issues and some of the questions they raise.

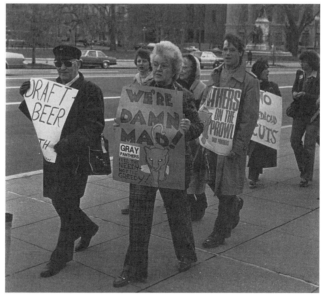

One of the many nonprofessional groups that affects social policy through its representatives and by testifying before legislative bodies

1. Morality of Social Services . . . Who shall receive services and on what terms? (p. 5)

Questions: Shall services be given to only those who are unable to work? What about (a) those who cannot find work or (b) those who cannot earn enough to stay above the poverty line? Should those who receive benefits be required to work in the community? Should those on welfare not receive increased benefits for additional children?

2. Nature of Social Obligations . . . For what needs and problems is society responsible and which shall receive priority? (p. 5)

Questions: Are we our brothers' keepers? Is society responsible for providing for all who cannot care for themselves? Should society provide for only food, shelter, clothing, and medical care? What about education, cultural enrichment, and economic needs?

3. Preferred Interventions . . . What kind of policy remedies should be chosen to address specific social problems? (p. 5)

Questions: Should drug abusers be jailed, or should drugs be legalized? Should society emphasize treatment and prevention of drug abuse, or should the focus primarily be on keeping drugs from entering the country and on enforcement of antidrug laws? Should society prohibit abortions or continue to allow them, and on what terms? Should there be gun control, and on what terms? Should society force the homeless into shelters or hospitals, or jail them if they refuse to go to either?

4. Compensatory Strategies . . . Should society give preferential assistance or treatment to members of specific groups that lag behind the rest of the population in economic and other conditions? (p. 5)

Questions: Does not society do this through welfare, affirmative action, and other programs? The real question is, To what extent and when does society provide assistance and treatment? Should society guarantee basic health care for those who cannot afford such care? Should affirmative action programs, which seek to guarantee jobs, education placements, and contract work to members of minorities, take precedence over equal opportunity programs? Should this involve quotas?

5. Magnitude of Federal Policy Roles . . . What policy powers should federal authorities possess, and what should be the magnitude of federal social spending? (p. 5)

Questions: Is the federal government too large? Are state and local governments better able to know and understand the needs of their people? Should the federal government step in to meet the needs of its citizens if state and local governments cannot? Does the federal government, through its policies and funding power, wield too much influence on state and local policies and practices? Should federal social spending be limited to maintaining a balanced budget or until additional taxes are needed?

The various interest groups continue to disagree in their answers to these and many other questions. A brief look, however, at just two specific issues dealing with welfare, life, and death will further exemplify the problem.

Welfare.   The proposals being considered by states to deny benefits to single mothers on welfare who then have additional children raise many moral issues. Conservatives feel that such benefits reward welfare mothers for having more children and so provide an incentive for them to become welfare dependent. They believe that it is basically irresponsible to bring children into the world if one cannot adequately provide for them. Should society support this perceived irresponsible behavior? Liberals argue that society has an obligation to take care of those in need and that children should not be punished for the behavior of their parents. They also question the assertion that denial of benefits for additional children is an effective way to help the mothers become more independent. They question whether the proposed cuts would really discourage these women from having additional children. Could not society find better ways of helping welfare mothers to become independent of the welfare system? Better yet, cannot society find a way to end poverty?

Euthanasia.   The issue of **euthanasia** was revived suddenly and sharply when a doctor recently helped a woman suffering with Alzheimer's disease commit suicide. The doctor was charged with murder, but the case was dismissed because there was no state law that prohibited assisted suicides.

The same doctor, through the use of devices he developed, assisted two other women to commit suicide ("2 Doctor-Assisted Suicides," 1991). In both instances, the doctor provided the means and the women committed the act. There was no doubt that the women wanted to die; however, several disturbing ethical questions remain. Should assisted suicides be allowed? If so, other questions need answering. Who is to assist, and under what circumstances? Should these decisions be made by the patient, family, doctor, community, all, or a combination of some of the above? What criteria should be used to justify active (assisted) or even passive (unassisted) euthanasia? Should the criteria be age, finances, quality of life, life expectancy, health, or any other condition? Should euthanasia be legalized (Bernards, 1989)? The Hemlock Society, a group that supports suicide and assisted suicide for the dying, strongly endorses the right to die and the legalization of euthanasia (Humphry, 1991).

Let us take a closer look at how the clash of values creates problems that directly affect human service workers, consumers, and people in general. In presidential campaigns and budget or legislative battles, past and present, one constantly heard contestants speak of American values or what is right. Are the American values of conservatives more valid than those of liberals? Who decides what values are American values? Do liberals know more about what is right than do conservatives? What about individuals, schools, churches and synagogues, or any other institutional perceptions of American values or of what is right or moral? How does one resolve these questions, for it is their attempted resolution that allows us to struggle somewhat successfully as a democratic society? Some issues that highlight this struggle, which were touched upon in previous chapters, follow.

For example, is it an American value or morally right both to perpetuate corporate welfare and significantly cut welfare to the poor? Some claim that each is an American value and morally right because it helps the poor get off welfare and helps the economy and effort to balance the budget in 2002. Others claim that corporate welfare should be cut because it is too costly and helps corporations and businesses rather than the individuals in need. Is it an American value or morally right to maintain a minimum wage that does not provide enough income to raise individuals and families above the poverty level? Some claim that to raise the minimum wage any higher will create inflation and cause the loss of jobs; therefore, it is better not to increase it. What about the shutdown of the government by Congress not appropriating funds unless its demands in a budget battle were met. Keeping government workers from working, who have no control or play no part in budget issues, is seen by many as not morally right or not an expression of American values. Others feel that such pressure is correct because it is for the good of the country. Completing the exercise on Ranking American Values at the end of this chapter might help clarify the many differences and issues regarding the use and frequent overuse, most often by political candidates and their supporters, of the concept of American values.

Aside from these being significant moral issues and sources of controversy in our society, they are perfect examples of how social policies are influenced through the interpretation of policies and laws (discussed in Chapter 7).

GOVERNMENT:
HOW MUCH SUPPORT FOR THE NEEDY?

In recent years, the annual struggle over the federal budget has highlighted a major controversy affecting human services workers and programs. The Reagan and Bush administrations and Congress have significantly reduced funding for some programs that provide a safety net to help the truly needy. Even in the 1960s, at the height of President Johnson's Great Society when the Democrats were in the majority in both houses, there was tremendous pressure to reduce domestic spending (Califano, 1994). The pressure was focused primarily on programs serving those in need. According to many liberals, there seems to be a pattern of primarily reducing domestic spending for the needy over defense or other needs whenever there is pressure to reduce spending. One needs only to look at the proposed and actual cuts in budgets over the years to see how direct and indirect support for those most in need are targeted for reduced aid.

The proposed cuts and reduced rate in spending for social programs starting in 1995 in an effort to achieve a balanced budget in 2002 have not been finalized as of yet. That there will be reductions in the rate of domestic spending is a certainty; however, what specifically will be cut and by how much are examples of a clash of values between conservatives and liberals. The question raised in the title of this section (i.e., how much support for the needy?) provokes further discord regarding values and morality. One might say that there is never enough support as long as over 35 million people live in poverty, over 37 million have no health insurance, and so on. Other conservatives and liberals point out that we cannot afford to help everyone. Although there is agreement in this regard, there is little agreement in how much we can afford, who should be helped, and by what means. We do know, however, that too many need health care, jobs, nutrition, shelter, vaccines, treatment for mental illness, and welfare, among many other needs.

The proposed changes in budgets of social programs raise key questions regarding the role of government in providing services. Who has the major and/or ultimate responsibility for the welfare of those in need? Is it the local, state, or federal government? Does government have responsibility for the welfare of only those who are poor? These and other questions will always be raised as long as there are people in need, funds are limited, and those in power make decisions that reflect their values and philosophies. A look at some of those who seek support and the issues they face will help identify the problems one must deal with as a human services worker.

TARGET POPULATIONS: THE STRUGGLE FOR SUPPORT

The struggle for support takes place on two major fronts. One is the struggle to gain the moral support of the public, the media, and professionals. That generally involves convincing others that your goals are just and good. The second front, closely related to the first, is the struggle to gain financial support.

Throughout the late 1980s and early 1990s, three populations have frequently made the headlines: welfare recipients, AIDS victims, and the homeless. The reason they are so often in the news is that we as a society are desperately trying to provide additional and more effective programs to help and to cope with these people. One major problem in trying to develop more successful programs for these groups is how they are perceived by others. Much of the public, much of the media, and many politicians, legislators, officials, and yes, human services workers have a negative attitude toward these people (Dye, 1987; Marin, 1987). Although many others have very positive attitudes and do whatever they can to help these groups, effective programs are difficult to develop without significant public, media, and professional support. A second major problem that makes the development of more successful programs very difficult is the diversity of values and points of view regarding the most effective ways of dealing with these groups. These two factors lead to the third problem, namely that of funding programs for these and other needy populations. The variety of possible solutions given by the professionals involved with developing programs, as well as those offered by the public and the media, reflect the different and often conflicting philosophies and values that create problems in shaping effective policies and programs. The first group to be considered here will be victims of AIDS.

The AIDS Epidemic.   The question of priorities in the funding of treatment and research programs of various social and medical problems has become quite controversial. Because there is a limited amount of funds provided for these programs, if funds are increased for one program, they must be reduced in another program. Such a conflict over delegation of funds has now become quite heated in the fight against AIDS. The now powerful AIDS lobby has been fighting for and demanding significant increases in funding for treatment and research for their constituents. However, there is significant controversy about the level of funding that should be supplied for various diseases. According to Califano (1994), the federal government reported that under 800,000 deaths were due to heart disease and over 500,000 were due to cancer in 1993, but 25,000 people died of AIDS.

Over the years, funding of approximately $1–1.5 billion or more was provided for the fight against each of these diseases. In spite of difference in the number of fatalities, which has been fairly consistent in recent years, Edmondson (1990) urged that the fight against AIDS should be funded at a much higher level than before for two reasons. First, two-thirds of those who die of cancer are over 65 years of age, and over half of those who die of heart disease are over 75 years of age. By comparison, most people who die of AIDS are under 40 years of age. Therefore, the lives of AIDS patients were cut short often before their real contributions to society could be made. Those who died at later ages had made their contribution and had lived fuller lives. The second reason given by Edmondson for increased funding for the fight against AIDS was that AIDS is infectious. What would you decide if it were in your power and you had to make such a decision?

There are two additional controversial practices regarding the AIDS issue, both aimed at reducing the spread of the virus: (a) exchanging dirty needles for clean ones for drug users and (b) distributing condoms to high school students. There was no guarantee, according to the critics, that the exchanged needles would not be shared among users. The feeling was that such a program also encouraged drug use. Meanwhile, the New Haven program of exchange, authorized by the Connecticut state legislature, provided evidence that such programs could be successful.

The distribution of condoms in high schools under specific conditions has been approved in Philadelphia, San Francisco, Los Angeles, and New York City, among other jurisdictions. The approval in each case was not attained without controversy and struggle. In New York City, for example, it was approved only after a long—and still continuing—struggle against the program by many parents, religious organizations, and others. Opponents of the program claim that none of the demonstration programs were actually proven effective, and there was no guarantee that the condoms provided would actually be used. Such programs, it was felt, encouraged young people to engage in sexual intercourse.

What can one do to help prevent the spread of AIDS?

+ Isolate victims from the uninfected population?
+ Prohibit children infected with the AIDS virus from attending regular school or day care centers?
+ Distribute free hypodermic needles to drug addicts to prevent the sharing of needles and thus the spread of the virus?
+ Teach contraceptive methods in elementary and secondary schools as a form of prevention of the spread of AIDS?
+ Mandate testing for the virus and specify who shall be tested?
+ Make the names of those who test positive available to the public?

The Homeless.   When one looks at the problems of the homeless, one finds many different attitudes and approaches to solving the problem. A conservative candidate in the 1992 presidential race recommended that the homeless be forcibly taken to shelters or jailed if they resisted and tried to sleep on the streets. Other candidates did not appear to feel that homelessness was an election-year issue, even though the problem seemed to be increasing (Holmes, 1991). Advocates for the homeless, however, strongly urge an increase in low-income subsidized housing. Others believe that deinstitutionalization is a major cause of homelessness and that mental patients make up the majority of the homeless. In some jurisdictions, the mentally ill become a political football. If, for example, most of the homeless are considered mentally ill, they become a state problem; if they are not, they are a local problem. Kozol (1988) and Johnson (1990) both made the point that poverty, not mental illness, is the major cause of homelessness, even though there are some homeless people who do need psychological treatment. Income and subsidized housing, they believe would resolve the issue.

For the homeless, should we and can we:

- Allow them to sleep in public places and on the streets?
- Allow them to use and sleep in abandoned buildings?
- Allow them in any business or residential neighborhood they choose?
- Allow them to forage in garbage for food or anything else of value to them?
- Force them off the streets and into shelters or hospitals against their will?
- Provide subsidized housing?

Welfare Recipients. The third group, welfare recipients, is also of major concern to society. Many taxpayers resent having to pay taxes to support welfare recipients who are all too frequently stigmatized and stereotyped as being lazy, cheats, and welfare dependent. However, few of these very same taxpayers and others realize how many people receive benefits from government in one way or another (Abramovitz, 1983). For example, tobacco, sugar, and dairy farmers, among others, are paid billions of tax dollars each year to limit production and to maintain price levels that assure profits. Are they the truly needy? What about all those who are able to take deductions on income taxes for health costs, interest on mortgages, entertainment for business, and other items? Although the government does not actually pay cash to these more affluent people, it is, in effect, telling them that they can keep the money they would have to pay were the deductions not allowed. These deductions total billions each year. Actually, it turns out that the more money one makes, the more benefits one may get through increased deductions (Abramovitz, 1991). What about community- and state-college students who obtain federal and state aid? Tax monies are supporting them in obtaining an education even if they are paying the full tuition. Do they and all the others mentioned really see themselves as "welfare recipients"? Clearly, we taxpayers have less problem with government aid dispensed to "us" rather than to "them," especially when the "others" are poor and in need of food, clothing, and shelter. The question really is: Why are these benefits acceptable and those for the truly needy less so?

For welfare recipients, should we and can we:

- Mandate that they take whatever jobs are available, including dead-end jobs?
- Mandate that they take jobs even if the wages would be less than their welfare benefits?

- Mandate that they take part in job-training programs?
- Mandate that all students in community and state colleges (they are all subsidized by state and local tax monies) pay the actual cost of their education?
- Mandate that they accept community work, if jobs are not available, in exchange for some of their benefits?
- Reduce additional benefits for additional children?

The many questions raised with each group are controversial enough in their own right. Additional questions arise that may be of particular concern to human services workers. One question has to do with the problem of individual rights versus rights of the public. Another question has to do with the apparent effort to control these target populations in some fashion. Are we not really attempting to devise behavioral and social controls for people who for the most part are victims of situations beyond their control, and who for the most part have not broken any laws? Other controversies in the human services center around the effects of a conservative government and/or a recession on social programs. The basic question is: Whose benefits shall be cut?

Regardless of who has control of the purse strings, be they liberals or conservatives, there will always be a limited amount of funds made available for social programs. This is clearly a political decision. The general trend has been that in times of prosperity and/or when liberals are in power, social programs are funded more generously. When conservatives are in power, support for social programs is usually significantly reduced. The major questions then become: Which programs shall be reduced or eliminated? Shall it be programs serving the elderly, or school lunch programs, or programs for people with disabilities? What about programs for the homeless, the mentally ill and retarded, or for the poor? Who shall make the decisions? What criteria would you use in making these choices? These kinds of questions and their answers create all kinds of tensions in the human services field. Peirce (1982) perhaps answered some of these questions when discussing budget cuts made by the local, state, and federal government. He pointed out that "the stark fact is that the budget cuts it makes are far deeper in subsidized housing, in job training, in welfare and education programs of primary benefit to poor people than to programs the middle class utilizes most—social security, Medicare, civil service, and military pension levels" (p. 14).

Wright (1991) describes how, in spite of increased domestic violence and need for services and shelters, the cuts in the 1991 New York State budget would end 70 programs. The state Department of Social Services reported that more than 12,000 women and children were turned away from shelters in 1990. A further example of how cuts in budgets affect human services is described by Hinds (1990). He tells of the problems states encounter in trying to carry out the recent changes in the federal welfare laws because of their tight budgets. The law mandates that the states must partially support child care and medical benefits to welfare clients who obtain jobs outside the home. Some states claim that, in order to do so, they would have to take the funds from other programs that serve the working poor who are getting child care benefits. With proposed changes in welfare funding and programs, the problems of the states regarding federal regulations might be ameliorated.

Although it is generally acknowledged that all of the groups receiving support have a legitimate claim to that support, it becomes clear that some programs will lose funding. Several things happen in situations like this. First, the agencies serving the different target populations, and the members of those populations, start competing strenuously with one another for available funds. The most articulate and organized of the various target populations, the ones with the most political influence, generally are more successful in gaining support and funds. As an example, the outcry some time ago by the recipients of social security about the threat of reduced benefits tempered efforts in benefit reduction.

When funds are cut and staff reductions occur, caseloads tend to increase. This then requires a screening process that assures that those in most need get service, while others are turned away. According to a report in the *NASW News* ("Child Abuse," 1983), child welfare agencies turned away clients that could have used prevention programs in child abuse so that active child abuse cases could be served. Without the prevention program, additional child abuse cases may occur. The increased caseload puts additional pressure on the workers, and services to the needy often suffer. Competition and struggle for existence shift the focus, energies, and resources away from a unified effort by target populations and the human services field to increase overall funding for social programs. This kind of competition seems to demand that the strong shall survive and the weak shall perish.

PROFESSIONALISM IN THE HUMAN SERVICES

Two major and muted struggles have developed among human services workers in the last two decades. Both struggles involve money, status, and levels of responsibility. One conflict occurs between generalist human services workers and traditional professional human services workers. The other conflict occurs among traditional professional human services workers. Fortunately, these quarrels have not had significant ill effects on the direct services provided by the human services workers themselves. It is nonetheless important to know and understand the different points of view of the various contestants, as well as to recognize that all is not sweetness and light in the helping professions. A brief description of the issues follows.

Since the introduction of indigenous community leaders as paraprofessionals in the war on poverty of the 1960s, the number of workers in the human services has grown steadily and rapidly. In addition, the responsibilities, knowledge, training, and competence of generalist human services workers have, from their point of view, increased to a level comparable to that of traditional professional human services workers. Furthermore, large numbers of generalist human services workers and some traditional professional human services workers believe strongly that many generalists outperform traditional professional workers. A trainer of generalist human services workers cited by Sobey (1970) stated that such workers are often superior to traditional professionals. These convictions on the part of generalist human services workers are the basis for strong feelings about the differences in pay, status, responsibilities, and opportunities for advancement between generalists and traditional professional human services workers. "Aides are expressing growing resentment at what they perceive as a system of double standards—one for them, the other for credentialed professionals," stated Birnbach (1981, p. 553).

Many educators believe that graduates of recognized undergraduate human services programs should be considered professionals. Generalist human services workers assert that, although they do not have graduate degrees, the combination of their life experiences and limited formal education are "credentials" equal to those obtained through advanced formal education.

Many human services educators are convinced that human services is a profession (Clubok, 1984) and that graduates of recognized college human services programs should be considered professionals. In addition, there are some who feel that human services is an evolving profession (Feringer & Jacobs, 1987). These and other human services educators assert that most criteria needed for the establishment of the traditional human services professions have been met in regard to the human services. These criteria include, among others: a professional membership organization, regional and nationwide annual professional conferences, journals, standards for approval of college human services curricula, and an organization to approve college programs (e.g., Council for Standards in Human Services Education). Furthermore, according to other human services workers and educators, the growth of graduate degree programs in human services is further proof of professionalism in the human services. On the other hand, human services workers with advanced degrees feel that their advanced intensive training provides them with greater knowledge and skill in providing specific services and enables them to function at a significantly higher level than can generalist human services workers. Professionalism, they assert, is based on the attainment of a specific body of knowledge unique to that field and gained only through traditional professional schools. Much of the knowledge and skills referred to by traditional professionals deals with clinical functions in addition to supervisory and educational responsibilities directly related to their specific profession. These professions might include psychology, occupational therapy, social work, and others described in Chapter 6.

In addition, these professionals feel strongly that until college human services programs are accredited by an organization sanctioned by the Council on Post Secondary Accreditation the human services is not yet a profession. The Council is the only organization sanctioned by the U. S. Department of Education to allow specific groups to provide recognized accreditation. It is also felt by these people that until the human services is recognized and incorporated into the Civil Service Systems as a profession it is not to be considered a profession. The struggle goes on, and you will be faced with this issue in one way or another, to one degree or another, as a human services worker.

Generalist human services workers' efforts to gain recognition and parity with traditional professionals are duplicated among the traditional professionals themselves. The issue centers around which traditional professionals shall be eligible for third-party payment without the need of being supervised by those with higher standing or credentials. **Third-party payment** is payment to the traditional professional by an insurance company, such as Blue Cross or by Medicare, for services provided to the client. Third-party payment permits many more individuals to obtain help that they previously could not afford. Third-party payment also significantly increases the amount of income for agencies and traditional professionals who provide services to the needy.

Who, then, among the traditional professionals, is eligible to receive these third-party payments? Most traditional human services professionals, particularly those in private practice, are eager to be included in these programs. Medical doctors and psychiatrists are included in all such programs. In some jurisdictions, psychologists are included and in others they are not. Social workers and other traditional human services professionals are also not included everywhere. In certain situations, some traditional professionals are included in these programs only if they are supervised by a traditional professional of another discipline. For example, a psychiatrist might supervise a psychologist or social worker. It goes without saying that professionals in one discipline object strenuously to being supervised by those in other disciplines. Competition for jobs has increased in recent years as a result of the growing number of professionals and cuts in programs and services. In 1990, for example, there were approximately 36,000 psychiatrists, 42,000 clinical psychologists, 80,000 clinical social workers, and 40,000 marriage and family counselors. It is obvious that large sums of money are at stake and that status and recognition by the public and the government regarding the competence of various professions are involved (Turkington, 1984). Unfortunately, little if any positive changes have occurred regarding these professional issues to date.

Acceptance into these insurance programs is achieved for the most part through legislative action at local, state, or national levels. Therefore, the professional organizations representing the different disciplines lobby to have their members included in these programs. Professional groups already included in the plans often oppose the inclusion of new groups, claiming that they are only trying to protect the public. Some think that there is enough to go around for everyone and that the constant competition for high status, recognition, and control does little for the image and dignity of human services workers.

Another professional issue that is being raised among many social workers involves whom social workers serve. Specht and Courtney (1994) stated the issue clearly:

> Today, a significant proportion of social workers are practicing psychotherapy, and doing so privately, with a primarily middle-class, professional, Caucasian clientele in the 20 to 40 year age group. The poor have not gone away; there are more of them now than at any time in recent memory . . . Certainly many professional social workers are still committed to the public social services, to helping poor people, and dealing with social problems . . . but a large part of the profession is "adrift in the psychiatric seas." (p. x)

They further claim that it is the former kinds of students and practitioners "that the profession needs if it is to realize its original mission" (p. x). There is little doubt from our point of view that such human services workers are in desperate need. Huff and Johnson (1993) support this view when they write:

> Since its birth, social work has been in the vanguard of many national reforms, often speaking on behalf of populations who are too beleaguered to forcefully represent themselves. Of late, too many social workers have abandoned the traditional mission as advocates for social justice . . . Social workers must rededicate themselves to leading a new reform movement dedicated to a more equitable redistribution of America's wealth. (p. 315)

We feel the same might be said regarding many other human services workers.

DEINSTITUTIONALIZATION: DOES IT WORK?

Deinstitutionalization, or decarceration, is the practice of releasing individuals who were inmates in institutions such as mental hospitals and prisons. The hope is that they will be released into a community with facilities and resources to help them live independently and/or to family or friends who will help them so that they will not need to be institutionalized again. The claims of those in favor of the deinstitutionalization policy are that (a) treatment and rehabilitation are more successfully achieved in the community; (b) it is more humane to treat people in the community in which they live; (c) because of overcrowding, grossly inadequate facilities, and inadequate numbers of personnel, prisons and mental hospitals in effect constitute cruel and inhumane punishment; and (d) it is less costly to provide the necessary services outside the institutions and in the community. Some believe that it is this last factor—less cost—that provided the main impetus for these programs (Mechanic, 1980). Regardless of motives, who can really argue with the concept of deinstitutionalization? The idea certainly sounded sensible and was hailed as the start of a new revolution in the human services.

What is the state of deinstitutionalization today? It is clear that too few communities in which released mental patients live have adequate facilities or resources for proper treatment or rehabilitation. Several years ago, the deaths of former mental patients in a rooming house fire triggered an investigation of the facilities and procedures for discharging mental patients. It was discovered that the residential facility was not the safest, but that a shortage of decent housing made moving difficult. The investigation also pointed out that the outpatient center was not given sufficient notice of patient discharges and that important information about the patients was not used. Lack of care leaves the released patient in limbo. Having little or no support in the community, the patient often reverts back to the kind of behavior that caused him or her to be institutionalized in the first place. In many instances, those individuals are refused readmission to the hospital and are found on the streets or in facilities not geared to help them.

Regardless of why communities do not have adequate resources or provide the necessary services—be it a lack of funds (the reason given by most human services workers) or "we don't want them in our neighborhood" (the reason given by most of the public)—it is clear that the results of releasing patients into the community have not met the expectations of the supporters of the program. Most of the released individuals are not only being denied treatment in one way or another, they are also often abused physically and emotionally and shunned by the public, often becoming increasingly desperate and in need of help. Some communities use "Greyhound therapy" (Cordes, 1984)—giving the patient a one-way ticket out of town. If and when the patient is accepted back into the institution, the cycle starts all over again. Stabilize them and get them out as quickly as possible is the order of the day. This is what is referred to as the revolving door policy.

There seem to be three realities. First, deinstitutionalization has not solved the problem of treating or rehabilitating mental patients. Second, treatment of the mentally ill in institutions has not improved significantly, and in many instances, it has deteriorated. Third, funding or the lack of funding has created even greater problems, not only for the mentally ill but for the community at large as well. We can only hope that facing these realities will provide a focus for further efforts.

What about releasing criminals from prisons? New York City recently released over 200 inmates. In this instance, there was no discussion about how criminals could be rehabilitated easier, faster, or better. They were let go because the court ordered relief from overcrowding in prisons. The court order was supported by families of inmates, human services workers, and prison officials, among others. The claim was that overcrowding, inadequate facilities, and insufficient staff created conditions that constituted cruel and unusual punishment. It was believed that such conditions had resulted in violent outbreaks among inmates and that violence would again erupt if conditions were not improved. One solution to a similar condition occurred in 1972. Massachusetts, riddled with scandals regarding the over-crowding and brutality of its juvenile institutions, without warning closed all of them within a month (Scull, 1977).

Today the public seems to be less concerned about the problem of over-crowding and inadequate facilities than about criminals out on the street. The public also is not as eager to pay for building new or additional pris-ons. Many a bond issue (the borrowing of money) and tax package for building additional space have been turned down by the voters. In many places, however, funds were made available for the building of additional prisons. The courts, on the other hand, are reluctant to sentence any but the worst offenders to already overcrowded settings. Parole and probation personnel are generally so swamped with parolees and probationers that they are unable to provide required services. The result is a revolving door situation with ever-growing numbers of criminals. While overall crime rates have in fact dropped in certain areas, the number of adjudicated criminals and delinquents in the community has increased in others. How-ever, there are now, for the first time, over 1 million individuals in prison and jails in the United States. The dilemma is clear. The public does not want criminals on the streets, but the public is not interested in paying for additional prisons and parole and probation services. What are the alternatives?

Other questions about deinstitutionalization arise when one also considers the plight of the mentally retarded, juvenile offenders, and the el-derly. What are the specific conditions that would make deinstitutionaliza-tion programs work? Are halfway houses, supervised residences, aftercare clinics, and similar community institutions the answer? Finally, is deinsti-tutionalization automatically preferred?

THE ROLE OF HUMAN SERVICES WORKERS

Is the role of the human services worker to help individuals solve their in-terpersonal problems? Is it to help them cope with the stress brought on by financial difficulties, physical disabilities, or other outside pressures? Or is it to try to help change those conditions that create the problems in the first place?

During the war on poverty in the latter part of the 1960s, agencies were formed to fight poverty, racism, and crime, among other problems. Federal, state, and local governments, as well as some private foundations, funded these agencies. The workers in an agency located in a high poverty and crime area helped local residents to learn their rights in the courts. The workers went to court with their clients to protest against police brutality when it occurred. They taught them how to organize and conduct rent strikes when the tenants were not getting service. They also defended people who were on welfare whenever they needed help (Krozney, 1966). The focus of human services workers during those years was mainly on helping people cope with injustice (Morales & Sheafor, 1980). The main concept was gaining and using power, and people did protest and fight against injustice. However, in one case, the protests and struggles aroused those who were threatened by these actions, and who in turn brought pressure on those in power to curtail the funding for such projects. This, in effect, changed the nature of the role of the workers. No longer able to use government funds to fight "the Establishment"—government agencies and supporters—human services workers shifted their focus to helping clients adjust to their situation.

There are still many human services workers who feel that helping people adjust to their problems is not a very useful activity. To adjust to poverty, racism, crime, mental illness, and similar problems rather than to make every effort to combat or prevent these problems is seen by many as a losing battle. Poverty still exists and is growing. Crime rates have increased tremendously during the last two decades, although some recent declines in some categories have been noted. The number of people in need of mental-health services has increased, even though mental hospitals have released large numbers of patients. Child abuse, wife abuse, and divorces all have increased. Treatment and living conditions of the elderly leave much to be desired. All this has occurred in spite of the efforts of human services programs to date.

What else, then, can a human services worker do? "Become more of an activist," urge the activists. "But activists are seen as radicals by the public, government officials, and other human services workers," is often the reply. It is true that activists in the human services do not often win a lot of friends. The activist role usually stirs controversy and involves some risk. A worker some years ago prevented clients from entering an unlicensed nursing home and was reprimanded by his agency. The worker, with the help of his union, not only had the reprimand withdrawn, but initiated action on a state level to change the rules regarding placing people in unlicensed nursing homes. The worker was successful in that instance. Activists, unfortunately, are not always successful; but if there is to be any chance for success in eliminating injustice, there must be activists.

WHOM DO HUMAN SERVICES WORKERS SERVE?

Whom do human services workers serve? The answer to this question seems obvious and simple. In theory, it might be. However, in practice, significant issues arise. For example, suppose you are a human services worker in a mental hospital. The policy is to discharge patients as quickly as possible. One of your patients has been selected for discharge and you are asked to follow through, but you are convinced that the patient is not able to function outside the institution. He is generally stabilized in the institution, however, and has been there for over 6 months without creating trouble, so "get him out" is the word. What do you do? You are working for the hospital, and they are under pressure to discharge as many patients as possible in the shortest time possible. You are also responsible for the well-being of the patient. What happens if you do not discharge the patient? What happens if you do discharge the patient? This situation has actually occurred not once but many times in state institutions.

There are several possible answers to the question whom do human services workers serve. They include the client, the agency for which one works, the government, society in general, or themselves. Some workers would claim that it is possible to serve all of the above but not at the same time or to the same degree. In any case, human services workers might soon be required to make difficult choices regarding whom they serve.

An even more complicated situation arises if and when workers who are paid by third parties such as insurance companies or Medicare must give detailed reports of service to the companies. These reports not only identify the individuals but also the nature of the problem and the course of treatment. In effect, this is a break of confidentiality and a way of influencing the treatment provided. The insurance companies and managed care organizations often may attempt to limit or control the course of treatment. Do you as a human services worker go along with this kind of program, thus serving yourself with regard to payment and future patients? Do you refuse such a program and patients enrolled in those programs? Do you work with the patient anyway, even though payment might be reduced? Whom do you really serve—yourself, the insurance company, the client, or all three?

What about the situation in which you might be serving the taxpayer? Such a situation came up when eligibility criteria for disability payments were revised and thousands of disabled persons were denied payments. The object here was to save the taxpayers money and to cut costs to help reduce the federal deficit. What do you do when asked to administer such a program? Where do your human services responsibilities lie? Do they override your fiscal or administrative responsibilities?

The last example involves a much broader issue. It raises the question of not only whom do we serve, but when do we serve them and at what cost. As stated previously, all the present efforts of human services have not been able to provide services for all those in need. Choices must be made. How do you, the human services worker, make them? Furthermore, if one chooses to become an activist or to work in prevention programs, those in need of specific help are denied your services. These kinds of choices affect those in need, other human services workers, professional organizations, legislators, and the public in general.

Without further description or comment, many other controversial issues in the following list and those already described should provide you with more than enough material to ponder at this point.

illegal immigration
legal immigration
poverty
violence in the media
unemployment
alcoholism
gambling
sexual harassment
criminal justice
hunger
mental illness
health crisis

All this may be confusing, but it can also be stimulating and exciting to struggle with these issues and discover your own way as a competent human services worker.

A BASIC READING AND THINKING SKILL*

Ranking American Values

This activity will give you an opportunity to discuss with classmates the values you and your classmates consider important and the values you believe are considered most important by the majority of Americans.

PART 1

Step 1.   The class should break into groups of four to six students and discuss the meaning of the Hägar cartoon.

Step 2.   Working individually within each group, each student should rank their values listed below, assigning the number 1 to the value he or she personally considers most important, the number 2 to the second most important value, and so on, until all the values have been ranked.

*The following is from *Opposing Viewpoint Series*. Copyright © Greenhaven Press Inc. Reprinted by permission.

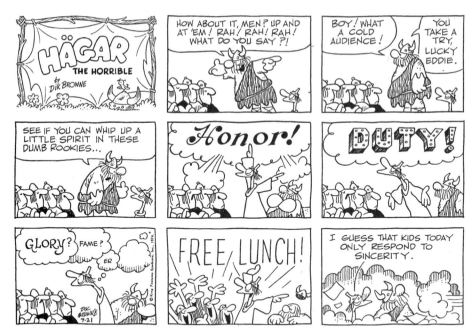

Reprinted with special permission of King Features Syndicate

Step 3.   Students should compare their rankings with others in the group, giving the reasons for their rankings.

_____ financial security
_____ freedom of speech
_____ equality of opportunity
_____ self-reliance
_____ loyalty to country
_____ tolerance of others
_____ freedom of religion
_____ individual initiative
_____ right to private property
_____ government by law and not people
_____ concern for the underdog
_____ fair play
_____ justice
_____ order in society

PART 2

Step 1.   Working in groups of four to six students, each group should rank the values listed in what the group considers the order of importance to the majority of Americans. Assign the number 1 to the value the group believes is most important to the majority of Americans, the number 2 to the second most important value, and so on until all the values have been ranked.

Step 2.   Each group should compare its ranking with others in a class-wide discussion.

Step 3.   The entire class should discuss the following questions.

1. What noticeable differences do you see between the personal rankings in part 1 and the perceived rankings of the majority of Americans in part 2?

2. How would you explain these differences?

3. What conclusions would you draw about America's future in light of your rankings in parts 1 and 2? ◆

REFERENCES

Abramovitz, M. (1983). Everyone is on welfare: "The role of redistribution in social policy" revisited. In I. Colby (Ed.), *Social welfare policy: Perspectives, patterns, insights.* Belmont, CA: Wadsworth.

Abramovitz, M. (1991). Putting an end to doublespeake about race, gender, and poverty: An annotated glossary for social workers. *Social Work, 36,* 380–384.

Bernards, N. (Ed.).(1989) *Euthanasia: Opposing viewpoints.* San Diego: Greenhaven Press.

Birnbach, D. (1981, August). Backward society: Implications for residential treatment and staff training. *Hospital and Community Psychiatry, 32,* 550–555.

Califano, J. A. (1994) *Radical surgery: What's next for america's health care.* New York: Times Books/Random House.

Child Abuse, neglect on the rise—Study finds links to unemployment. (1983, September). *NASW News,* p. 12.

Clubok, M. (1984, October). Four-year human service programs: How they differ from social work. *Journal of the National Organization of Human Services Education,* 1–6.

Cordes, C. (1984, February 15). The plight of homeless mentally ill. *APA Monitor,* pp. 1, 3.

Cunningham, S. (1984, March). Social programs asked to tighten belts again: Block grants mean less money. *APA Monitor,* p. 2.

Duffy, J. J., Jr. (1993, May). Gentrification read with interest [Letter to the editor]. *Social Work, 38*(3), 359.

Dye, T. R. (1987). *Understanding public policy* (6th ed.). Englewood Cliffs, NJ: Prentice Hall.

Edmondson, B. (1990, March). Why AIDS deserves what it gets. *American Demographics,* p. 28.

Feringer, R., & Jacobs, E. (1987, February). Human services: Is it a profession? *The Link,* pp. 1, 7, 8.

Fulton, R. (1981, Fall). Federal budget making in 1981: A watershed in federal domestic policy. *New England Journal of Human Services, 1,* 21–31.

Hinds, de C. (1990, April 2). Pulling families out of welfare is proving to be an elusive goal. *The New York Times*, p. A1.

Holmes, S. A. (1991, December 25). Homelessness rises, but not as issue. *The New York Times*, p. 9.

Huff, D. D., & Johnson, D. A. (1993, May). Phantom welfare: Public relief for corporate America. *Social Work, 38*(3), 311–315.

Humphry, D. (1991). *Final exit: Practicalities of self-deliverance and assisted suicides for the dying.* Eugene, OR: The Hemlock Society.

Is deinstitutionalization working? (1983, January 25). *Human Services*, p. 3.

Jansson, B. S. (1988). *The reluctant welfare state: A history of American social welfare policies.* Belmont, CA: Wadsworth.

Johnson, A. B. (1990). *Out of bedlam: The truth about deinstitutionalization.* New York: Basic Books.

Kozol, J. (1988). Mental illness does not cause homelessness. In L. Orr (Ed.), *The homeless: Opposing viewpoints.* San Diego: Greenhaven Press.

Krozney, H. (1966). Beyond welfare: Poverty in the super city. New York: Holt, Rinehart & Winston.

Marin, P. (1987, January). Helping and hating the homeless: The struggle at the margins of America. *Harper's Magazine*, pp. 39–49.

Mechanic, D. (1980). *Mental health and social policy* (2nd ed.). Englewood Cliffs, NJ: Prentice Hall.

Morales, A., & Sheafor, B. W. (1980). *Social work: A profession of many faces* (2nd ed.). Boston: Allyn & Bacon.

Peirce, N. R. (1982, Summer). New federalism and the social services: Friends or foes? *New England Journal of Human Services, 2*, 13–19.

Scull, A. T. (1977). *Decarceration: Community treatment and the deviant—A radical view.* Englewood Cliffs, NJ: Prentice Hall.

Sobey, F. (1970). *The nonprofessional revolution in mental health.* New York: Columbia University Press.

Specht, H., & Courtney, M. (1994). *Unfaithful angels.* New York: Free Press.

Tolchin, M. (1988, June 13). Welfare revision: Moynihan seeking to stand system on its head. *The New York Times*, p. B6.

Turkington, C. (1984, February). Preferred providers please and puzzle private practitioners. *APA Monitor*, pp. 10–11.

Turkington, C. (1985, December). More research funds sought at ADAMHA. *APA Monitor*, p. 9.

2 doctor-assisted suicides ruled homicides. (1991, December 19). *The New York Times*, p. A29.

Wright, G. (1991, May 18). Women who need to escape men: After the state cuts where will they find shelter? *The New York Times*, p. 23.

GLOSSARY

acceptance Viewing another's thoughts, feelings, and attitudes as worthy, even if one doesn't agree with them.

acupuncture A traditional Chinese medicine in which needles are placed at key points along energy pathways of the body in order to restore energy balance.

advocacy Representing a client to obtain needed services.

advocate One who supports clients in obtaining services.

AFDC Aid to Families with Dependent Children: Public assistance to families with children who have little or no income.

affective disorder A type of psychological disorder that is characterized by recurrent episodes of mania, depression, or both.

ageism Negative attitudes toward older people based on prejudices and stereotypes.

almshouse (poor house) A type of shelter created by the government of England during the 1600s to house the disadvantaged.

alternative medicine Various approaches to diagnosis and treatment that fall outside of conventional medical treatments.

Alzheimer's disease A chronic and progressive brain disorder characterized by loss of cognitive functions, such as short-term memory.

amphetamines Stimulant drugs that initially produce an energizing or euphoric effect, sometimes followed by sudden "crashes" and depression.

anecdotal records Information or events recorded but unsupported by hard evidence.

animism The belief first held by primitive peoples that spirits inhabit inanimate objects such as rivers, volcanoes, or rocks, as well as living things.

Antabuse (trade name for disulfiram) A drug used in the treatment of alcoholism that causes an unpleasant reaction when alcohol is consumed.

antianxiety agent A medication that is used to reduce anxiety, tension, and restlessness.

antidepressant A type of drug used to elevate mood in depressed persons.

antipsychotic agent A type of psychoactive drug used to control agitation, delusions, hyperactivity, and other symptoms associated with schizophrenia and the psychotic states.

archetypes According to Jung, the thought forms common to all people that are inherited from our ancestral past and contained in the collective unconscious.

assertion training A behavioral approach that is designed to help people stand up for their rights in socially appropriate ways.

assessment Determining the scope of someone's problem, disability, or disorder.

asylum A place of refuge that provides food, shelter, and protection. The term came to be applied to a place of refuge for the unsound of mind.

attending The ability of the helper to be free from distraction and fully focused on the client. To "be there" for and with someone.

authenticity The act of being oneself or being real and not a phony.

aversive therapies Treatment methods that employ punishment or noxious stimulation to reduce the frequency or strength of an undesirable behavior; for example, the use of Antabuse to control alcoholism.

barbiturates A class of sedative-hypnotic compounds, sometimes used to treat insomnia, epilepsy, and anxiety.

behavior therapy The application of the principles of learning and conditioning theory to treatment of psychological and behavioral problems.

belongingness and love needs A feeling of closeness to others; third level of human needs on Maslow's hierarchy of needs.

benzodiazepine A class of chemically related compounds that is used to reduce tension and anxiety, of which diazepam (Valium) is an example.

biofeedback A technique that is used to help people gain voluntary control over a physiological function, such as blood pressure, by means of a device that provides a visual or auditory signal reflecting the strength of the response.

block grant Federal funds given to states to provide programs for a wide range of service needs.

budget An estimate of the income and expenses needed to carry out programs for a fiscal year.

cannabis The plant from which marijuana is derived.

catatonic state A state of stupor and muscular rigidity.

central nervous system (CNS) The part of the body that contains the brain and spinal cord.

child abuse   Actions involving physical or emotional injury to a child, as well as neglect of the child's basic needs.

classical conditioning   The kind of learning that takes place when a neutral stimulus is paired with a stimulus that automatically produces a reflex response; the neutral stimulus comes to elicit the response.

clinical psychology   The branch of psychology that specializes in the diagnosis and treatment of mental and emotional disorders.

cocaine   A drug derived from the coca plant that generally acts as a behavioral stimulant and may also produce anxiety and addictive cravings.

code of ethics   A set of beliefs and standards of behavior/practice that serves to clarify and unify a particular field.

collective bargaining   Negotiating union contracts on an industrywide basis.

collective unconscious   In Jung's theory, the part of the unconscious that is inherited and common to all humans and that is distinguished from the personal unconscious, which includes the individual's repressed thoughts and memories.

coma   A long period of unconsciousness due to disease or injury.

community mental health   The provision of a coordinated program of mental-health care to a specified population in a community setting, usually contrasted with provisions of service in a large institution that is removed from the community.

community organizing   The process of working toward the provision of a new or improved program for an underserved population in the community.

compensation   The process of attempting to overcome real or imagined defects and weaknesses.

compulsion   A strong desire to perform a senseless, ritualized form of behavior.

confrontation   The process of presenting various information/feedback to the client for his or her personal benefit; often viewed as a challenge.

congruence   A characteristic of genuineness that refers to behavior in which a person's words and behavior seem to match.

conservative perspective   A philosophy that emphasizes traditional American values including self-reliance, personal liberty, and respect for private property, often accompanied by a distrust of government's efforts to help the needy.

constituents   People who select or elect others to represent or serve them in some manner.

conversion disorder   A class of disorders in which a physical disability has no known physical cause but is related to psychological problems.

counseling A process that helps people to consider their choices and options in life.

crack A street name for a smokable form of concentrated cocaine that may be highly addictive.

creative arts therapy The use of creative activities such as music, art, dance to facilitate personal insight, self-expression, and social awareness.

crime An act committed in violation of a law.

crisis intervention A type of help designed to meet the needs of a person faced with an unusually difficult life situation.

criteria Standards.

daily hassles Everyday annoyances or mishaps of a minor kind.

data Collected information or facts, usually for purposes of analysis.

defense mechanisms Tactics and strategies, such as denial and rationalization, that an individual may use to reduce awareness of guilt, anxiety, or other unpleasant feeling states.

deinstitutionalization The practice of discharging inmates from large institutional settings to the community, particularly of those chronically mentally ill patients who would otherwise be kept in a hospital for extended periods of time.

demonology A system of beliefs first practiced by prehistoric people in which behavior was thought to be influenced by evil spirits (demons).

detoxification The process of eliminating accumulations of alcohol or other drugs from the body, often under medical supervision and as a first step in treatment of addiction.

developmentally disabled Individuals with a significant delay in one or more of the following areas of development: cognitive, language, and psychosocial skills.

diagnosis The act of identifying a disease on the basis of its signs and symptoms.

discrimination Unfair treatment against certain groups of persons in matters of employment, housing, and education based on prejudicial attitudes.

dissociative disorder A disorder, such as multiple personality, in which one part of the personality seems separated or screened from another.

diversion program A program that aims to keep juvenile and adult law violators out of court and prison.

drug tolerance The tendency of a user to experience progressively reduced responsiveness to a given dose of a drug.

due process A constitutional right guaranteeing a hearing process in a case of grievance.

dysfunction A state of abnormal functioning during which one is unable to fulfill the expectations of society.

economic policies Plans or strategies that deal with the finances of individuals, groups, or states.

efficacy Effectiveness, efficiency.

ego In psychoanalytic theory, the rational part of the personality that mediates between the demands of instinctual urges, conscience, and reality.

electroconvulsive therapy (ECT) A therapy, used primarily to treat severe depression, in which an electrical current is passed through the brain for a brief period.

Elizabethan Poor Laws An official policy, created under the rule of Henry VIII of England in 1601, that established a system of shelter and care for the poor.

empathy The ability to see things from another's point of view.

esteem needs The desire to be a respected, competent, or even superior person.

euthanasia A way of causing a painless death, usually to end the suffering of people dying of an incurable disease.

existentialism A philosophy that emphasizes the freedom to choose one's own values and way of life.

extended family A family including not only parents and children, but also grandparents and other relations.

extinction The decrease in the strength of a learned response caused by withholding of reinforcement.

feedback The process of conveying information between client and helper.

felony A serious criminal offense.

food stamps A government program designed to offset some of the food expenses of poor people who qualify.

free association A technique used in psychoanalytic therapy in which the client is asked to speak freely, saying whatever comes to mind without concern about the effect on the listener.

generalist A human services worker concerned with a wide range of individual problems rather than a specific or specialized area of concern.

genuineness The ability to express true and honest feelings.

geographic decentralization A psychiatric hospital procedure in which patients are placed in hospital wards based on their last place of residence in the community prior to admission.

ghetto An inner-city area inhabited by minorities.

hallucinogen A psychedelic drug, such as mescaline, that produces marked distortions in perceptual experience.

hardiness Personality traits that enable an individual to withstand stress.

heroin An opiate, used for its sedative effects, that is produced by a chemical modification of morphine.

holistic perspective The viewpoint that assumes that the whole is greater than the sum of its parts or that the whole has properties that cannot be inferred from the parts.

human services Organized activities that help people in the areas of health, mental health, criminal justice, recreation, education, and related spheres.

human services model The theoretical view that emphasizes unfulfilled needs as major causes of human disorders. It employs a treatment approach based on satisfaction of human needs as a means of preventing and ameliorating dysfunction.

humanistic perspective A school of psychology that emphasizes subjective experience and the desire of each person to realize his or her full human potential.

id In psychoanalytic theory, the part of the personality that contains the basic instincts, urges, and desires.

immune system The body's first line of defense against disease consisting of complex mechanisms that detect and destroy foreign invaders such as bacteria and viruses.

implementation Putting a plan or program to work.

incidence The number of new cases of a condition reported during a given period of time, such as the previous year.

indigenous worker One who lives in the community in which he or she works.

industrialization The widespread utilization of factory and machine-based methods of production, as opposed to earlier reliance on hand tools.

inferiority feelings According to Adler, negative feelings derived from childhood and based on unfavorable comparisons with others.

inpatient One who lives in an institution 24 hours a day, where treatment is provided.

Inquisition A religious tribunal (court), established in the 13th century under Pope Innocent III, that was given the primary responsibility of seeking out and punishing all crimes associated with witchcraft and heresy.

intelligence The ability to learn, to think logically, and to behave adaptively.

intelligence quotient (IQ) A score or value given to intelligence that is based on test performance, with a score of 100 indicating average ability.

interest group An organization focusing on a single area of concern and attempting to influence others to take steps favorable to its agenda.

intervening The act of stepping in and attempting to change or modify a person's behavior or situation.

interviewing Specialized pattern of communication with specific goals.

involuntary service A decision that a service is necessary for an individual made by another individual, an agency, or court.

jurisdiction Usually a geographical area in which legal power is exerted.

LaBicetre A mental institution in France in the late 1790s in which the director, Phillipe Pinel, expressed the notion that some of the insane could be cured and that forcible restraint in the management of the mentally ill was not always useful or necessary.

laissez-faire economy A doctrine first introduced by Adam Smith in 1776 in his book *The Wealth of Nations* that held that an economic system functions best when there is no interference by government.

laudatory Praiseworthy.

law of effect The theory that a response that consistently results in a reward will be "stamped in" or become part of the organism's repertoire.

learning The process by which experience brings about a relatively permanent change in behavior.

least restrictive alternative A client's right to treatment in settings that interfere the least with his or her personal freedoms.

less-eligibility A concept established by the government of England in 1830 that created guidelines for assistance to the disadvantaged; any assistance given to these people must be lower than the lowest wage given to any working person.

liberal perspective A philosophy that emphasizes the role of government in providing services to those who are unable to be self-supporting.

life-sustaining needs Needs such as food, clothing, and shelter.

lithium carbonate A metallic element that is used in the treatment of mania and depression.

living system In systems theory, cells, organisms, and human organizations are defined as living systems; that is, they are open to the environment, act as if motivated to achieve goals, and have some degree of self-control.

lobbyist One who is paid to represent the interests of an organization, usually regarding some form of legislation.

lobotomy (prefrontal lobotomy)   A surgical procedure used to treat severely disturbed mental patients in which the frontal lobes of the brain are severed from the deeper centers; now rarely performed.

lysergic acid diethylamide (LSD)   A synthetic hallucinogenic drug.

major tranquilizer   A type of medication used in the treatment of schizophrenia and other psychotic states.

managed care   Health care insurance systems that contract with a network of hospitals, clinics, and doctors who agree to accept set fees or flat payments per patient.

mandated policy   A policy ordered by a court or legislative body to be followed.

mandated program   A program ordered by a court or legislative body to be carried out.

mania   A mood disorder characterized by elation, extreme talkativeness, and generally increased behavioral activity.

MAO inhibitors   Drugs that act to allow the neurotransmitter, norepinephrine, to build up and thereby alleviate depression. These drugs require that the patient follow a special diet, and may have undesired effects.

marijuana   The crushed leaves, flowers, and small buds of the hemp plant (*Cannabis saliva*) that contain a mild hallucinogen and may produce feelings of euphoria.

Medicaid   A government insurance program that pays some medical expenses for low-income people who qualify.

medical model   The view that behavioral and emotional problems are analogous to physical diseases.

Medicare   A public health insurance program designed to help pay some medical and hospital expenses of the elderly.

mental illness   Psychological, emotional, or behavioral disorders and the view that these disorders are diseases of the mind.

mental retardation   A state of intellectual impairment that is shown in delayed maturation, a less-than-average capacity to learn from experiences, and a lowered ability to maintain oneself independently.

mescaline   A psychedelic drug that is derived from the peyote cactus.

methadone (dolophine)   A synthetically produced opiate narcotic used to treat heroin addiction but which is itself addictive.

minimum wage laws   Wage and hour standards for workers established by law.

minor tranquilizer   A type of drug that is used primarily to reduce tension and anxiety.

morphine   A pain-relieving drug that is derived from opium.

motive A specific need or desire, such as hunger or achievement, that energizes and directs behavior.

multicultural perspective To see, hear, or understand information from another's culture free of judgment or cultural comparisons; the ability to see things from another person's racial or ethnic background.

narcotic antagonists A relatively new type of drug that blocks the euphoric effects produced by heroin or other opiates.

narcotics Potentially addicting drugs derived from opium, including heroin, morphine, and codeine.

natural disaster An event in which forces of nature, including earthquakes and hurricanes, have a destructive effect on a human population.

neuroses A class of disorders in which anxiety is the characteristic feature or the avoidance of anxiety seems to be the dominant motive of the disturbed behavior.

New Deal A system of social and economic legislation government aid programs designed to benefit the mass of working people; established by President Franklin Delano Roosevelt in the 1930s.

new federalism The tendency of the federal government to transfer power and control over programs, such as welfare, to the states.

nonjudgmental attitude Behavior that does not impose one's own personal values and standards on others.

objectivity To note the verifiable facts of an event.

obsession A disturbing, unwanted repetitive thought.

occupational therapy The selective and purposeful therapeutic use of activities to aid in the treatment of physical or mental disorders.

operant conditioning A type of learning in which the likelihood of a voluntary behavior is increased or decreased by reinforcement or punishment.

opiates A class of addictive drugs—including opium, heroin, and morphine—that dulls the senses, reduces pain, and induces feelings of well-being.

opium The crude resinous substance taken from the opium poppy.

outpatient A person who receives treatment for a mental or physical disorder outside the hospital setting and usually in an office or clinic setting.

paraphrase To reword a message using one's own words rather than the words of others.

paraprofessional One who works alongside a professional but does not possess an advanced (graduate) academic degree.

parole Release of an inmate from prison after part of the sentence has been served. The person is then supervised by a parole officer for the remainder of the sentence.

partial hospitalization A program, usually for mental patients, in which part of the day is spent in an institution and the remainder is spent in a community setting.

personal unconscious According to Jung, the part of the unconscious mind that contains the person's repressed thoughts and forgotten experiences.

phobia An exaggerated or extreme fear of a stimulus or situation.

physical dependence A state in which a person needs a certain drug in order to function normally; the state becomes apparent when withdrawal of the drugs leads to distressing symptoms.

physiological needs Basic needs for physical survival; the lowest level on Maslow's hierarchy of needs.

plea bargaining A practice in which a defendant pleads guilty to a lesser offense in return for a reduction in charges or other considerations.

poverty line The level of income that the federal government considers sufficient to meet basic requirements for food, shelter, and clothing.

power structure Those who control the sources of power—usually economic and political power.

prejudice Negative feelings or attitudes toward certain racial, religious, or ethnic groups based on overgeneralizations about these groups.

preliterate societies Societies that existed prior to the introduction of writing or written records.

prevalence The total number of existing cases of a particular disorder or condition.

primary prevention Programs and activities designed to prevent people from developing a physical or psychological disorder.

primary social supports The network of social relationships, including friends and family, that provides gratification of a person's needs.

privatization Arranging for private companies to take on certain jobs and functions that were formerly done by government.

probation Suspending the sentence of a convicted offender and placing him or her under the supervision of a probation officer.

prognosis The expected outcome of an illness or disorder.

prosthesis An artificial device used to replace a missing body part.

protestant work ethic A social philosophy that supports the accumulation of wealth as a reward for hard work and condemns idleness as almost sinful.

psychedelic drug Any drug that causes marked alterations in perceptual experience, possibly including hallucinations.

psychiatric nursing The specialization within the broad field of nursing that places emphasis on treatment of the physical and mental well-being of patients in psychiatric settings.

psychiatry The medical specialty that investigates, diagnoses, and treats mental, emotional, or behavioral disorders.

psychoactive drug Any compound that alters mood, feeling state, or behavior.

psychoanalysis A school of psychology originated by Freud and the treatment method derived from his theories.

psychological dependence A strong desire to use a drug for its pleasurable effects that may lead to both continued use and eventual physical dependence.

psychological needs Basic needs such as love, self-esteem, and self-actualization.

psychopharmacology The development and utilization of drugs to treat mental illness.

psychosurgery Brain surgery, such as prefrontal lobotomy, used to modify severely disturbed behavior.

psychotherapy The treatment of personal, emotional, and behavior problems by psychological means.

quarantine Isolating people to prevent the spread of disease.

recidivism Repetition of a crime by someone who was previously incarcerated, and their possible rearrest and return to prison.

recipients In the human services field, those who receive benefits from a human services agency.

redistribution of power In the human services field, to politically empower those with no power.

rehabilitation A helping process designed to assist people with disabilities to achieve the highest possible level of productive functioning.

reinforcement An event that increases the probability that a given response will recur.

reliable data Data that consistently give the same results when used in the same way.

safety needs Human needs for a stable, predictable, and secure environment.

St. Mary's of Bethlehem One of the earliest public asylums incorporated in 1547 in London; this first English "lunatic asylum" became popularly known as "Bedlam," a term later synonymous with states of frenzy and excitement.

second-generation antidepressants Drugs that may alleviate depression by enhancing the sensitivity of neurotransmitter receptors and by increasing the activity of serotonin. They are considered as effective as the earlier tricyclics and have fewer side effects.

secondary prevention Early detection and intervention to keep beginning problems from becoming more severe.

sedative hypnotic drug Any chemical that has a general depressant action on the nervous system.

self-actualization In Maslow's hierarchy of needs, the desire to fully express one's inner nature and talents.

self-awareness The quality of knowing oneself.

self-concept The set of positive and negative attitudes that one uses to evaluate oneself.

self-help groups Individuals who meet without professional help to provide mutual support for shared problems.

settlement house movement Begun in the period of the late 1800s to early 1900s, a reflection of early human services philosophy. Each individual settlement house offered a variety of human services to the disadvantaged. Newly arrived immigrants were the initial population served.

sexism Discrimination against a person on the basis of gender.

side effect Any drug-induced effect, often undesirable, that accompanies the primary effect for which the drug was intended.

single-issue groups Groups that lobby for one particular issue to the exclusion of all others.

Social Darwinism A group of ideas first expressed by Herbert Spencer as an interpretation of Charles Darwin's writings on evolution. Spencer applied Darwin's theory of natural selection to human beings and supported the premise that disadvantaged people who are unfit for society should not be helped.

social interest According to Adler, the awareness of being part of the human community and striving to build a better future for humanity.

social learning theory The study of learning that takes place by observing others rather than by firsthand experience of the learner.

social policies Plans that deal with the quality of life and of society in general.

social welfare A series of programs and/or services aimed at helping people who need help in supporting themselves.

social work The field that focuses on helping individuals realize their potential to live as fully and successfully as possible.

status quo The existing conditions or situations.

stereotype   A set of beliefs or perceptions about groups of people, or ideas shared by a number of people, often not based on fact.

stigmatize   To characterize or identify as disgraceful, negative, or harmful.

stress   The condition that comes about when the demands of a situation place a strain on a person's resources.

subjectivity   A personal, private, possibly biased view of an event.

summarize   A skill or technique of restating what the client has expressed during a series of counseling/therapy sessions.

superego   In psychoanalytic theory, the part of personality that contains the moral standards of society as interpreted by the parents to the child.

Supplemental Security Income (SSI)   A public program that provides a minimum income for blind, disabled, and elderly persons who have little or no financial resources.

systematic desensitization   A therapy designed to gradually reduce fear about a particular stimulus by substituting a relaxed response for the fear response.

systems theory   A holistic approach that assumes that the human being is made up of smaller subsystems, such as cells and organs, but that the human being is in turn part of larger systems, such as family and society.

Tardive dyskinesia   A disorder produced by prolonged treatment with antipsychotic drugs that manifests itself in uncontrolled muscular movements and sometimes memory losses.

target population   A group of people, such as the poor or the elderly, that has been selected for help by human services.

technological disaster   An event in which a malfunction in plant or machinery, such as a nuclear power plant, causes destruction to human habitat.

tertiary prevention   Efforts to rehabilitate those affected with severe mental disorders and return them to the community.

theory   A concept that attempts to explain the relationships between events and that may be used to predict or control those events.

therapeutic recreation   Selected use of recreational activities as an aid in the treatment, correction, or rehabilitation of physical or mental disorders.

third-party payment   Payment to a professional from a client/patient's insurance coverage.

token economy   A procedure in which tokens are used to reward members of a group or community for performing certain desirable behaviors; the method may be used in schools, prisons, and mental hospitals.

transference   In psychoanalytic therapy, the tendency of the client to displace feelings, attitudes, and defenses originating in a previous relationship onto the therapist.

trephining   A primitive medical treatment first practiced by certain prehistoric people in which a hole is bored into the skull to allow evil spirits a route to leave the body.

tricyclics   A class of medications that may reduce depressive symptoms by blocking neurotransmitter reuptake mechanics, thereby increasing the activity of norepinephrine and serotonin. They are considered to have higher success rates than the MAO inhibitors.

underemployment   The condition in which people are working at jobs below their level of skill and/or are working part-time because they cannot get full-time jobs.

undocumented worker   An individual from a foreign country coming illegally into this country in search of employment.

unemployment insurance   A government program that provides an unemployed worker with a weekly cash benefit for a limited time, usually 26 weeks.

union movement   Organized efforts to improve working conditions and wages started by groups of workers who banded together in the latter half of the 19th century.

valid data   Data that when examined provide the information sought after.

voluntary agencies   Agencies that are private and profit making; nongovernmental institutions.

voluntary service   A client's decision that some form of help is needed and he or she contracts for such service.

withdrawal syndrome   The often distressing symptoms that occur when a heavy user stops ingesting alcohol or other drugs.

NAME INDEX

SUBJECT INDEX

IN-BOOK SURVEY

At Brooks/Cole, we are excited about creating new types of learning materials that are interactive, three-dimensional, and fun to use. To guide us in our publishing/development process, we hope that you'll take just a few moments to fill out the survey below. Your answers can help us make decisions that will allow us to produce a wide variety of videos, CD-ROMs, and Internet-based learning systems to complement standard textbooks. If you're interested in working with us as a student Beta-tester, be sure to fill in your name, telephone number, and address. We look forward to hearing from you!

In addition to books, which of the following learning tools do you currently use in your counseling/human services/social work courses?

_____ **Video** _____ in class _____ school library _____ own VCR

_____ **CD-ROM** _____ in class _____ in lab _____ own computer

_____ **Macintosh disks** _____ in class _____ in lab _____ own computer

_____ **Windows disks** _____ in class _____ in lab _____ own computer

_____ **Internet** _____ in class _____ in lab _____ own computer

How often do you access the Internet? _____

My own home computer is:

_____ Macintosh _____ DOS _____ Windows _____ Windows 95

The computer I use in class for counseling/human services/social work courses is:

_____ Macintosh _____ DOS _____ Windows _____ Windows 95

If you are NOT currently using multimedia materials in your counseling/human services/social work courses, but can see ways that video, CD-ROM, Internet, or other technologies could enhance your learning, please comment below:

_____

_____

_____

Other comments (optional): _____

_____

Name _____

Address _____

Telephone number (optional): _____

You can fax this form to us at (408) 375-6414; e:mail to: info@brookscole.com; or detach, fold, secure, and mail.

CUT ALONG DOTTED LINE

FOLD HERE

NO POSTAGE
NECESSARY
IF MAILED
IN THE
UNITED STATES

BUSINESS REPLY MAIL

FIRST CLASS   PERMIT NO. 358   PACIFIC GROVE, CA

POSTAGE WILL BE PAID BY ADDRESSEE

ATTN: _MARKETING_____

Brooks/Cole Publishing Company
511 Forest Lodge Road
Pacific Grove, California 93950-9968

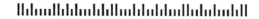

FOLD HERE

TO THE OWNER OF THIS BOOK:

We hope that you have found *Human Services in Contemporary America,* Fourth Edition, useful. So that this book can be improved in a future edition, would you take the time to complete this sheet and return it? Thank you.

School and address: ——————————————————————————————

Department: ——————————————————————————————————

Instructor's name: —————————————————————————————

1. What I like most about this book is: —————————————————

——

——

2. What I like least about this book is: —————————————————

——

——

3. My general reaction to this book is: —————————————————

——

4. The name of the course in which I used this book is: ———————————

——

5. Were all of the chapters of the book assigned for you to read? ———————

   If not, which ones weren't? ————————————————————————

6. In the space below, or on a separate sheet of paper, please write specific suggestions for improving this book and anything else you'd care to share about your experience in using the book.

——

——

——

——

Optional:

Your name: _____ Date: _____

May Brooks/Cole quote you, either in promotion for *Human Services in Contemporary America* or in future publishing ventures?

Yes: _____ No: _____

Sincerely,

Paul Schmolling, Jr.
Merrill Youkeles
William R. Burger

FOLD HERE

NO POSTAGE
NECESSARY
IF MAILED
IN THE
UNITED STATES

BUSINESS REPLY MAIL
FIRST CLASS   PERMIT NO. 358   PACIFIC GROVE, CA

POSTAGE WILL BE PAID BY ADDRESSEE

ATT: *Paul Schmolling, Jr., Merrill Youkeles, William R. Burger*

Brooks/Cole Publishing Company
511 Forest Lodge Road
Pacific Grove, California 93950-9968

FOLD HERE